Topical Diagnosis in Neurology

Anatomy · Physiology · Signs · Symptoms

Peter Duus, M.D.

Professor of Neurology and Psychiatry
Former Director of Neurology Department
Academic Hospital Northwest
Johann Wolfgang Goethe University
Frankfurt/Main, Germany

Translated by Richard Lindenberg, M.D.

Third, revised edition
432 illustrations, most in color

Illustrated by Gerhard Spitzer

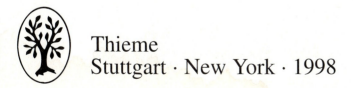

Thieme
Stuttgart · New York · 1998

Library of Congress Cataloging-in-Publication Data

Duus, Peter, 1908–
 [Neurologisch-topische Diagnostik. English]
 Topical diagnosis in neurology : anatomy, physiology, signs, symptoms / Peter Duus ; translated by Richard Lindenberg ; illustrated by Gerhard Spitzer. -- 3rd, rev. ed.
  p. cm.
 Translation of the updated and rev. 6th German ed. 1995.
 Includes bibliographical references and index.
 ISBN 3-13-612802-8 (Georg Thieme Verlag). -- ISBN 0-86577-305-X (Thieme Medical Publishers)
 1. Nervous system--Diseases--Diagnosis. 2. Nervous system--Anatomy. 3. Anatomy, Pathological. 4. Nervous system--Pathophysiology. I. Title.
 [DNLM: 1. Nervous System--Diseases--diagnosis. 2. Nervous System--anatomy & histology. 3. Nervous System--physiology. WL 141 D981n 1998a]
RC347.D8813 1998
616.8'04754--dc21
DNLM/DLC
for Library of Congress   97-31483
                                                            CIP

1st German edition 1976
6th German edition 1995
1st English edition 1983
1st Brazilian (Portugese) edition 1985
2nd Brazilian (Portugese) edition 1990
1st Italian edition 1987
1st Japanese edition 1982
3rd Japanese edition 1988
1st Korean edition 1990
1st Polish edition 1990
1st Spanish edition 1985
1st Greek edition 1992
1st Indonesian edition 1996
1st Chinese edition 1996
1st Russian edition 1996

This book is an authorized translation of the updated and revised 6th German edition published and copyrighted 1995 by Georg Thieme Verlag, Stuttgart, Germany. Title of the German edition: Neurologisch-topische Diagnostik: Anatomie–Physiologie–Klinik

Any reference to or mention of manufacturers or specific brand names should not be interpreted as an endorsement or advertisement for any company or product.

Some of the product names, patents and registered designs referred to in this book are in fact registered trademarks or proprietary names even though specific reference to this fact is not always made in the text. Therefore, the appearance of a name without designation as proprietary is not to be construed as a representation by the publisher that it is in the public domain.

This book, including all parts thereof, is legally protected by copyright. Any use, exploitation or commercialization outside the narrow limits set by copyright legislation, without the publisher's consent, is illegal and liable to prosecution. This applies in particular to photostat reproduction, copying, mimeographing or duplication of any kind, translating, preparation of microfilms, and electronic data processing and storage.

Important Note: Medicine is an ever-changing science undergoing continual development. Research and clinical experience are continually expanding our knowledge, in particular our knowledge of proper treatment and drug therapy. Insofar as this book mentions any dosage or application, readers may rest assured that the authors, editors and publishers have made every effort to ensure that such references are in accordance **with the state of knowledge at the time of production of the book.**

Nevertheless this does not involve, imply, or express any guarantee or responsibility on the part of the publishers in respect of any dosage instructions and forms of application stated in the book. **Every user is requested to** examine carefully the manufacturers' leaflets accompanying each drug and to check, if necessary in consultation with a physician or specialist, whether the dosage schedules mentioned therein or the contraindications stated by the manufacturers differ from the statements made in the present book. Such examination is particularly important with drugs that are either rarely used or have been newly released on the market. **Every dosage schedule or every form of application used is entirely at the user's own risk and responsibility.** The authors and publishers request every user to report to the publishers any discrepancies or inaccuracies noticed.

© 1998 Georg Thieme Verlag, Rüdigerstrasse 14
70469 Stuttgart, Germany
Thieme Medical Publishers, Inc.
333 Seventh Avenue
New York, N.Y. 10001

Printed in Germany by Druckhaus Götz, GmbH
Ludwigsburg

ISBN 3-13-612803-6 (GTV, Stuttgart)
ISBN 0-86577-711-X (TMP, New York)
                                              1 2 3 4 5 6

Foreword

It can be safely stated that this book has gained the reputation of being a classic. It is now referred to in many countries as "THE DUUS." This third English edition represents a revised form of the book's sixth German edition of 1995.

The many experts who reviewed previous editions of this book praise the clarity and simplicity with which the author has organized and presented the very complex and difficult subject matter of what I call *basic* neurology. They agree with the author that it should be read straight through, as one reads a novel, starting with page one. They comment on the wealth of information contained in each chapter and on the ease with which it is written. One wrote that the book is a joy to read, and another that it is difficult to become bored reading it. All praise the copious drawings by Gerhard Spitzer, Professor of Medical Graphic Arts, which are both instructive and beautiful, and recognize their share in the growing popularity of "THE DUUS."

Most reviewers agree with me that the book, originally written as an introduction to the broad and intricate field of *special* neurology for medical students, interns, and residents, is recommended reading also for the general practitioner and the accomplished, practicing, or researching specialist in any of the many fields dealing with the nervous system.

Some may question this, in view of the incredible, almost explosive advances made in the various modes of diagnostic imaging during the last few years. One may ask whether it still pays to learn all the minutiae of anatomy and physiology and the signs and symptoms of every segment of the nervous system. I believe it does! I believe it is simply elementary for any educated dealing with the nervous system to know at least as much about it as what "THE DUUS" offers. This holds true, without question, for the daily practice of neurology and psychiatry, and equally applies to that of neuroimaging and neuropathology, and of the most recent field of endeavor, psychoneuroimmunology.

Richard Lindenberg

Preface to the Third Edition

Eight years have passed since the second edition was published, and a new edition has become necessary. The book has been revised and updated. The text has been expanded and new illustrations added. Meanwhile the book has been translated into even more languages. It was always my intention to write a book that would be both readable and easily understood by prospective doctors; numerous and instructive illustrations were necessary to fulfill this objective.

Didactically, the book is structured so that each chapter builds on the material presented in the preceding chapters; I therefore recommend reading the book straight through, as one reads a novel, to maximize comprehension of the contents.

It is my hope that the present third edition will meet with as warm a welcome from its readers as the earlier editions.

I am very grateful to Professor Gerhard Spitzer for his cooperation.

I also want to thank Dr. Günther Hauff and his colleagues, in particular, Gert Krüger, at Thieme for their support and willingness to realize my wishes.

Peter Duus

Editor's note: this preface has been adapted from the author's preface to the sixth German edition. The author died in August 1994.

Preface to the First Edition

"If clinical neurological work in the future is to bring results of value, it is essential that the neurologist understands the major principles in the organization of the nervous system, and that he has a fair knowledge of its structure and function." A. Brodal

It is the purpose of this small book on topical neurologic diagnostics to acquaint students, interns and residents with the specialty of neurology by keeping the text concise and by using the greatest possible number of illustrations for conveying much information. Perhaps, the book offers valuable suggestions also to the practicing physician interested in neurology.

A well-based knowledge of the structural and functional relationships within the nervous system is requisite for the understanding of signs, symptoms, and syndromes of the various diseases and injuries of the nervous system and for bringing them into proper perspective for diagnosis.

Differential diagnosis is based on such knowledge and also on data collected from pointed anamnestic questioning and on the results of physical and neurologic examination conducted in search for focal as well as neighborhood signs. The conclusions drawn after differential diagnostic elaborations determine which further procedures should be used and which of the various technical diagnostic tools can most effectively be applied. The result of one or the other technical examination may corroborate what was tentatively diagnosed before or may suggest to employ additional methods.

The use of technical diagnostic procedures alone is liable to fail without carefully collecting anamnestic data and performing a routine neurologic checkup. This is particularly true when dealing with an incipient disease process. One reason for neurology being so fascinating and attractive is the possibility to deliberate on differential diagnosis just by analysing anamnestic data and basic clinical findings.

Presenting an overview of the very large field of neurology within the framework of a small book required not always easy decisions. In order to keep the descriptive text concise, illustrations had to be more numerous than usual and had to be as instructive as possible. Since the material to be presented had to be selective, certain subjects, however important, could only be touched upon or had to be omitted. These concessions notwithstanding, it is hoped that the description of those structural and functional features of the nervous system, which are important to know in the daily practice of neurology, have come out clearly and comprehensibly.

To illustrate the book so richly required tireless assistance of an expert in graphic arts, very astute in medical matters. He is Mr. Gerhard Spitzer of Frankfurt/Main. I am grateful to him for his most pleasant cooperation, his support and, particularly, for the patience he had with me.

I also want to thank very much Professor Dr. Rolf Hassler, Max Planck Institute for Brain Research, Frankfurt/Main, for reviewing text and illustrations in spite of being burdened by his own work. He gave me important suggestions and valuable stimuli.

Frankfurt/Main, July 1976 *Peter Duus*

Table of Contents

1 Sensory System 1

Receptors 1
The Peripheral Nerve 3
Neurons of the Central Nervous System 6
Proprioception 7
   Peripheral Servo Mechanism 7
      Monosynaptic Proprioceptive Reflex 7
      Other Reflexes 10
   Spinocerebellar Tracts 14
      Posterior Spinocerebellar Tract 14
      Anterior Spinocerebellar Tract 14
Posterior Funiculi 15
   Syndromes of Injury of Posterior Funiculi 16
Spinothalamic Tracts 17
   Anterior Spinothalamic Tract 17
   Lateral Spinothalamic Tract 17
Spinal Cord and Peripheral Innervation 21
Syndromes of Interruptions of Sensory Pathways 26

2 Motor System 29

Corticospinal or Pyramidal Tract 30
Corticonuclear or Corticobulbar Tract 32
Extrapyramidal Motor System 32
   Damage to Pyramidal and Extrapyramidal Pathways 35
   Syndrome of Central Spastic Paralysis 36
Peripheral Neuron, Motor and Sensory 38
   Syndrome of Radicular Nerve Damage 42
Segmental and Peripheral Muscle Innervation 43
   Disorder of the Motor Unit 43
      Syndrome of Flaccid Paralysis 46
      Damage to Plexuses 47
      Frequent Syndromes of Peripheral Nerve Damage 48
      Syndrome of Spinal Cord and Peripheral Nerve Damage 49
      Spinal Radicular Syndromes Caused by Diseases of the Disk (Osteochondrosis, Disk Protrusion, Prolapse, or Herniation) 59
Blood Supply of the Spinal Cord 63
   Arterial Supply 63
   Venous Drainage 65
   Syndromes Caused by Spinal Vascular Lesions 66
Spinal Tumors 66
   Extramedullary Tumors 66
   Intramedullary Tumors 68
   Hourglass Tumor 68
Disorders of Neuromuscular Junctions and Muscles 69
   Myopathies 69

3 Brainstem ... 70

External Structure ... 70
  Medulla Oblongata ... 70
  Pons ... 72
  Midbrain ... 73
Cranial Nerves ... 74
  Origin, Constituents and Function ... 74
  Olfactory System (I) ... 75
  Optic System (II, III, IV, VI) ... 81
    The Visual Pathway (II) ... 81
  Oculomotion (III, IV, VI) ... 85
    Paralysis of Eye Muscles ... 90
    Voluntary and Reflex Innervation of the Eye Muscles ... 94
    Convergence and Accommodation ... 97
    Light Reflex ... 99
    Sympathetic Innervation of the Eye ... 101
  Trigeminal Nerve (V) ... 103
    Facial Pain ... 106
  Facial and Intermediate Nerves (VII) ... 108
    Facial Nerve Proper ... 109
    Intermediate Nerve ... 110
    Frequent Types of Damage to VII ... 113
  Auditory System (VIII) ... 114
    Impairments of Hearing ... 119
  Vestibular or Equilibrium System (VIII) ... 120
    Impairment of the Vestibular System ... 124
  Vagal System (VII Intermediate, IX, X, Cranial XI) ... 125
    Glossopharyngeal Nerve (XI) ... 125
  Vagus Nerve (X) ... 128
  Accessory Nerve (Cranial XI) ... 129
  Nucleus Ambiguus ... 129
  Parasympathetic Motor Nuclei ... 129
  Visceral Afferent Fibers of IX and X ... 130
  Somatic Afferent Fibers of IX and X ... 131
  Accessory Nerve (Spinal XI) ... 131
  Syndrome of impairment of accessory nerve ... 131
  Hypoglossal Nerve (XII) ... 132
    Combined Impairment of IX through XII ... 134
Internal Structure of the Brainstem ... 134
  Medulla Oblongata ... 136
  Pons ... 140
  Mesencephalon (Midbrain) ... 141
Blood Supply of the Brainstem ... 145
  Arteries ... 145
  Veins ... 148
Syndromes Caused by Circulatory Disorders ... 148
Syndromes Caused by Tumors ... 154
Syndromes of Tentorium and Foramen Magnum Impaction ... 156
    Decerebrate Rigidity ... 162
    Apallic Syndrome ... 163

4 Cerebellum ... 164

External Architecture ... 164
Internal Architecture ... 165
Function ... 170
  Signs of Neocerebellar Dysfunction ... 171
Blood Supply of the Cerebellum ... 172
  Arteries ... 172
    Superior Cerebellar Arteries ... 173
    Inferior Anterior Cerebellar Arteries ... 174
    Inferior Posterior Cerebellar Arteries ... 174
Veins ... 174
Circulatory Lesions ... 174
  Obstruction of Superior Cerebellar Artery ... 174
  Compression of Superior Cerebellar Arteries along Tentorial Margin ... 174
  Cerebellar Hematoma ... 175
Cerebellar Tumors ... 176
  Cerebellar Astrocytoma ... 176
  Medulloblastoma ... 176
  Angioblastoma (Lindau's Disease) ... 177
  Metastatic tumors ... 177
  Acoustic Neurinoma ... 177
  Ependymoma ... 179
Other Cerebellar Diseases ... 179
  Addendum ... 179

5 Diencephalon 180

Thalamus 181
    Function 187
    Blood Supply 187
Syndrome of Thalamic Disorders 188
    Syndromes of Thalamic Circulatory
    Disorders 189
    Tumors of the Thalamus 190
    Inflammatory Disease of the
    Thalamus 191
Epithalamus 192
Subthalamus 193
Hypothalamus 194
    Structure 194
    Hypothalamus and Hypophysis 197
    Function of Hypothalamus 200
    Limbic System 202
        Entorhinal Area 203

Amygdaloid Nuclear Complex 204
Hippocampus 205
    Limbic System as a Circuitry for
    Mechanisms of Expression,
    Formation of Emotions,
    Dispositions, and Instinctive
    Drives 205
    Damage to the Hypothalamus 208
    Tumors 209
Peripheral Autonomic Nervous System . 213
Control by the Hypothalamus 213
    Function 213
    Sympathetic Nervous System 215
    Parasympathetic Nervous System 217
    The Sacral Component 217
    Referred Pain 222

6 Basal Ganglia and Extrapyramidal System 225

Basal Ganglia 225
Extrapyramidal System 226
    Signs Caused by Lesions in Extra-
    pyramidal Grisea 232
        Hypokinesia-Hypertonia
        Syndrome 232

    Hyperkinesia-Hypotonia
    Syndrome 234
    Other signs 236

7 Meninges, Ventricles and Cerebrospinal Fluid 239

Meninges 239
    Dura mater 239
    Arachnoid 240
    Pia mater 241
    Subarachnoid Space 241

Ventricles and Cerebrospinal Fluid 243
    Ventricles 243
    Cerebrospinal Fluid 244
    Blockages of Cerebrospinal Fluid
    Flow 247

8 Telencephalon or Cerebral Cortex 256

External Characteristics 256
Internal Characteristics 259
    Cortex 259
    White Matter 264
        Projection Fibers 264
        Association Fibers 266
        Commissural Fibers 268
Functional Organization of the Cortex ... 268
    Primary Receptive Fields of Parietal,
    Occipital, and Temporal Cortex 274
        Primary Somatosensory Cortex 274

    Primary Visual Cortex 275
    Primary Auditory Cortex 277
    Primary Gustatory Cortex 277
    Primary Vestibular Cortex 277
    Frontal Lobe 277
        Primary Somatomotor Cortex
        (Precentral Gyrus) 278
        Premotor Cortex 278
        Motor Speech Cortex (Broca) 279
        Prefrontal Cortex (Frontal
        Association Areas) 281

Secondary Receptive Cortical Fields (Parietal, Occipital, Temporal Association Areas) 284
   Focal Signs Caused by Lesions in Association Territories 285
Sensory or Wernicke's Aphasia 294
   Additional Remarks 297
General Signs and Symptoms Accompanying Diseases of the Cerebrum 297
   Meningiomas 299
   Epileptic Seizures 300
Circulatory System of the Cerebrum 301
   Arterial Supply 301
      Internal Carotid Arteries 302
      Vertebral Arteries 302
      Arterial Circle of Willis 302

      Cerebral Arteries Proper 304
      Peripheral Anastomoses of Cerebral Arteries 308
Signs and Syndromes of Cerebral Circulatory Deficiencies 308
   Vertebrobasilar Insufficiency 309
   Internal Carotid Artery Insufficiency 311
   Arterial Aneurysms 316
   Hypertensive Arterial Disease and Intracerebral Bleeding 318
Veins and Dural Sinuses 320
   External Veins 320
   Internal Veins 322
   Symptomatology of Venous and Sinus Thromboses 324

References 328

Index 337

1 Sensory System

Receptors

Receptors are specialized sensory organs capable of registering certain changes in their vicinity and within the organism and of transmitting these stimuli as impulses. They are the end-organs of afferent nerve fibers. One can subdivide them according to their functions into *exteroceptors,* which tell the body what is going on in its ambient environments and *teleceptors,* such as those in eyes and ears, which register stimuli originating in the more distant environment.

Proprioceptors, among them the receptors in the labyrinth, provide information about the position and movement of the head in space, about tension in muscles and tendons, about the position of joints, about muscular strength, and about other movements and positions of the body. Finally, there are *entero-* and *visceroceptors,* which report on events taking place within the organism. They are *osmo-, chemo-, baroceptors,* and others. For the various receptors to react, stimuli must be appropriate.

Skin receptors will be discussed first (Fig. 1.1). They are subdivided into *mechanoceptors* (touch, pressure), *thermoceptors* (cold, heat), and *nociceptors* (pain). These receptors are abundant in the skin, particularly between the epidermis and connective tissue. Consequently, the skin may be looked upon as a sensory organ covering the entire surface of the body.

Skin receptors consist of two large groups: (1) free nerve endings and (2) encapsulated end-organs. *Free nerve endings* occur in the spaces between the epidermal cells and between structures of neural origin, such as Merkel's *tactile menisci* (menisci tactus). Free nerve endings are present over almost the entire surface of the body and transmit pain and temperature impulses produced by injury to the cells. The tactile menisci are located mainly at the fingertips and react upon active touching or passively being touched.

Hair cuffs take an intermediary position. They are present wherever there is hairy skin, and transmit touch stimuli. Meissner's *touch corpuscles* (corpuscula tactus) are present only in hairless skin, such as the palms of the hands and soles of the feet (as well as the lips, tip of the tongue, and genital mucosa). They are very sensitive to active and passive touch. The *Vater-Pacini lamellar corpuscles* (corpuscula lamellosa) are situated in deeper layers of the skin, particularly between the cutis and subcutis. They transmit pressure sensations. *Krause's corpuscles* (corpuscula bulboidea) have been considered cold receptors, and *Ruffini's corpuscles* (corpuscula lamellosa), receptors of warmth.

This is now questioned. The free nerve endings are also capable of registering temperature. The cornea, for example, has only free nerve endings, and they pick up cold as well as heat.

Aside from the receptors mentioned, there is a variety of other receptors in the skin, the functions of which have not been clarified.

A second group of receptors consists of those that are located in deeper tissues of the body: in muscles, tendons, fasciae, and joints (Fig. 1.2).

1 Sensory System

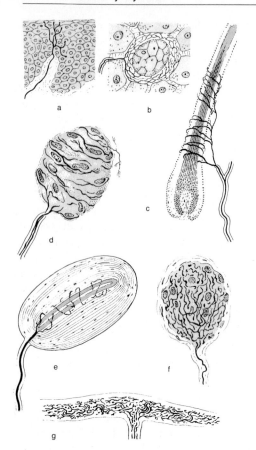

Fig. 1.1 Endings of afferent nerve fibers (receptors) in the skin. **a** Free ending (pain, temperature); **b** Merkel's tactile meniscus; **c** hair cuff (touch); **d** Meissner's touch corpuscle; **e** Vater-Pacini's corpuscle (lamellated corpuscle; (pressure); **f** Krause's bulboid corpuscle (cold?); **g** Ruffini's corpuscle (heat?).

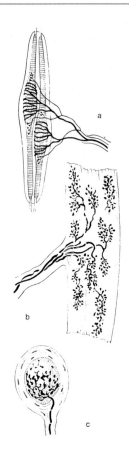

Fig. 1.2 Receptors in muscles, tendons and fasciae. **a** Anulospiral ending of muscle spindle (stretching); **b** Golgi tendon organ (tension); **c** Golgi-Mazzoni's corpuscle (pressure).

Muscle receptors consist of several types, the most important of which are the *neuromuscular spindles*. They respond to passive stretching of the muscle and are responsible for the *stretch* or *myotactic reflex*. These thin, spindle-shaped structures are ensheathed by a layer of connective tissue and are located between striated muscle fibers of the skeletal musculature. They contain 3 to 10 very thin striated fibers called *intrafusal muscle fibers* (*fusus* means spindle) in contrast to the other or *extrafusal fibers*. The polar endings of the connective tissue capsules are tied to the diffuse connective tissue stroma that invests fibers, fascicles, and the entire muscle. In this way the spindles participate in the movements of the muscle. Afferent fibers, called *anulospiral endings* or *primary endings*, are spun around the middle of a muscle spindle. These fibers have rather thick myelin sheaths and belong to the fastest-conducting fiber group the so-called Ia fibers. The equatorial, noncontractile portion of a spindle contains 40 to 50 small nuclei in so-called *nuclear-bag fibers*. Attached to them are *nuclear-chain fibers* each harboring a row of individual nuclei. For more detail, see pages 7–14 (monosynaptic proprioceptive reflex and polysynaptic reflexes).

The *tendon organs of Golgi* are delicate nerve endings or branches of thickly myelinated nerve fibers that are wrapped around groups of collagenous tendon fibers. They are surrounded by a connective tissue capsule, are located at the transitional area between tendon and muscle, and are arranged in series with the muscle fibers. Like muscle spindles, they respond to tensile stimuli, but their threshold is higher (see Fig. 1.**10**).

In addition to muscle spindles and tendon organs of Golgi, there are still other types of receptors in this region that transmit pressure, pain, and other stimuli. The *Vater-Pacini lamellar corpuscles, corpuscles of Golgi-Mazzoni*, and *terminal nerve endings* are some of them.

All these receptors in skin and deeper tissues are attached to a collateral of an axon. Several axonal collaterals converge toward the axon of a sensory neuron. Every cutaneous stimulus impinging on the skin activates not merely one but several types of receptors. The sum total of stimuli is transmitted to the central organ as an impulse of varying velocity.

The encapsulated, more differentiated terminal corpuscles likely transmit epicritic qualities, such as light touch, discrimination, vibration, and pressure. The free nerve endings are probably responsible for transmitting protopathic qualities, such as differences in pain or temperature.

Receptors are the peripheral endings of afferent nerve fibers, which are the peripheral processes of *pseudounipolar spinal ganglion neurons*. Each neuron of the ganglion gives off a short axon, which soon branches like a T. One branch runs to the periphery, joining the receptors. The other branch connects, via the posterior root, with the spinal cord, in which it proceeds in different directions, depending on the quality of the sensory impulse it carries (see Fig. 1.**19**).

The Peripheral Nerve

A nerve consists of one or more bundles of nerve fibers (axons). A nerve of medium size may contain thousands upon thousands of nerve fibers, some unmyelinated and others surrounded by myelin sheaths of different thickness. Fig. 1.3 shows a nerve on cross

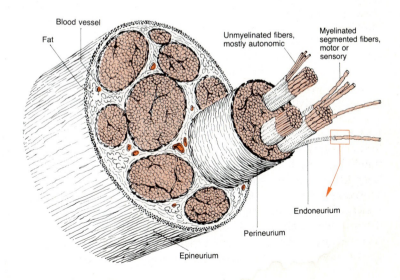

Fig. 1.3 Cross-section of a peripheral mixed nerve.

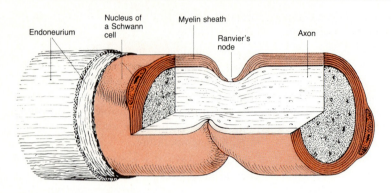

Fig. 1.4 Myelinated nerve fiber. Enlargement of fiber passing through rectangle in Figure 1.3.

section. Fig. 1.4 illustrates a single myelinated nerve fiber, cut crosswise and lengthwise, and shows that the centrally located axon is surrounded by a sheath of myelin (myelin is a mixture of lipids and protein). The nuclei of two Schwann cells can be seen. According to electron micrographs, the surface membranes of these cells are spirally wrapped around the axon, forming multiple layers enclosing lamellae of myelin, which are part of the Schwann cells. The myelin sheaths may be thought of as layers of insulating material.

The sheaths of Schwann and the myelin they contain are interrupted at 1 to 2 mm intervals by ring-shaped constrictions called *nodes of Ranvier*. These nodes play an important role in the propagation of stimulus effects from receptor to spinal cord or vice versa by facilitating fast conduction of the impulses through saltatory conduction of action potentials. The thicker the myelin sheaths, the faster the nerve fiber conducts. Both myelinated and unmyelinated or poorly myelinated fibers are surrounded by the protoplasmic membranes of the Schwann cells, only one of these cells serving the nerve fiber segment between two nodes of Ranvier.

The Schwann cells are enveloped by a layer of connective tissue, the *endoneurium*. The connective tissue surrounding several bundles of nerve fibers is called the *perineurium* and the one wrapped around larger nerves, the *epineurium*. These connective tissue coverings protect the nerve from mechanical injury and direct contact with nerve-damaging agents. The connective tissue carries the blood vessels nourishing the nerve fibers.

The peripheral nerve contains afferent as well as efferent, myelinated as well as unmyelinated, and somatic as well as vegetative or autonomic fibers. The somatic fibers connect receptors with the spinal cord, and the motor cells of the anterior horns with the musculature. The autonomic fibers are also both afferent and efferent and innervate the viscera, blood vessels, and glands.

Somatic and autonomic fibers, whether afferent or efferent, do not run in separate bundles within a mixed nerve. They are intermingled until they approach the point of destination. Then they separate again, as nerves for skin, muscles, joints, and viscera.

The nerve fibers are classified according to the thickness of their myelin sheaths and the velocity of their conduction. Table 1.1 provides examples.

The *posterior roots* contain only afferent nerve fibers. All impulses originating in receptors in skin, muscles, joints, and internal organs have to pass through the posterior roots to enter the spinal cord. *These afferent fibers are the central branches of the pseudounipolar spinal ganglion cells. The impulses are not switched or transferred to neurons of the spinal ganglia.*

Table 1.1 Classification of Nerve Fibers According to Thickness of Myelin Sheaths and Velocity of Conduction.

Type of Fiber	Diameter (μ)	Velocity (m/sec)
Ia fibers (A, α) From anulospiral endings	Approx. 17	70–120
Ib fibers (A, α) From tendon organs of Golgi	Approx. 16	70–100
II fibers (A, β, and γ) From flower-spray endings and Merkel's touch menisci	Approx. 8	15–40
III fibers (A, δ) Pain, temperature, pressure	Approx. 3	5–15
IV or C fibers Pain, temperature, heavy touch	Approx. 0.2–1	0.2–2

The nerve fibers transmitting impulses from the various sensory receptors are intermingled in the peripheral nerve. As the nerve approaches the spinal ganglion, the fibers separate into groups according to their specific functions and take definite positions within the dorsal root (Fig. 1.5). The nerve fibers that originate in the neuromuscular spindles

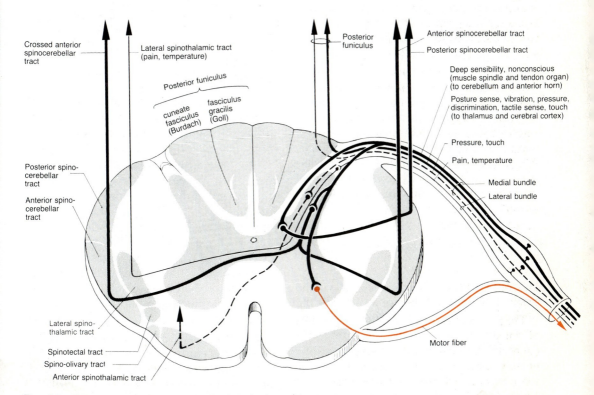

Fig. 1.5 Course of posterior root fibers in spinal cord.

and have the thickest myelin sheaths occupy the most medial part of the root. The midportion of the root is taken up by fibers that derive from encapsulated receptors and transmit, among other sensations, those of touch, vibration, pressure, and discrimination. The most lateral fibers are the ones that are almost unmyelinated and carry pain and temperature impulses.

The nerve fibers with the thickest myelin sheaths conduct deep sensibility (*proprioception*). Only some of the impulses coming from muscles, joints, fasciae, and other tissues reach the level of awareness; most serve the automatic control of motor activity needed for walking and standing.

Upon passing through the *entrance zone* of the posterior roots into the spinal cord, the individual fibers divide into numerous collaterals, which secure synaptic connections with other neurons in the spinal cord. Fig. 1.5 shows that the nerve fibers join different tracts within the cord, depending on the sensory modality they serve. It should be noted that all afferent fibers when passing through the entrance zone of the posterior root, also called the Redlich-Obersteiner area, become momentarily devoid of myelin sheaths. The transition from peripheral to central nerve fiber thus is rather abrupt. Schwann cells characteristic of the peripheral nerve cease to exist, and oligodendrocytes take over. This physiological lack of myelin in the transitional area is said to render the nerve fibers vulnerable to disease, such as tabes dorsalis.

Neurons of the Central Nervous System

We must briefly discuss the neurons of the central nervous system before we describe the further course of the fibers that carry impulses from diverse sensory modalities into the spinal cord via spinal ganglia and posterior roots.

Fig. 1.6 shows the afferent fiber of a pseudounipolar neuron of the spinal gan-

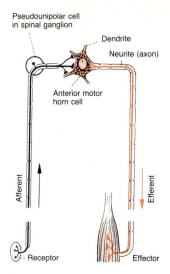

Fig. 1.6 Simple monosynaptic reflex arc.

glion forming a simple *monosynaptic reflex arc* with a highly specialized motor neuron in the anterior horn of the spinal cord.

The structure of these neurons is so complicated that we can give only a brief description. The body or *perikaryon* of a cell of this type has numerous processes of different lengths. One of them is particularly long and carries the discharges of the cell to the periphery. It is called the *axon* or *neurite*. The others are shorter, branch extensively, and are called *dendrites*.

The neurons produce and conduct action potentials. A neuron can transmit excitation to another neuron via one or multiple points of contact, or *synapses*. Synapses are separated from the surface of the other cell by a very small space. As an excitation reaches the synapse (presynaptic), a transmitter substance is set free into the space and either enhances (acetylcholine) or inhibits (γ-aminobutyric acid) the postsynaptic element of the other neuron.

A single nerve cell receives impulses not from only one or two neurons, but from many and even thousands of neurons. A great number of *boutons terminaux* (synaptic end-feet) are attached to the outside of the

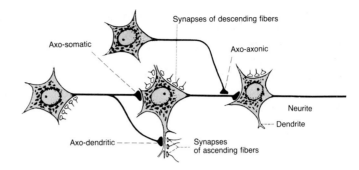

Fig. 1.7 Polysynaptic circuits in the central nervous system.

cell body, axon, and dendrites of a neuron. Some have a stimulating, others an inhibiting effect on the activity of the specific neuron (Fig. 1.7). An excitation always travels in the same direction: from the cell body to the synaptic junction. The synapses are switch-like contacts where impulses can be either reinforced or reduced.

Thus, a nerve cell simultaneously receives a great number of signals, of which some are stimulating and others are inhibiting. The cell adds the number of positive impulses, subtracts the sum of the inhibiting ones, and then transmits the balance. The impulse carried by a nerve fiber can travel via synaptic connections with a chain of neurons in various ways, determined by the pattern it meets of stimulating and inhibiting junctions. This is the reason why the influence of a stimulus differs greatly, depending on which of the various possible directions it takes.

Proprioception

Impulses deriving from muscular spindles and tendon organs are transmitted by the most richly myelinated fast-conducting fibers, Ia fibers. Other impulses of proprioception originating in receptors of fasciae, joints, and deeper layers of connective tissue travel in less myelinated fibers.

Only a small number of the proprioceptive impulses reach the cerebral cortex and, therefore, enter consciousness. Most travel in feedback circuits or servo systems and do not reach the level of awareness. They are elements of reflexes basic to voluntary and other movements, and of static reflexes, which counteract the gravity of the earth.

Peripheral Servo Mechanism

A few words must be said about the function of the diverse peripheral feedback systems before we continue to describe the course of the various fiber groups carrying the sensations of pain, temperature, pressure, touch, and so on in spinal cord and brain.

Fig. 1.5 illustrates that the thick afferent fiber which comes from the neuromuscular spindle divides at the entrance zone of the posterior root, and that one part of the fiber enters into direct contact with a neuron in the anterior horn. This is a *motoneuron*, which is located in the gray anterior horn and gives off an efferent fiber. These efferent motor fibers leave the spinal cord via the anterior root, and after bypassing the spinal ganglion, join the peripheral nerve on their way to the skeletal muscle. Consequently, the afferent and efferent fibers form an arc, which extends from the muscle spindle to the anterior horn motoneuroń and from here back into the skeletal musculature. This is called a *simple monosynaptic reflex arc*, consisting of two neurons joined by synapses.

Monosynaptic Proprioceptive Reflex

Figs. 1.9 and 1.10 illustrate *neuromuscular spindles* near their tendons. Every muscle contains a great number of these encapsulated, complex *stretch receptors* in charge of keeping the length of the muscle under control. They are made up of modified muscle fibers, called *intrafusal* fibers, and of bag-like structures in their central or equatorial segments each containing 40–50 spherical nuclei, hence the term *nuclear bags*. The intrafusal fibers are thinner than the ordinary, *extrafusal* fibers. They are subdivided into nuclear-bag and nuclear-chain fibers. These two types of fibers are shown separately in Figs. 1.9 and 1.10 for didactic reasons. In reality, the shorter and thinner nuclear-chain fibers

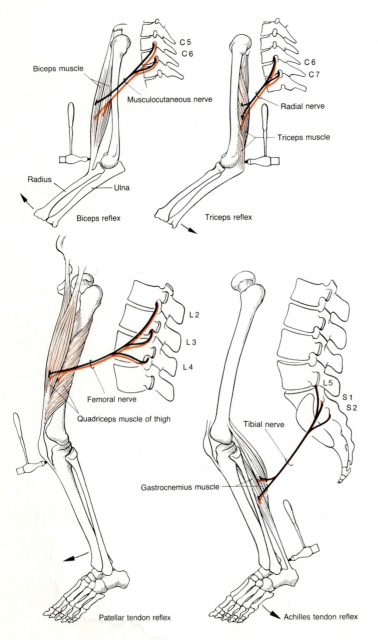

Fig. 1.8 The most important proprioceptive reflexes.

are attached to the longer nuclear-bag fibers. In general, a spindle contains two nuclear-bag and four or five nuclear-chain fibers.

Both extrafusal and intrafusal muscle fibers are innervated with motor fibers, the intrafusal ones via gamma fibers (fusimotors) from small motoneurons accompanying the large motoneurons in the anterior horns. The nuclear bag of each spindle is enmeshed in a net of fine sensory nerve fibers, the *anulospiral endings* (anulus, latin: ring-like structure). These endings are extremely sensitive to stretching of the muscle. Therefore, the spindle is considered to be a *stretch receptor* in charge of keeping the muscle at a constant length.

The extrafusal muscle fibers are of a definite length when at rest. The organism always tries to maintain this length. As the muscle is stretched, so is the spindle. The anulospiral nerve endings immediately respond to the stretching with action potentials, which are transmitted to the large motoneuron in the spinal cord via the fast-conducting afferent Ia fibers and from here via the also fast-conducting, thick $alpha_1$ efferent fibers to the extrafusal musculature. As the muscle contracts, its original length is restored. Any stretching of the muscle promptly initiates this mechanism.

A light tap on the tendon of a muscle – for example the tendon of the quadriceps muscle – momentarily stretches the homonymous muscle. The spindles react immediately. As their impulse is transmitted to the anterior horn motoneuron, this neuron fires causing immediately a brief contraction. This *monosynaptic reflex* is basic to all proprioceptive reflexes.

The reflex arc involves not more than 1 or 2 segments of the spinal cord, a fact of great diagnostic value in determining the location of a lesion.

Fig. 1.8 shows the segments of the spinal cord involved in the four most important proprioceptive reflexes. The very brief stretchings of the muscles caused here by taps with the reflex hammer rarely occur under ordinary circumstances.

The servo mechanism maintaining the length of a muscle can be adjusted to maintain a different length by a particular motor system acting on the intrafusal muscle fibers of the spindles.

Fig. 1.9 demonstrates that the large alpha motor cells of the anterior horn are accompanied by smaller, gamma motoneurons. Very delicate gamma fibers extend from these gamma neurons to the intrafusal muscle fibers. Impulses carried by these gamma

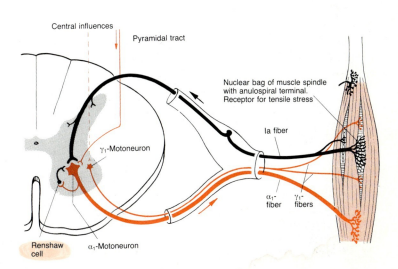

Fig. 1.9 Feedback circuit for maintaining length of muscle.

fibers produce contraction of the intrafusal musculature at both poles of the spindle, causing a stretching of the equatorial midportion. This change is instantly picked up by the anulospiral endings. Their action potentials increase the tension of the working musculature.

The gamma motoneurons are under the influence of fibers descending from motoneurons located in rostral portions of the central nervous system in pathways such as the pyramidal, the reticulospinal, and the vestibulospinal tracts. Thus, muscle tension can be influenced directly by the brain, an influence that is important for every voluntary movement. The efferent action of gamma fibers makes it possible for voluntary movements to be modified and finely tuned to their purposes. Because of the efferent gamma action, it is possible to regulate the responsiveness of the stretch receptors through what can be called a *gamma neuron-spindle system*. Contraction of the intrafusal muscles brings about a lowering of the action threshold of the stretch receptors; in other words, a minor stretching of the musculature in itself causes an activation of the stretch receptors. Under normal circumstances, the length of the muscles is automatically adjusted by the fusimotor innervation via this reflex arc.

If primary and secondary receptors are slowly stretched, the response of the spindle receptors is *static*. If the stretching is fast, their answer is strong, *dynamic*. Both static and dynamic reactions are controlled by efferent gamma neurons.

Presumably, there are two types of efferent gamma neurons. One consists of gamma-dynamic cells innervating predominantly the intrafusal nuclear-bag fibers. The other represents gamma-static cells predominantly stimulating the intrafusal nuclear-chain fibers. A stimulation of the nuclear-bag fibers by the gamma-dynamic neurons provokes a strong dynamic and very little static response. Conversely, if the gamma-static neurons excite the intrafusal nuclear-chain fibers, the reaction will be static, tonic, and barely dynamic.

Other Reflexes

The fast-conducting Ia fibers transmit action potentials from primary endings of nuclear-bag fibers and nuclear-chain fibers in a central direction. Many muscle spindles, particularly nuclear-chain fibers, have not only primary but also *secondary endings*, known as *flower-spray terminals*. These terminals also respond to tensile stimuli, and they transmit

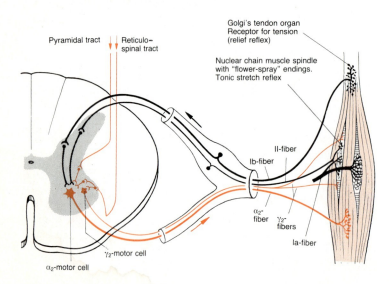

Fig. 1.10 Feedback circuit for maintaining tension of muscle.

their action potentials centrally via thin II fibers connecting with intercalated (inserted in between) neurons capable of reciprocal actions. Through these neurons they may activate flexor or extensor muscles, simultaneously inhibiting the respective antagonist muscles.

Fig. 1.**10** shows muscle spindles and a *tendon organ of Golgi*. These organs respond to the tension in the homonymous muscles, whether caused by active or by reflexive contraction, with inhibitory impulses traveling over one or two intercalated neurons. These impulses are transmitted by the fast-conducting Ib fibers. It is the primary task of the organs of Golgi to measure the effort of the individual muscles on the basis of returning signals and to maintain muscle tension within physiologic limits by sending out inhibiting impulses.

Thus, every muscle is under the control of two feedback systems: (1) its length is controlled by a system in which the muscle spindles act as the measuring sensors, and (2) its tension is controlled by another system, in which the tendon organs of Golgi are the measuring sensors.

Our bodies are continuously exposed to the gravitational forces of the earth. We would not be able to stand upright or walk if certain muscles, such as the quadriceps muscles, the muscles of the neck, and the long muscles of the back, did not counteract gravity by having a correspondingly high tone. The normal level of this tension is not sufficient, however, if one wants to lift a load. The quadriceps muscles, for example, would not be sufficiently strong to prevent falling to the knees unless the increased stretching caused the muscle spindles to activate instantaneously the reflex that increases the tone of the musculature to an appropriate level. It is by this mechanism that the muscle tone is automatically adjusted to that required for a given situation. It is a *servo mechanism* based on

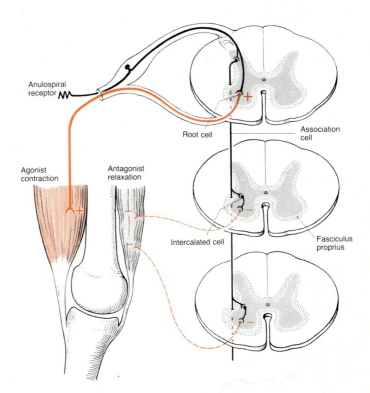

Fig. 1.**11** Monosynaptic reflex with polysynaptic inhibiting effect on antagonists.

feedback circuits that continuously carry action potentials for retaining the muscle tone necessary for standing and walking.

Every muscle has a certain tone, a so-called *resting tone*, even when totally relaxed. This tone can be noticed when one passively bends or stretches one of the limbs. To abolish the tone completely it is necessary to transect all anterior roots containing the motor fibers of the muscles. Transection of the posterior roots has the same effect. Thus, the resting tone is produced not by the musculature itself but by the reflex arcs mentioned earlier.

The so-called monosynaptic reflex is, strictly speaking, not monosynaptic. It has a polysynaptic component. For a reflexive movement of a limb to occur, there must be a contraction of the prime moving muscle, or *agonist*, and simultaneously a relaxation of the opposing muscle, or *antagonist*. The contraction as described, is the result of an afferent impulse from stretch receptors producing excitation of the motoneuron in the anterior horn of the cord.

The afferent fibers, however, give off collaterals to intercalated or internuncial (*internuncio* means messenger) neurons of the neuronal apparatus proper of the spinal cord, and these connect with the motoneurons responsible for the antagonist. The message of

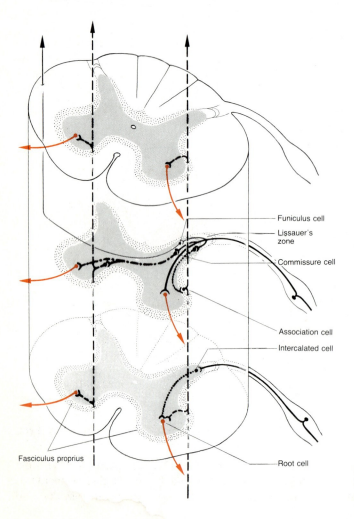

Fig. 1.12 Intrinsic neuronal system of the spinal cord; polysynaptic relay stations.

the internuncial cells is not facilitative but inhibitory. This inhibitory effect explains why the stretching of the antagonist from contraction of the agonist does not produce a simultaneous contraction of the antagonist, which would make any movement impossible (Fig. 1.**11**).

Another reflex arc is instrumental in causing the important *flexor reflex*. This is a protection or *flight reflex*. It is also a polysynaptic use of many intercalated neurons as stations in impulse transmission. For example, when one touches a hot stove with a finger, the hand withdraws with lightning speed even before one becomes aware of pain.

In this instance the receptor is a *nociceptor* (pain receptor). Its action potentials ascend to the *substantia gelatinosa* of the spinal cord, where the afferent fibers synapse with numerous intercalated nerve cells of the *intrinsic neuronal system of the cord* (tract cells, internuncial cells, association cells, and root cells), shown in Fig. 1.**12**. The initial impulse is transmitted to all muscles participating in retracting the hand from the pain-producing object. It must initiate numerous impulses causing, on one side, contraction and, on the other side, relaxation of certain muscles in certain sequence and intensity. The reflex system proper of the spinal cord is not unlike the wiring system of a modern computer.

For example, stepping on a sharp, pointed stone causes pain, which immediately sets off a programmed sequence of movements (Fig. 1.**13**). The smarting foot is lifted by flexion, and the weight of the body is thus transferred to the other leg. The sudden shift would lead to a fall if the muscles of the trunk, shoulders, neck, and arms did not immediately compensate for the breakdown of equilibrium and secure the upright position of the body. This event requires the existence of a rather complex circuitry within the spinal cord, which connects with areas in brainstem and cerebellum. This entire sequence happens within a fraction of a second, and it is not until afterward that pain is felt, that one looks for its cause, and that one

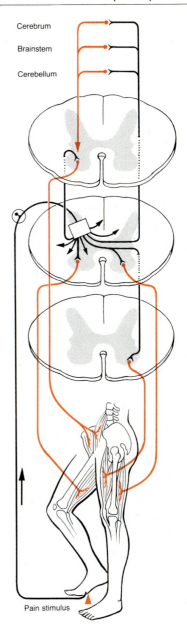

Fig. 1.**13** Flexor reflex with polysynaptic connections.

checks to see whether the foot has been injured.

Events like these take place, for the most part, in the spinal cord. Higher segments of the central nervous system are usually also linked with the spinal circuits. In the last example involvement of higher segments was necessary to prevent the loss of equilibrium. Part of the impulses from muscles, tendons, joints, and deeper tissues went to the cerebellum, the organ controlling equilibrium. To get there, the impulses traveled along the *spinocerebellar tracts*.

Spinocerebellar Tracts

Posterior Spinocerebellar Tract

The fast-conducting Ia fibers coming from muscle spindles and tendon organs split up into several collaterals after they enter the spinal cord. Some collaterals proceed to the large alpha anterior horn cells representing part of the monosynaptic reflex arc mentioned earlier (see Fig. 1.5). Another group of collaterals connects with neurons of the thoracic nucleus (Stillings' nucleus, Clarke's column) which is located in the medial base of the posterior horn and extends longitudinally through the cord from the level of C8 to the level of L2. These cells represent the "second neurons." Their axons form the *posterior spinocerebellar tract*, and they are among the fastest-conducting fibers. They ascend ipsilaterally in the posterior portion of the lateral funiculus near the surface of the cord to the inferior pontocerebellar peduncle and to their destination, the cortex of the vermis of the paleocerebellum (Fig. 1.14). The collaterals of cervical posterior roots ascend via the cuneate fascicle to their own nucleus, the *accessory cuneate nucleus*, from where the "second neurons" connect with the cerebellum (see Fig. 1.19).

Anterior Spinocerebellar Tract

A third contingent of collaterals of the afferent Ia fibers form synapses with neurons in the posterior horns and in the medial portions of the spinal gray matter (see Figs. 1.5, 1.14, 1.19). These "second neurons", which are present throughout the entire cord, the lumbar cord included, extend to form the *anterior spinocerebellar tract*. It ascends in the anterior peripheral portion of the lateral funiculi of both sides until it reaches the cerebellum. Unlike the posterior spinocerebellar tract, the anterior tract passes through the tegmentum of medulla oblongata, pons, and midbrain and reaches the vermis via the superior cerebellar peduncle (brachium conjunctivum) and the superior medullary velum.

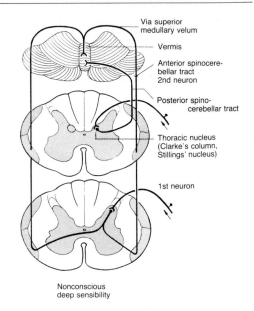

Fig. 1.14 Anterior and posterior spinocerebellar tracts.

The paleocerebellum receives information about all afferent stimuli of deep sensibility and influences the tone of the muscles through polysynaptic conduction of impulses. It also controls the collaboration between agonists and antagonists which is basic to standing, walking, and any other form of movement. Thus, a circuit of higher function is superimposed on the lower feedback circuit of the spinal cord and influences the musculature by acting via extrapyramidal pathways on the gamma motor cells of the anterior horn and the gamma efferent impulses. All these activities do not reach the level of consciousness.

Posterior Funiculi

What we are aware of is the position of our extremities and the tone of their muscles. We feel the ground beneath our feet or, more correctly, the pressure of our body on the soles of our feet. We are aware of movements in our joints. This is evidence that some of the proprioceptive impulses reach the cerebral cortex.

As mentioned earlier, the impulses producing proprioceptive sensations originate in receptors in muscles, tendons, fasciae, capsules of joints, deep connective tissue, and skin. They travel to the spinal cord through axons of pseudounipolar neurons of the spinal ganglia. After giving off collaterals to neurons in the posterior and anterior horns of the gray matter, the main portions of the central axonal branches enter the posterior funiculus.

Some branches descend, and the others ascend in two tracts making up each funiculus: the medial *fasciculus gracilis* of Goll and the lateral *fasciculus cuneatus* of Burdach. They terminate in their own nuclei, the *nucleus gracilis* and the *nucleus cuneatus*, located in the dorsal tegmentum of the lower medulla oblongata (Figs. 1.15 and 1.16; see Fig. 1.19).

The fibers that ascend in the posterior funiculi are arranged in somatotopic order. Those carrying the impulses of the perineal saddle region, legs, and lower trunk run in the fasciculus gracilis, commencing next to the posterior median septum. Those carrying the impulses from chest, arms, and neck are arranged in the fasciculus cuneatus, the fibers from the neck being located most laterally (see Fig. 1.15).

The nerve cells in the nuclei gracilis and cuneatus represent the "second neurons." Their axons form the *bulbothalamic tract* and connect with the "third neurons" in the *thalamic posterolateral ventral nucleus*. Starting at the nuclei gracilis and cuneatus, the bulbothalamic tracts proceed at first anteriorly on

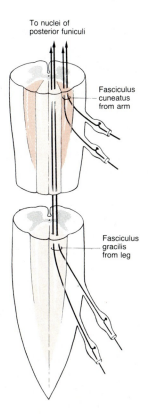

Fig. 1.15 Posterior funiculus.

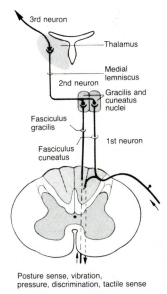

Fig. 1.16 Posterior funiculus.

either side of the so-called central gray matter of the lower medulla oblongata just above the decussation of the descending pyramidal tracts. Thereafter they travel as *medial lemnisci* across the midline (decussation of the medial lemnisci) and ascend posteriorly to the pyramids and medially from the inferior olives through the tegmentum of the upper medulla and that of pons and midbrain to the thalamus (see Fig. 1.**16**). (Mnemonic suggestion: m<u>e</u>dial lemniscus for <u>s</u>ensory, l<u>a</u>teral lemniscus for <u>a</u>coustic stimuli.)

The nerve cells of the posterolateral ventral thalamic nucleus are the "third neurons" in this chain (see Fig. 1.**16**). Their axons form the *thalamocortical tract*, which passes through the posterior portion of the posterior limb of the internal capsule (posterior to the pyramidal tract) and through the *corona radiata* of the cerebral white matter to the posterior central convolution (postcentral gyrus). This is the reason the sensory impulses are consciously noticed. The somatotopic arrangement as described for the fibers in the spinal cord continues during their entire course to thalamus and cerebral cortex. In the latter, their projection corresponds to the body scheme of a homunculus standing on its head (see Fig. 8.**20a**).

The posterior funiculi transmit predominantly impulses that originate in proprioceptors and receptors of the skin. If they are damaged it becomes impossible to determine the position of one's extremities and to recognize objects by touch. Numbers and letters written on the skin can no longer be identified. Discrimination of two simultaneous stimuli on the skin is abolished. Sensations of pressure are reduced; therefore, one does not feel the ground beneath one's feet and is insecure (ataxic) while standing or walking, particularly in the dark or with eyes closed. These dysfunctions are pronounced if the posterior funiculi are damaged. They are usually less severe when the gracilis and cuneate nuclei, the medial lemnisci, the thalami, or the posterior central gyri are damaged.

Syndromes of Injury of Posterior Funiculi

1. *Loss of posture and locomotion sensation:* With eyes closed the patient cannot identify how his limbs are positioned.
2. *Astereognosis:* With eyes closed the patient cannot recognize and describe the shape and material of objects he touches.
3. *Loss of two-point discrimination.*
4. *Loss of vibratory sense:* The patient does not feel the vibration of a tuning fork held against bone.
5. *Positive Romberg's sign:* With eyes closed the patient is not able to stand securely when his feet are put together. He sways and may fall. With eyes open he can compensate greatly for the loss of deep esthesias. This compensation is not seen in a patient with cerebellar ataxia.

In addition to the posterior tracts, two separate afferent pathways of the spinal cord also terminate in the thalamus. These are the anterior and lateral spinothalamic tracts. They

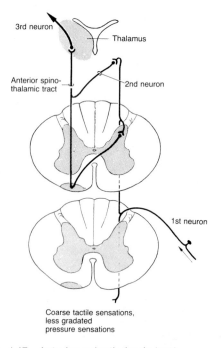

Fig. 1.**17** Anterior spinothalamic tract.

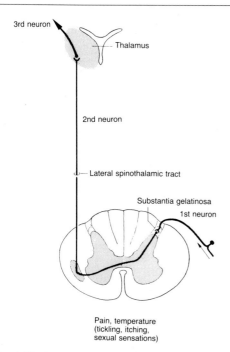

Fig. 1.18 Lateral spinothalamic tract.

represent axons of "second neurons" and not of the pseudounipolar nerve cells of the spinal ganglia (see Figs. 1.17 and 1.18).

Spinothalamic Tracts

Anterior Spinothalamic Tract

The first neurons are again the pseudounipolar nerve cells of the spinal ganglia. Their moderately thick, myelinated peripheral fibers conduct tactile and not particularly differentiated pressure sensations from skin receptors, such as hair baskets and tactile corpuscles. The central branches of these axons pass through the posterior roots into the posterior funiculi of the cord. Here they may ascend for 2 to 15 segments and may send collaterals downward for 1 to 2 segments. At a number of levels they synapse with neurons of the posterior horns (Fig. 1.17). These nerve cells constitute the "second neurons" that form the anterior spinothalamic tract. This tract crosses in the *anterior commissure* in front of the central canal to the opposite side and continues to the anterior peripheral area of the anterolateral funiculus. From here it ascends to the thalamic posterolateral ventral nucleus together with the lateral spinothalamic tract and the medial lemniscus (see Fig. 1.19). The nerve cells of the thalamus are "third neurons" projecting the impulses into the postcentral gyrus via the thalamocortical tract.

The fact that the central branches of the first neurons run up and down within the posterior funiculus and communicate via many collaterals with the "second neurons" is the reason that injury to the lumbar and thoracic portions of the spinothalamic tract usually causes no essential loss of tactile sensation. The impulses can simply bypass the area of injury. If the damage involves the cervical portion of the anterior spinothalamic tract, it may produce a light hypesthesia in the contralateral leg.

Lateral Spinothalamic Tract

This tract carries *pain and temperature* sensations. The peripheral receptors are the free nerve endings in the skin. They are end-organs of peripheral branches of the pseudounipolar spinal ganglion neurons that represent thin group A fibers and almost unmyelinated C fibers. The central branches enter the spinal cord via the lateral portion of the posterior roots. Within the cord they divide into short, longitudinal collaterals, which over 1 or 2 segments have synaptic contact with nerve cells of the *substantia gelatinosa* (Rolandi). These are the "second neurons" that form the lateral spinothalamic tract (Fig. 1.18). The fibers of this tract also cross through the anterior commissure and proceed to the lateral portion of the lateral funiculus and upward to the thalamus. Like the fibers of the posterior funiculi, those of both spinothalamic tracts are also arranged in somatotopic order: those coming from the legs are most peripherally and those arriving from the neck are most centrally (medially) located (see Fig. 1.21).

1 Sensory System

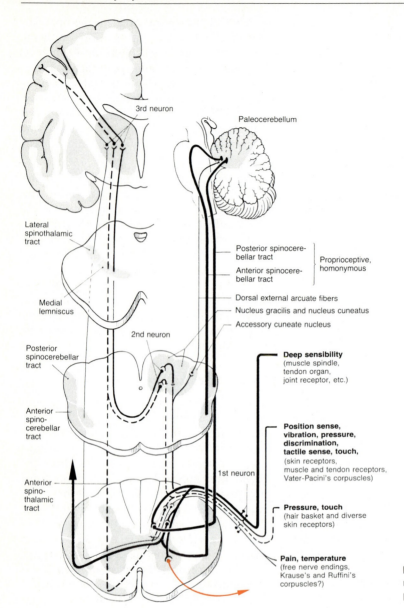

Fig. 1.19 Spinal cord with most important ascending pathways.

The lateral spinothalamic tract accompanies the medial lemniscus as the spinal lemniscus through the brainstem. It terminates at the ventral posterolateral nucleus of the thalamus (see Fig. 5.5 *VPL* and *V.c.e.*). From here the "third neurons" form the thalamocortical tract, which proceeds to the cortex of the posterior central gyrus (see Fig. 1.**20**). The fibers that carry pain and temperature sensations run in the spinothalamic tract so tightly side by side that it is not possible to separate them anatomically. If the lateral spinothalamic tract is injured, pain as well as temperature sensations are impaired, although not always to the same degree.

The lateral spinothalamic tract is the main pathway for pain and temperature. If the

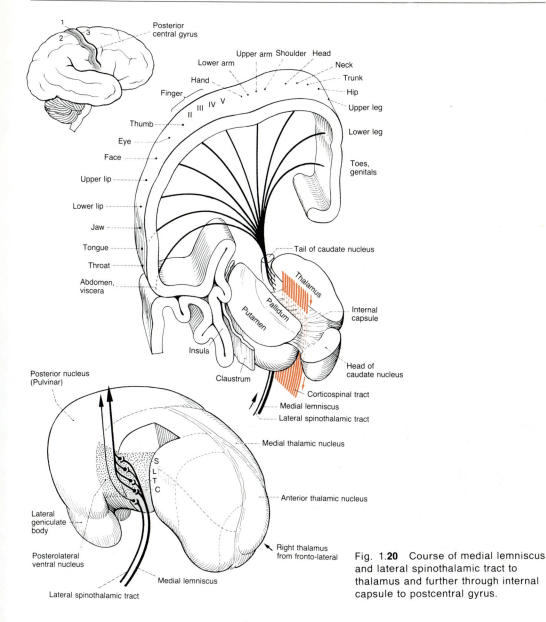

Fig. 1.20 Course of medial lemniscus and lateral spinothalamic tract to thalamus and further through internal capsule to postcentral gyrus.

tract is transected (chordotomy), an operation occasionally performed bilaterally for treatment of intractable pain, the pain may not be abolished totally. This result suggests that pain stimuli may be transmitted also via internuncial neurons along the intrinsic pathways of fasciculi proprii of the spinal cord.

Transection of the lateral spinothalamic tract in the ventral white matter of the cord abolishes pain and temperature sensation contralaterally about 1 to 2 segments below the level of the operation.

Pain and temperature impulses reaching the thalamus are felt but are indistinct. Once the impulses reach the cerebral cortex, differences in pain can be distinguished.

Fig. 1.**19** shows schematically the topography of the sensory pathways we have thus far mentioned, as they extend from the posterior roots to areas where they terminate. All sensory "third neurons" connecting thalamus and cerebral cortex pass through the posterior limb of the internal capsule posterior to the pyramidal tract and go to the receptive sphere for body sensations in the posterior central convolution (*gyrus postcentralis*: Brodmann's cytoarchitectonic areas 3a, 3b, 2 and 1). Here the "third neurons" project superficial sensations such as pain, touch, pressure, and temperature and, to some extent, deep sensations (Figs. 1.**20** and 5.**5**).

Not all afferent impulses are transmitted by the thalamus to the sensory cortex. A number of them terminate in the motor cortex of the *precentral gyrus*. It is possible to elicit from the postcentral gyrus not only sensory but also motor reactions. The motor and sensory cortical fields overlap to some extent. Therefore, one may speak of the central gyri as a *sensorimotor region*. Sensory signals can be immediately transformed into motor reactions in this region, because of sensorimotor feedback circuits to be discussed later. The pyramidal fibers of these short closed circuits usually terminate directly at the anterior horn cells without the presence of intercalated neurons.

Although there is some overlapping of connections and functions between pre- and postcentral gyri, the precentral gyrus should still be considered a predominantly motor region, and the postcentral gyrus a predominantly sensory territory.

The impulses carried by the afferent fibers of the "third neurons" arrive in the cerebral cortex in somatotopic order corresponding to the scheme of a sensory homunculus standing on its head. Furthermore, the different qualities of sensation have a definite spatial order: Brodmann's area 3a carries impulses from muscle spindles; area 3b, those of pain and

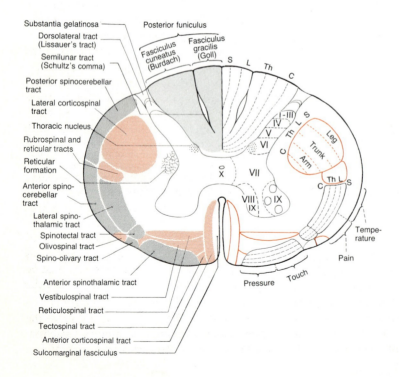

Fig. 1.**21** Cross-section of spinal cord showing topography of ascending and descending pathways and cytoarchitectural lamination according to Rexed (1954).

temperature; area 1, tactile sensations; and area 2, posture sensations (see Figs. 1.20 and 5.5).

Thalamically, pain, temperature and other stimuli are felt as dull, indistinct sensations, as we have stated. When they reach the cortex, they can be consciously distinguished as different qualities. Higher functions, such as two-point discrimination and exact determination of the location of individual stimuli, are cortical activities. Damage to the sensory cortex causes some decrease in sensations of pain, temperature, and touch but abolishes discrimination and posture sensation in the respective portion of the body contralateral to the lesion, because all sensory pathways have crossed before reaching the cortex.

Functions such as recognition of objects by touch (*stereognosis*) require additional association areas. These areas are located in the parietal lobe, where the many individual sensations of size, shape, and physical property (sharpness, dullness, softness, hardness, coolness, warmth and so forth) become integrated and can be compared with recollections of formerly experienced touch sensations. A lesion of the lower parietal lobe may result in loss of the ability to recognize objects by touching on the side opposite to that of the lesion. This loss of ability is called *astereognosis*.

The spinal cord contains not only afferent pathways and its own intrinsic fiber connections, such as the *fasciculi proprii*, but also a number of efferent pathways. There are the pyramidal tracts subserving voluntary movements and, in addition, numerous so-called extrapyramidal tracts, which have an effect on the complicated reflex mechanisms of the cord. Fig. 1.21 illustrates, on a cross-section of the cord, the distribution of the various sensory pathways and also the descending motor fiber bundles and their relationship to one another. Pathways of sensory "second neurons" are shown. The cells are located in the posterior horn, and their axons occupy the anterolateral funiculus, from which they ascend to neurons of the brainstem.

These pathways are, for example, the spinoreticular, the spinotectal, the spino-olivary, and the spinovestibular tracts (Fig. 1.21). They belong to the group of afferent pathways that are connected with the feedback circuits of the extrapyramidal system, to be discussed later. The *spinovestibular tract* is located in the cervical cord above C4 and adjacent to the *vestibulospinal tract*. It is probably a collateral of the dorsal spinocerebellar tract.

Comments on a few important features of the spinal cord are now in place.

Spinal Cord and Peripheral Innervation

In the adult the spinal cord is shorter than the spinal column. It terminates approximately at the level of the intervertebral disk between the first and second lumbar vertebrae (Fig. 1.22). Before the age of 3 months the segments of the spinal cord, indicated by its roots, directly face their corresponding vertebrae. Thereafter, the column grows more than the cord. The roots remain attached to the original intervertebral foramina and become increasingly longer toward the end of the cord (*conus terminalis*), eventually located at the level of the 2nd lumbar vertebra. Below this level the bag-like subarachnoid space contains only anterior and posterior roots that form the *cauda equina* (see Fig. 2.34). Occasionally, the *conus terminalis* may reach down to the level of the third lumbar vertebra.

Except for the segmental origin of its nerve roots, the cord itself shows no morphologic markings of its metameric subdivisions (see Fig. 1.22). The discrepancy between the location of spinal cord segments and that of their respective vertebrae, which increases as one approaches the conus terminalis, must be taken into account in attempts to localize the level of a spinal disease process.

The roots of segments C1 to C7 leave the spinal canal through the intervertebral foramina situated at the superior or rostral side

22   1 Sensory System

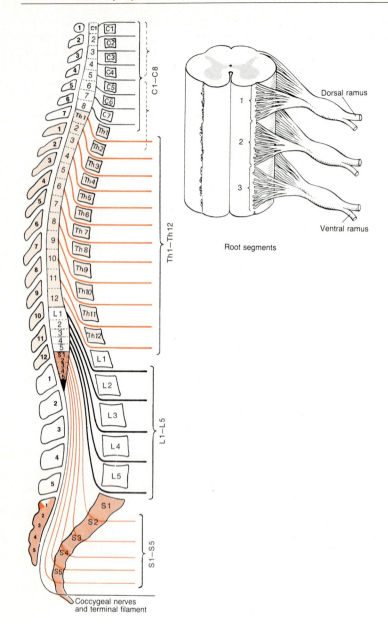

Fig. 1.22 Relationship of spinal root segments to vertebral bodies.

of each vertebra. Because the cervical cord has one segment more than there are cervical vertebrae, the roots of the 8th segment leave the canal through the foramina located between the 7th cervical and the 1st thoracic vertebrae. From here downward, the nerve roots leave through the foramina of the lower aspects of the corresponding vertebrae.

Between C4 and T1 and also between L2 and S3, the diameter of the cord is enlarged. These *intumescentiae cervicalis* and *lumbalis* exist because the roots of the lower half of the cervical cord give rise to the brachial plexus, innervating the upper extremities, and those of the lumbosacral region form the lumbosacral plexus, innervating the lower extremities (see Fig. 1.22).

The formation of plexuses permits the fibers of each pair of roots to branch into different peripheral nerves; in other words, each peripheral nerve is made up of fibers from several adjacent segmental roots (Figs. 1.23, 1.24, and 1.25). Toward the periphery of the nerves the afferent fibers deriving from one posterior root rejoin and supply a specific segmental territory of the skin, called a *dermatome* or *dermatomic area* (Fig. 1.26).

There are as many dermatomes as there are root segments. Fig. 1.28 shows all dermatomes of the body as seen from the front and from the rear. The metameric order of the dermatomes is best seen in the thoracic area. Fig. 1.26 demonstrates that the dermatomes overlap each other so that the loss of only one root can hardly be detected. There must be a loss of several adjacent roots for a sensory loss of segmental character to occur. Because the dermatomes correspond to the various root segments of the cord, they have great diagnostic value in determining the altitudinal level of cord damage. Fig. 1.27 is intended to be a mnemonic device to simplify learning the borders of the cervical, thoracic, lumbar, and sacral areas of innervation.

Of course, if part of a plexus or an individual peripheral nerve is damaged, the pattern of distribution of sensory loss is different from that caused by damage to roots. Involvement of a plexus predominantly produces motor deficits, which may represent typical syndromes to be discussed later in the section on motor functions (pages 47f.).

It may be repeated once more that the fibers making up a peripheral nerve come from various roots. If the nerve is damaged, the fibers innervating one part of a dermatome are unable to rejoin fibers supplying the other portion of the dermatome, because these fibers run in different peripheral nerves.

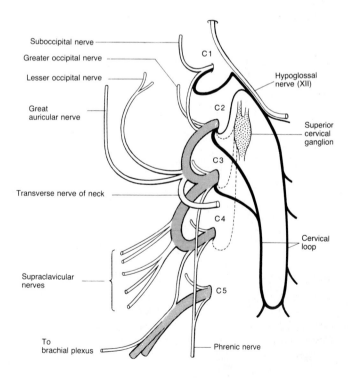

Fig. 1.23 The cervical plexus.

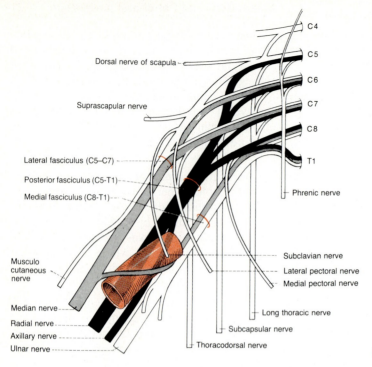

Fig. 1.24 The brachial plexus.

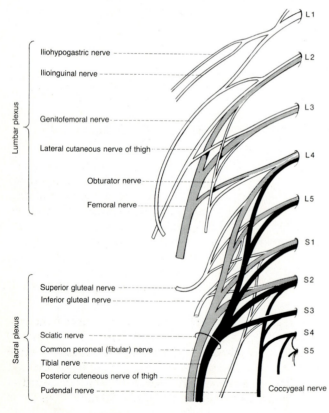

Fig. 1.25 The lumbosacral plexus.

Spinal Cord and Peripheral Innervation   25

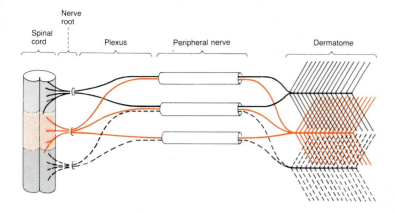

Fig. 1.26 Nerve roots in plexus divide into peripheral nerves having segmental arrangement in the skin (dermatomes). The segments overlap.

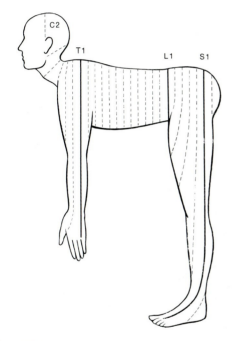

Fig. 1.27a
Simplified diagram of segmental borders.

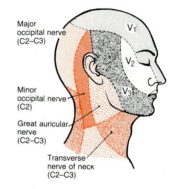

Fig. 1.27b
Skin innervation of head and neck by branches of V and of upper cervical segments.

Consequently, the sensory loss produced by damage to a peripheral *nerve* shows a pattern completely different from that caused by damage to a spinal *root*. Overlapping of the sensory areas of adjacent nerves is rather limited in comparison with that of radicular sensory territories. This greatly facilitates detection of the presence of a sensory disorder.

In dermatomic areas, regions for touch sensation overlap more than do those for sensation of pain. Therefore, damage to only one or two roots will produce a hardly recognizable decrease in sensitivity to touch, whereas such decreases in pain and temperature sensitivity are more easily spotted. One thus has to be watchful for the presence of hypalgesia or analgesia if root damage is suspected.

If the peripheral nerve is damaged, the area of hypesthesia is generally larger than that of hypalgesia. Therefore, hypesthesia is more easily recognized. What may be difficult on occasion is differentiating sensory disorders caused by a radicular C8 lesion from those

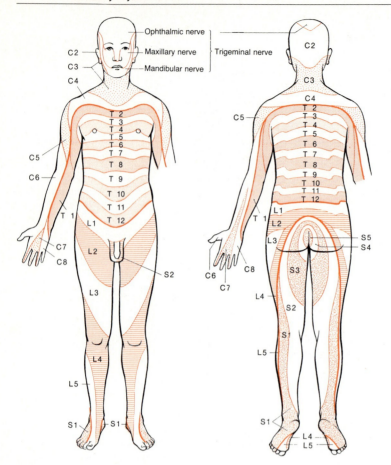

Fig. 1.28 The segmental innervation of the skin (after Hansen–Schliack).

produced by damage to the ulnar nerve, and sensory disorders from a radicular L5 to S1 lesion from those caused by damage to the peroneal nerve. In both instances the areas involved are almost the same, as can be seen by comparing Figs. 1.28 and 1.29.

Each peripheral sensory nerve has its well-defined area of innervation, making it possible to identify the damaged nerve by careful examination. For example, one may find that the area of dysesthesia corresponds to the territory of the *lateral femoral cutaneous nerve* (N. cutaneus femoris lateralis) and that this nerve is responsible for the *meralgia paresthetica*.

Syndromes of Interruptions of Sensory Pathways

The syndromes of sensory deficits vary, depending on the location of damage along the course of the sensory pathways. In Fig. 1.30 ten different locations are indicated by small red bars which are identified alphabetically (*a* through *k*).

Location a or b: A cortical or subcortical lesion in the sensorimotor area for arm (*a*) or leg (*b*) produces paresthesias (tingling, formication, etc.) and numbness in the respective extremity of the opposite side, most pronounced distally. The paresthesias may

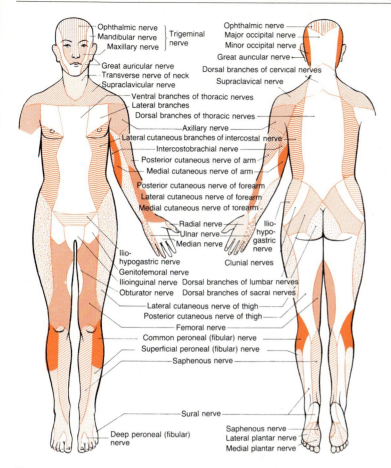

Fig. 1.29 Pattern of innervation of skin by peripheral nerves.

occur as focal sensory seizures. Because of the location of the motor cortex, a motor seizure discharge is not unusual (Jacksonian attack).

Location c: A lesion involving all sensory pathways just beneath the thalamus abolishes all sensory qualities in the contralateral half of the body.

Location d: If sensory pathways other than those for pain and temperature are damaged, hypesthesia is noted contralaterally in face and body. Pain and temperature sensations remain intact.

Location e: If the damage is limited to the trigeminal lemniscus and the lateral spinothalamic tract in the brainstem, there is absence of pain and temperature sensation in the contralateral face and body; all other sensory qualities remain undisturbed.

Location f: Involvement of the medial lemniscus and the anterior spinothalamic tract abolishes all sensory qualities in the contralateral portion of the body except pain and temperature.

Location g: Damage to the spinal trigeminal nucleus and tract and to the lateral spinothalamic tract produces loss of pain and temperature sensation ipsilaterally in face and contralaterally in body.

Location h: Damage to the posterior funiculi causes loss of posture, vibration, discrimination and other sensations associated with ipsilateral ataxia.

28   1 Sensory System

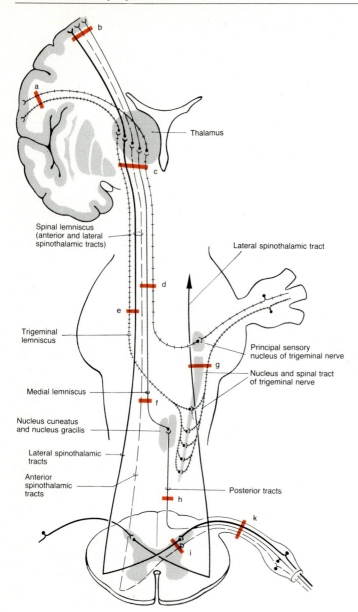

Fig. 1.30 Clinical syndromes of lesions interrupting sensory pathways at sites of red bars marked by letters. (See text for details.)

Location i: A lesion in the posterior horn abolishes pain and temperature sensations ipsilaterally; all other qualities remain intact (*dissociated disorder of sensibility*).

Location k: Injury to several adjacent posterior roots is followed by radicular paresthesias and pain and also by a decrease in or loss of all sensory qualities in the respective segment of the body. If the injured roots supply the nerves for arm or leg, there will also be hypotonia or atonia, areflexia, and ataxia.

2 Motor System

The voluntary use of muscles is linked to long nerve fibers that originate from cortical neurons and extend all the way down to the anterior horn cells of the spinal cord. These fibers form the *corticospinal* or *pyramidal tract*. The fibers are axons of neurons located in the motor region, the *precentral gyrus*, more specifically in Brodmann's cytoarchitectonic area 4 (Fig. 2.1). This area is a rather narrow field which extends all along the central fissure from the lateral or sylvian fissure dorsomedially to the dorsal margin of the hemisphere and from here into the anterior portion of the paracentral lobule at the medial aspect of the hemisphere. It runs just in front of the sensory cortex of the postcentral gyrus.

The neurons innervating pharynx and larynx are located at the lower end, next to the sylvian fissure. In ascending order follow those for face, arms, trunk, and legs (Fig. 2.2). This somatotopic order is that of a homunculus standing on its head with its face in the upright position. The scheme corresponds to that of the sensory homunculus in the postcentral gyrus mentioned earlier (see Fig. 8.20). The motoneurons are not restricted to area 4; they are also found in adjacent cortical fields. The great majority, however, occupy the 5th cortical layer of area 4. They are responsible for distinct and aimed single movements. The neurons include the giant pyramidal Betz's cells, which give off axons with thick myelin sheaths (Fig. 2.3). These fast-conducting fibers represent only 3.4 to 4% of all fibers making up the pyramidal tract. Most pyramidal tract fibers originate in small pyramidal or fusiform cells in motor areas 4 and 6. Those deriving from area 4 represent approximately 40% of all tract fibers, the rest coming from other areas of the sensorimotor region (see Fig. 2.1).

The motoneurons of area 4 control the finely tuned voluntary movements of the skeletal musculature of the *contralateral* half of the body, because most of the fibers of the pyramidal tract cross to the opposite side in the lower medulla oblongata (Fig. 2.4). Stimulation of area 4 results in general movements of individual muscles, whereas stimulation of area 6 causes more complex movements, such as a movement of an entire arm or leg.

Impulses in the pyramidal cells of the motor cortex in fact travel by two pathways contained in the rostral portion of the

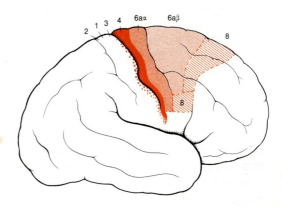

Fig. 2.1 Sensorimotor area with primary motor area 4 in precentral gyrus and premotor areas 6 and 8.

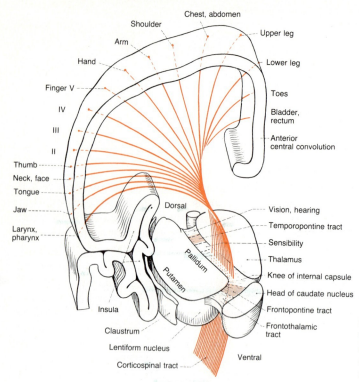

Fig. 2.2 Pyramidal tract. Passing through corona radiata its fibers converge toward posterior limb of internal capsule in somatotopic order.

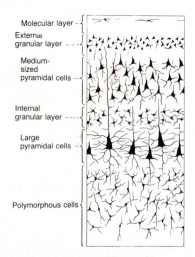

Fig. 2.3 Cytoarchitecture of motor cortex (Golgi stain). Large cells form pyramidal tract.

pyramidal tract. One is the *corticonuclear bundle*, which terminates at the nuclei of the cranial motor nerves in the brainstem. The other is the much thicker *corticospinal bundle*. It terminates in the anterior horns of the spinal cord at intercalated neurons which, in turn, are connected by synapses with the large motoneurons of the anterior horns. These nerve cells transmit the impulses along anterior roots and peripheral nerves to the motor end-plates of the skeletal musculature (see Fig. 2.4).

Corticospinal or Pyramidal Tract

As the fibers of the corticospinal tract leave the motor cortex, they converge through the corona radiata of the cerebral white matter

Corticospinal or Pyramidal Tract

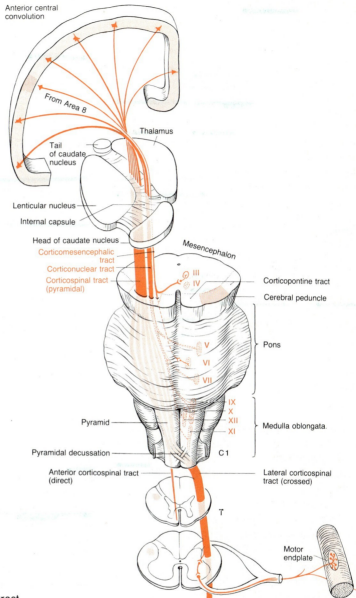

Fig. 2.4 Course of pyramidal tract.

toward the posterior limb of the internal capsule. Tightly packed, they pass through the internal capsule in somatotopic order and enter the midportion of the peduncle of the midbrain. They are now a compact bundle which descends through the center of each half of the base of the pons surrounded by the numerous nerve cells of the nuclei pontis and by fibers of various systems. At the pontomedullary junction the tracts become visible from the outside and form elongated, inverted pyramids on either side of the frontal midline of the medulla—hence the name *pyramidal tracts*. At the lower end of the medulla oblongata, 80 to 85% of the fibers of each pyramidal tract cross to the opposite side in the pyramidal decussation and become the *lateral corticospinal tract*. The remainder of the fibers continue to descend uncrossed in the anterior funiculus as *anterior corticospinal tracts*. These fibers cross at segmental levels through the anterior commissure of the cord (see Fig. 2.6). In the cervical and thoracic segments of the cord, some fibers probably connect with anterior horn cells of the same side, so that the muscles of neck and trunk receive cortical innervation from both sides.

The mass of fibers that crosses at the site of the pyramidal decussation descends as the *lateral corticospinal tract* through the lateral funiculus, becoming smaller and smaller toward the lumbar cord as fibers continually branch off. Approximately 90% of the fibers synapse with internuncial neurons, which in turn connect with the large alpha anterior horn cells as well as with the gamma motor cells (see Figs. 1.10 and 2.4).

Corticonuclear or Corticobulbar Tract

The fibers forming the corticonuclear tract leave the rostral pyramidal tract at the level of the midbrain and take a somewhat dorsal course, as indicated in Figs. 2.4, 3.49a, and 3.50a. On their way to the nuclei of the cranial motor nerves, some of these fibers cross, and some remain uncrossed (for details see the section on cranial nerves). The nuclei involved are those of the cranial nerves that control the voluntary innervation of facial and oral muscles: the trigeminal (V), facial (VII), glossopharyngeal (IX), vagus (X), accessory (XI), and hypoglossal (XII) nerves.

Another fiber bundle deserves mention. It originates in the *eye field* of Brodmann's area 8 and not in the precentral gyrus (see Figs. 2.4 and 2.5). Its impulses produce conjugate movements of the eyes. It has been called the *corticomesencephalic tract*, but there is consensus that it constitutes part of the corticonuclear tract.

As the fibers of this bundle leave area 8, they join the fibers of the pyramidal tract in the corona radiata. Thereafter they run more ventrally in the posterior limb of the internal capsule until they turn caudally on their way to the nuclei of the motor nerves of the eye: the oculomotor (III), trochlear (IV), and abducens (VI) nerves. Impulses from area 8 cannot innervate the eye muscles individually. They react synergistically in the form of conjugate movements to the opposite side (déviation conjuguée). It is not clear where the fibers of the corticomesencephalic tract terminate. It is only known that they do not synapse directly with the neurons in the oculomotor nuclei. (See the section on cranial nerves for details, p. 74.)

For a good understanding of the action of the peripheral motoneurons in brainstem and cord, other motor pathways must be discussed first. They represent what is called the *extrapyramidal motor system*.

Extrapyramidal Motor System

The term *extrapyramidal motor system* simply represents all motor pathways that do not pass through the pyramids of the medulla (Fig. 2.5) and are essential in that they influence regulatory motor feedback circuits in spinal cord, brainstem, cerebellum, and cerebral cortex. These are, for example, the *corticopontocerebellar tracts*, which connect the cerebral cortex with the cerebellum. Also part of this system are those fiber bundles that connect the cerebral cortex with extrapyramidal grisea (gray structures) such as the striatum, the red nucleus, and the substantia nigra, and with the reticular formation and several other tegmental nuclei of the brainstem. In these structures the impulses are transmitted to additional neurons which, via intercalated nerve cells, descend as *tectospinal, rubrospinal, reticulospinal, vestibulospinal*, and other tracts to the motoneurons of the anterior horns (see Fig. 2.5). These are the pathways by which the extrapyramidal system influences the spinal motor actions.

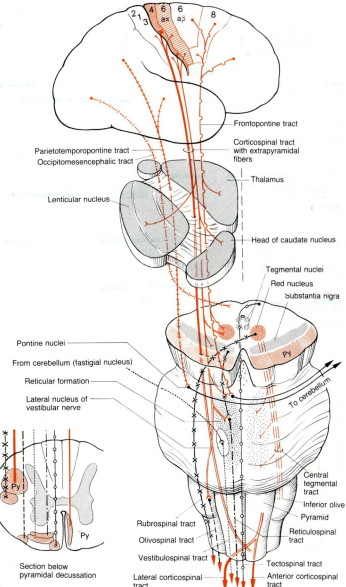

Fig. 2.5 The extrapyramidal tracts.

Fig. 2.5 illustrates that the cortex of the frontal, parietal, temporal, and occipital lobes has fiber connections with the pons. These fibers are the axons of the "first neurons" of the various corticopontocerebellar tracts. The frontopontine fiber bundles are located in the anterior limb of the internal capsule, just in front of those pyramidal fibers that innervate the facial muscles. In the midbrain they occupy the medial fourth of the peduncle next to the interpeduncular fossa. The fibers coming from the parietal, temporal, and occipital cortex pass through the posterior portion of the posterior limb of the internal capsule and the posterolateral part of the peduncle. All these *corticopontine fibers* synapse with groups of neurons in the base of the pons. These "second neurons" send their axons to the contralateral cerebellar cortex. Because of these connections, the cerebellar cortex receives, so to speak, a copy of all motor impulses that originate in the cerebral cortex. The cerebellum also receives information about all motor activities taking place in the periphery. It is thus in a position to exert a controlling and balancing influence on voluntary movements via the extrapyramidal system. More details are discussed in Chapter 4 (Cerebellum).

The extrapyramidal system supplements the cortical system of voluntary motor actions, raising its functioning to a higher level at which each voluntary movement is finely tuned and smooth in its performance.

The pyramidal tract (over intercalated neurons) and the extrapyramidal chain of neurons ultimately meet at the motoneurons of the anterior horns, at the alpha cells, and at the smaller gamma cells, and influence them in part by activation and in part by inhibition (Fig. 2.6).

The individual fiber groups occupy as tracts well-defined areas of the white matter in the cord. Fig. 2.7 shows the afferent pathways in gray and the efferent tracts in red. Within the various pathways the fibers are arranged in somatotopic order; the borders of the individual tracts are not sharply separated from one another, however, because marginal fibers mingle with those of neighboring tracts. The pyramidal tracts are free from any admixture of other fiber groups except for the pyramids of the medulla oblongata. Damage to the pyramidal tracts in areas other than

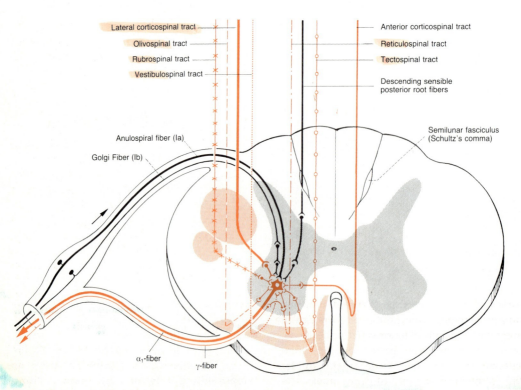

Fig. 2.6 Descending motor tracks synapsing with anterior horn neurons.

2. Aufbau der **Sprunggelenke?**

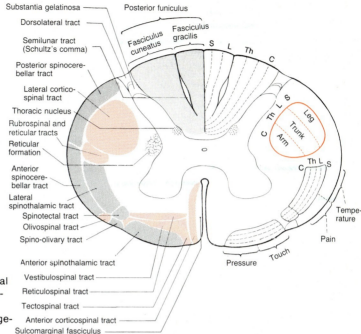

Fig. 2.7 Cross-section of spinal cord showing topography of ascending and descending pathways and the somatotopic arrangement of their fibers.

the pyramids always also involves extrapyramidal fibers.

These anatomical facts are of clinical significance. If only pyramidal fibers are interrupted, as is the case with alterations involving area 4 or the pyramids, the ensuing paralysis is flaccid. Because in other locations damage to the pyramidal tracts also involves extrapyramidal fibers, particularly those of the reticulospinal and vestibulospinal tracts, the resulting paralysis is always spastic.

Damage to Pyramidal and Extrapyramidal Pathways

An interruption of the pyramidal tract abolishes the transmission of all stimuli of voluntary movement from the motor cortex to the anterior horn cells. The result is a paralysis of the muscles supplied by these cells. If the interruption of the pyramidal tract is sudden, the stretching reflex of the muscles is suppressed. This means that the paralysis is flaccid at first. It may be days or weeks until the stretching reflexes return. When they do, the muscle spindles are more sensitive to stretching than they were before. This is particularly true for the flexors of the arms and the extensors of the legs.

This hypersensitivity of the stretch receptors is caused by damage to extrapyramidal pathways that terminate at the anterior horn cells and activate the fusimotor fibers of gamma motoneurons innervating intrafusal fibers of the muscle spindles. As a result, the feedback circuit controlling the length of the muscle is influenced in such a way that flexors of the arms and tensors of the legs become fixed at a particularly short length. The patient is no longer able to influence the length of the muscles, because he cannot voluntarily inhibit the overactivated fusimotors.

It is helpful to differentiate inhibiting and activating fibers. The inhibiting fibers are supposedly tightly interwoven with pyramidal fibers. This is the reason they, too, are always damaged by lesions involving the pyramidal tract. The activating fibers are less involved and can still exert their influence on the muscle spindles. The sequelae are spasticity and hyperreflexia associated with clonus.

A spastic paralysis is always evidence that the damage involves the central nervous system, in other words, the brain or spinal cord. The result of a pyramidal tract lesion is a loss of the most subtle voluntary movements. The loss can best be observed in hands, fingers, and face.

As was mentioned earlier, damage to the pyramidal tract interrupts all voluntary impulses along its course from cerebral cortex down to the respective motoneurons of the anterior horn. The muscles innervated by these motoneurons are no longer subject to voluntary control. A small lesion in the internal capsule may interrupt all tightly packed pyramidal fibers and cause a spastic paralysis of the entire opposite side. The paralysis is contralateral because the pyramidal fibers cross further down in the lower medulla oblongata. A lesion of the same dimension, when located in the corona radiata, may produce only a limited paralysis, for example, one of the arm or the leg. If the pyramidal tract is injured below the decussation, a hemiplegia results, this time involving the ipsilateral limbs. Bilateral damage in brain or upper cervical cord produces *tetraplegia*.

Spastic palsies are characterized by the appearance of spastic finger or toe signs, such as *Babinski's sign*. Although its neural mechanism is not fully understood, its presence is unequivocal proof of pyramidal tract injury. Another, less reliable sign consists of the absence of skin reflexes, such as abdominal and cremasteric reflexes.

Syndrome of Central Spastic Paralysis

General signs

1. decrease in strength associated with loss of subtle movements
2. spastic increase in tone (hypertonia)
3. exaggerated proprioceptive reflexes with or without clonus
4. decrease in or loss of exteroceptive reflexes (abdominal, cremasteric, plantar reflexes)
5. appearance of pathologic reflexes (Babinski's, Oppenheim's, Gordon's, Mendel-Bechterew, and others)
6. no degenerative muscular atrophy

Specific syndromes

The symptomatology varies according to the location of the lesion along the course of the pyramidal tract. Fig. 2.**8** shows involvement of the tract at eight different levels, indicated by black bars identified by the letters *a* through *h*.

a) *Subcortical lesion* (tumor, hematoma, infarct etc.): Contralateral paresis of hand or arm results. Subtle, skilled voluntary movements are most often involved. *Monoparesis*, not monoplegia, occurs. The paresis results from the almost total preservation of extrapyramidal fibers. A small lesion of the cortex of area 4 produces flaccid paresis and quite often focal epileptic attacks (Jacksonian epilepsy). It is of diagnostic importance to determine where the attack commences (see p. 290).

b) *Internal capsule lesion:* Contralateral spastic hemiplegia occurs, because the pyramidal and extrapyramidal fibers are close to each other. Because the corticonuclear tract is also involved, there is contralateral paralysis of facial and possibly of hypoglossal nerves. Most cranial motor nuclei are bilaterally supplied by the tract, either fully or partially (see the section on cranial nerves). A lesion causing rapid damage produces a contralateral paralysis, which is flaccid at first because the lesion has a shock-like effect on the peripheral neurons. It becomes spastic after hours or days because the extrapyramidal fibers are also damaged.

c) *Peduncle lesion:* The result of this lesion is a contralateral spastic hemiplegia, which

2. Aufbau der **Articulatio sternoclavicularis** und **acromioclavicularis**?

Extrapyramidal Motor System

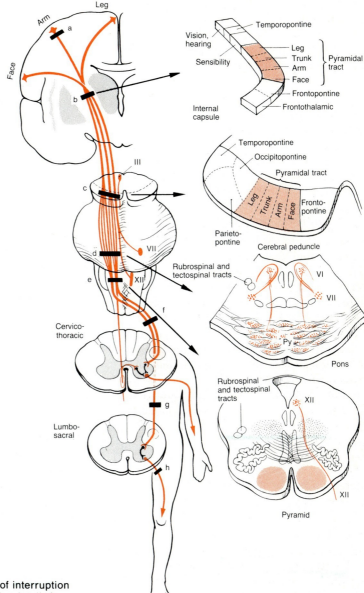

Fig. 2.8 Clinical syndromes of interruption of motor pathways. (See text for details.)

may be associated with ipsilateral paralysis of the oculomotor nerve (see discussion of *Weber's syndrome*, p. 152 [Fig. 3.63]).

d) *Pons lesion:* The result of this lesion is a contralateral and possibly bilateral hemiplegia. Often, not all pyramidal fibers are damaged. Because the fibers descending to the facial and hypoglossal nuclei are more dorsally located, the facial or hypoglossal nerves may be spared. On the other hand, there may be an ipsilateral paralysis of abducens or trigeminal nerves (see Figs. 3.60 and 3.61).

e) *Pyramid lesion:* Such a lesion produces a flaccid contralateral hemiparesis. There is no hemiplegia, because only pyramidal fibers are damaged. Extrapyramidal pathways are located more dorsally in the medulla and remain intact.

f) *Cervical lesion:* Involvement of the lateral pyramidal tract stemming from diseases such as amyotrophic lateral sclerosis or multiple sclerosis produces a spastic hemiplegia that is ipsilateral because the pyramidal tract has already decussated. The paralysis is spastic because extrapyramidal fibers, which are mixed with the pyramidal fibers, are also damaged.

g) *Thoracic lesion:* Interruption of the lateral pyramidal tract caused by diseases such as amyotrophic lateral sclerosis or multiple sclerosis results in a spastic ipsilateral monoplegia of the leg. Bilateral damage causes paraplegia.

h) *Anterior root lesion:* The palsy resulting from this lesion is ipsilateral and flaccid as a result of the damage of the peripheral or lower motoneurons.

A lesion involving the decussation of the pyramidal tract produces the rare syndrome of a *hemiplegia cruciata* (alternate hemiplegia). Its mechanism is illustrated in Fig. 2.9.

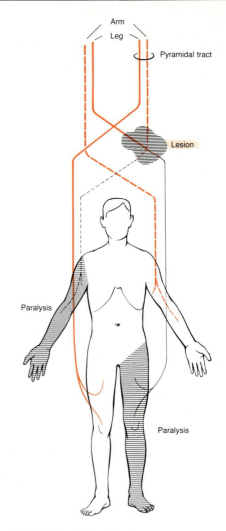

Fig. 2.9 Alternate hemiplegia.

Peripheral Neuron, Motor and Sensory

The fibers of the pyramidal tract and of various extrapyramidal pathways (reticulospinal, tectospinal, vestibulospinal, rubrospinal, and others), and afferent fibers entering the spinal cord via the posterior roots, terminate at cell bodies or dendrites of large and small alpha motoneurons and at small gamma cells directly or via internuncial, association, and commissural neurons of the intrinsic neuronal apparatus of the spinal cord. In contrast to the pseudounipolar neurons of the spinal ganglia, the neurons of the anterior horns are multipolar. Their dendrites have numerous synaptic connections with the various afferent and efferent systems. Some of these are facilitory and others inhibitory in their action.

Within the anterior horns the motoneurons form groups arranged in columns not subdivided into segmental units (Fig. 2.10). These columns show some *somatotopic* order. In the cervical cord the motoneurons of the lateral anterior horns innervate hands and arms, whereas the medial columns are responsible for the muscles of neck and

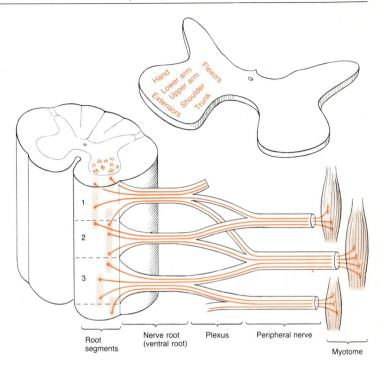

Fig. 2.10 Radicular and peripheral muscle innervation.

thorax. In the lumbar cord the neurons innervating feet and legs also occupy the lateral portion of the anterior horns. However, those responsible for the trunk are medially located.

The neurites or axons of the anterior horn cells leave the cord ventrally as radicular fibers (fila radicularia), which assemble at segmental levels to form the *anterior or ventral roots*. Each anterior root adjoins the posterior root just distal to the *spinal ganglion*, and the two together form the *spinal peripheral nerve* (see Fig. 2.6). Thus each segment of the body has its own pair of spinal nerves. The nerves consist not only of afferent sensory (somatic) and efferent motor (somatic) fibers, but also of efferent autonomic fibers arising from the lateral horns of the spinal gray matter and afferent autonomic fibers.

The richly myelinated, fast-conducting axons of the large alpha motor cells are called alpha 1 fibers (see Fig. 1.9); they go directly to the extrafusal musculature and give off more and more branches as they proceed distally. In varying numbers the fibers terminate at the motor end-plates of a corresponding number of muscle fibers. The anterior horn cells, the axons, and the muscle fibers innervated by them are called *motor units* (Sherrington). This *final common pathway* carries impulses from the pyramidal and extrapyramidal tracts and from intrasegmental as well as intersegmental reflex neurons to the muscle fibers.

Muscles performing delicate, refined movements have many anterior horn cells at their disposal, and each of them innervates not more than five to twenty muscle fibers. Conversely, large muscles that perform somewhat crude, simple actions, such as the gluteal muscles, are supplied by relatively few anterior horn cells, each of which innervates as many as 100 to 500 muscle fibers. Thus, motor units come in small as well as very large sizes.

Aside from large and small alpha motoneurons, the anterior horns contain numerous smaller gamma motoneurons with thin,

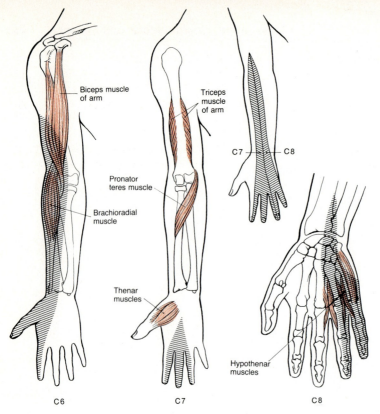

Fig. 2.11 Syndrome of root damage at C6, C7 and C8 with indicator muscles and dermatomes (after Mumenthaler and Schliack).

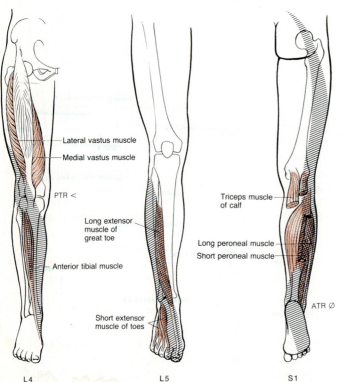

Fig. 2.12 Syndrome of root damage at L4, L5, and S1 with indicator muscles and dermatomes (after Mumenthaler and Schliack).

poorly myelinated or unmyelinated axons. They innervate the intrafusal muscle spindles, as was mentioned in Chapter 1 (see Fig. 1.9). Of the other internuncial neurons of the anterior horns, the Renshaw cells must be mentioned. As illustrated in Fig. 1.9, a large alpha motoneuron gives off a collateral to a small Renshaw cell. This cell in turn connects again with the anterior horn cell, producing some inhibition of its action. This is an example of the spinal negative feedback circuits that inhibit the action of the large motoneurons.

Fig. 2.10 demonstrates that the individual muscles are innervated by fibers of several

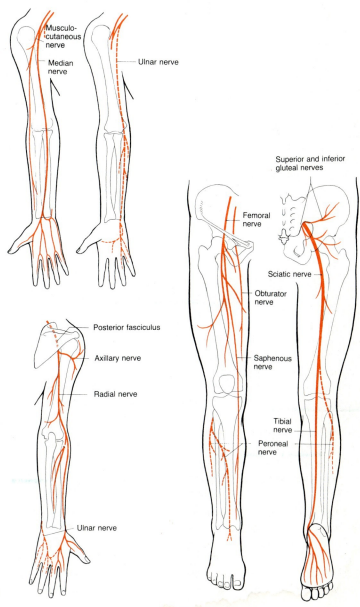

Fig. 2.13 Course of important peripheral motor nerves.

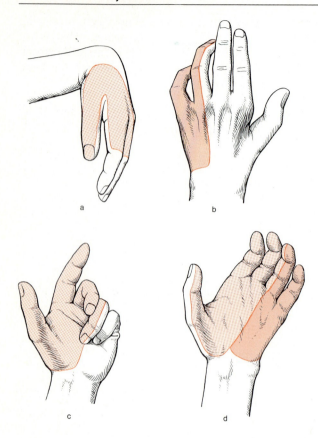

Fig. 2.14 Syndrome of flaccid paralysis: **a** wrist drop (radial nerve); **b** claw hand (ulnar nerve); **c** benediction hand (median nerve); **d** monkey paw (median and ulnar nerves).

ventral spinal roots (plurisegmental innervation). Consequently, if one root is transected, there is no definite loss of function, as is also the case with transection of just one posterior root. A paralysis of a radicular pattern occurs only if several adjacent roots are damaged. Each motor root has its own *indicator muscle*, however, making it possible to diagnose root damage by the fibrillation of the muscle in the electromyogram, particularly if cervical or lumbar areas are involved. The indicator muscles of the upper and lower extremities are illustrated in Figs. 2.11 and 2.12.

If a mixed peripheral nerve is severed, only the muscle innervated by this nerve will be paralyzed, and the paralysis will be associated with a sensory disorder caused by the interruption of the afferent fibers. The paralysis will be flaccid. Fig. 2.13 demonstrates the topography of several typical peripheral nerves quite often damaged in mechanical trauma. Fig. 2.14 shows four patterns of atrophy of hand muscles as a result of damage to the radial, median, and ulnar nerves.

Syndrome of Radicular Nerve Damage

1. The pain radiates according to the dermatome involved.
2. The algesia is more involved than the other sensory modalities.
3. There is decreased strength of the indicator muscles. With more severe damage, a muscle atrophy develops in rare instances (e.g., of the anterior tibial muscle).
4. Reflex disorders correspond to the damage of radicular nerves (see Fig. 1.8).

5. Autonomic signs (sweating, piloerection, vasomotor disorders) are absent.

Segmental and Peripheral Muscle Innervation

Table 2.1 lists the function and the peripheral as well as segmental innervation of each of the individual muscles. Such a classification permits determination of the nerve or root segments damaged, if a paralysis of a muscle is found.

Disorder of the Motor Unit

As we have mentioned earlier, flaccid paralysis is the result of an interruption of the motor unit somewhere along its course. The alteration may involve the anterior horns, several ventral or anterior roots, a plexus, or peripheral nerves themselves. The muscles involved show neither voluntary not involuntary, or reflex, innervation. The muscles are not only paralyzed but also hypotonic and areflexic because of the interruption of the monosynaptic stretch reflex. Atrophy of the

Table 2.1 Function and Peripheral and Segmental Innervation of Muscles.

Function	Muscles	Nerve
I. Plexus Cervicalis C1–C4		
Flexion, extension, rotation and lateral bending of neck	Mm. colli profundi (+ M. sternocleidomastoideus + M. trapezius)	Cervical nerves C1–C4
Lifting of upper thorax; inspiration	Mm. scaleni	C3–C5
Inspiration	Diaphragm	Phrenic nerve C3–C5
II. Plexus Brachialis C5–T1		
Adduction and internal rotation of arm and dorsoventral lowering of shoulder	M. pectoralis major and minor	Anterior thoracic nerve C5–T1
Fixation of scapula during lifting of arm (anterior movement of shoulder)	M. serratus anterior	Long thoracic nerve C5–C7
Elevation and adduction of scapula toward spinal column	M. levator scapulae Mm. rhomboidei	Dorsal scapular nerve C4–C5
Lifting and outward rotation of arm Outward rotation of arm in shoulder joint	M. supraspinatus M. infraspinatus	Suprascapular nerve C4–C6 C4–C6
Inward rotation of shoulder joint; adduction from ventral to dorsal; lowering of elevated arm	M. latissimus dorsi M. teres major M. subscapularis	Dorsal thoracic nerve C5–C8 (from dorsal portion of plexus)

Table 2.1 (continued)

Function	Muscles	Nerve
Lateral lifting (abduction) of arm up to the horizontal line	M. deltoideus	Axillary nerve C5–C6
Outward rotation of arm	M. teres minor	C4–C5
Flexion of upper and lower arm and supination of lower arm	M. biceps brachii	Musculocutaneous nerve C5–C6
Elevation and adduction of arm	M. coracobrachialis	C5–C7
Flexion of lower arm	M. brachialis	C5–C6
Flexion and radial deviation of hand	M. flexor carpi radialis	Median nerve C6–C7
Pronation of lower arm	M. pronator teres	C6–C7
Flexion of hand	M. palmaris longus	C7–T1
Flexion of fingers II–V in middle phalanges	M. flexor digitorum superficialis	C7–T1
Flexion of end phalanx of the thumb	M. flexor pollicis longus	C6–C8
Flexion of end phalanges of index and middle finger	M. flexor digitorum profundus (radial portion)	C7–T1
Abduction of metacarpal I	M. abductor pollicis brevis	C7–T1
Flexion of proximal phalanx of thumb	M. flexor pollicis brevis	C7–T1
Opposition of metacarpal I	M. opponens pollicis brevis	C6–C7
Flexion of proximal phalanges and extension of other joints	Mm. lumbricales Index and middle fingers	Median nerve C8–T1
Flexion of proximal phalanges and extension of other joints	Fourth and little fingers	Ulnar nerve C8–T1
Flexion and ulnar bending of hand	M. flexor carpi ulnaris	Ulnar nerve C7–T1
Flexion of proximal phalanges of fourth and little fingers	M. flexor digitorum profundus (ulnar portion)	C7–T1
Adduction of metacarpal I	M. adductor pollicis	C8–T1
Abduction of little finger	M. abductor digiti V	C8–T1
Opposition of little finger	M. opponens digiti V	C7–T1
Flexion of little finger in metacarpophalangeal joint	M. flexor digiti brevis V	Ulnar nerve C7–T1
Bending of proximal phalanges; stretching of fingers III, IV, & V in middle & distal joints as well as spreading & closing of these fingers	Mm. interossei palmares and dorsales Mm. lumbricales 3 and 4	C8–T1
Extension of elbow	M. triceps brachii & M. anconeus	Radial nerve C6–C8
Flexion of elbow	M. brachioradialis	C5–C6
Extension and radial abduction of hand	M. extensor carpi radialis	C6–C8
Extension of proximal phalanges II–V Extension and dorsoflexion of hand; stretching and spreading of fingers	M. extensor digitorum	C6–C8

Table 2.1 (continued)

Function	Muscles	Nerve
Extension of proximal phalanx of little finger	M. extensor digiti V	C6–C8
Extension and ulnar deviation of hand	M. extensor carpi ulnaris	C6–C8
Supination of forearm	M. supinator	C5–C7
Abduction of metacarpal I; radial extension of hand	M. abductor pollicis longus	C6–C7
Extension of thumb in proximal phalanx	M. extensor pollicis brevis	C7–C8
Extension of distal phalanges of thumb	M. extensor pollicis longus	C7–C8
Extension of proximal phalanx of index finger	M. extensor indicis proprius	C6–C8
Elevation of ribs; expiration; abdominal compression; anteroflexion and lateroflexion of trunk	Mm. thoracis and abdominalis	Thoracic nerves T1–L1

III. Plexus lumbalis
T12–L4

Function	Muscles	Nerve
		Femoral nerve
Flexion and outward rotation of hip	M. iliopsoas	L1–L3
Flexion and inward rotation of lower leg	M. sartorius	L2–L3
Extension of lower leg in knee joint	M. quadriceps femoris	L2–L4
		Obturator nerve
Adduction of thigh	M. pectineus	L2–L3
	M. adductor longus	L2–L3
	M. adductor brevis	L2–L4
	M. adductor magnus	L3–L4
	M. gracilis	L2–L4
Adduction and outward rotation of thigh	M. obturatorius externus	L3–L4

IV. Plexus sacralis
L5–S1

Function	Muscles	Nerve
		Superior gluteal nerve
Abduction and inward rotation of thigh	M. gluteus medius and minimus	L4–S1
Flexion of upper leg in hip; abduction and inward rotation	M. tensor fasciae latae	L4–L5
Outward rotation of thigh and abduction	M. piriformis	L5–S1
		Inferior gluteal nerve
Extension of thigh in hip	M. gluteus maximus	L4–S2
Outward rotation of thigh	M. obturatorius internus	L5–S1
	Mm. gemelli	
	M. quadratus	L4–S1
		L4–S1
		Sciatic nerve
Flexion of lower leg	M. biceps femoris	L4–S2
	M. semitendinosus	L4–S1
	M. semimembranosus	L4–S1

Table 2.1 (continued)

Function	Muscles	Nerve
Dorsiflexion and supination of foot	M. tibialis anterior	Deep peroneal nerve L4–L5
Extension of toes and foot	M. extensor digitorum longus	L4–S1
Extension of toes II–V	M. extensor digitorum brevis	L4–S1
Extension of large toe	M. extensor hallucis longus	L4–S1
Extension of large toe	M. extensor hallucis brevis	L4–S1
Lifting and pronation of outer portion of foot	Mm. peronei	Superficial peroneal nerve L5–S1
Plantar flexion of foot in supination	M. gastrocnemius M. triceps surae M. soleus	Tibal nerve L5–S2
Supination and plantar flexion of foot	M. tibialis posterior	L4–L5
Flexion of distal phalanges of toes II–V (plantar flexion of foot in supination)	M. flexor digitorum longus	L5–S2
Flexion of distal phalanx of big toe	M. flexor hallucis longus	L5–S2
Flexion of middle phalanges of toes II–V	M. flexor digitorum brevis	S1–S3
Spreading, closing, and flexing of proximal phalanges of toes	Mm. plantaris pedis	S1–S3
Closing of sphincters of bladder and rectum	Perineal and sphincter musculature	Pudendal nerve S2–S4

paralyzed muscle commences after a few weeks; it may be so severe that only connective tissue remains after months or years. The atrophy demonstrates that the anterior horn cells have a trophic influence on the muscle fibers that is basic to maintaining normal muscle function.

Syndrome of Flaccid Paralysis

The syndrome of flaccid paralysis is composed of the following symptoms:

1. decrease in overall strength
2. hypotonia or atonia of the muscle
3. hyporeflexia or areflexia
4. neurogenic muscle degeneration

An additional loss of sensory function suggests that the damage is located in the plexus or in the peripheral nerves. By using electromyography to assess the damage, it is usually possible to determine whether the anterior horns, the anterior roots, the plexus, or the peripheral nerves are involved.

It may be advisable to repeat here what has been stated before in regard to the anterior (ventral) and posterior (dorsal) roots of the spinal nerves. The posterior roots consist predominantly of afferent neurites, whereas the anterior roots consist predominantly of efferent nerve fibers. At every segment, each root takes its course to its respective intervertebral foramen. Here the dorsal root shows local enlargement, called the *spinal ganglion*. The anterior root passes the ganglion before it joins the posterior root to form the peripheral nerve.

There are, all in all, 31 pairs of spinal nerves. The uppermost pair leaves the spinal canal between the occipital bone and the atlas; the lowest pair does so between the first and second coccygeal vertebrae. As the roots are passing through the intervertebral foramina, they may be exposed to damage, predominantly caused by diseases of the intervertebral disks. Atrophy of the disks is frequent in the cervical region and may produce a stenosing process, that is a narrowing of the intervertebral foramina. Protrusion and prolapse of disks exerting pressure on the roots are more frequent, however, in the lumbar area (see Fig. 2.35). Actually, there is a whole series of disease processes that may endanger the spinal roots as they exit from the spinal canal, among them inflammatory diseases of the vertebrae and adjacent tissues, tumors, and trauma.

As ventral and dorsal roots join, they form the peripheral nerves. Those made up of thoracic segments will continue more or less as individual nerves. Their main branches are the *intercostal nerves*. In contrast, the peripheral nerves deriving from the roots of C2–C4 immediately form the *cervical plexus*, and those from C5–T1 form the *brachial plexus*, made up of three primary trunks: a superior (C5, C6), a middle (C7), and an inferior (C8, T1) trunk. The nerves deriving from T12–L4 form the *lumbar plexus*, and those from L5 and S1–S3 and possibly also those from L4 make up the *sacral plexus*.

Damage to Plexuses

The location of the cervical plexus (see Fig. 1.23, p. 23) offers so much protection that injury to this plexus is rare. A unilateral or bilateral involvement of the phrenic nerve (C3–C5) is more often caused by mediastinal disease than by damage to the plexus itself.

The situation is different with the *brachial plexus* (see Fig. 1.24, p. 24). Its superior trunk (C5, C6) is vulnerable to birth injury, causing *superior plexus paralysis* (Erb-Duchenne paralysis). Paralyzed are the deltoid, biceps, brachial, and brachioradial muscles. The small hand muscles are not involved. A sensory disorder extends over the area of the deltoid muscle and the radial aspect of forearm and hand.

Inferior plexus paralysis (Klumpke's paralysis) is caused by damage to the roots of C8 and T1 or the inferior primary trunk by a lesion such as Pancoast's tumor (pulmonary sulcus tumor). Inferior plexus paralysis is relatively rare and most often results from pressure exerted, for example, by a cervical rib (Fig. 2.15). Involved are the small hand muscles as well as the flexor of the hand. Occasionally, this paralysis is associated with Horner's syndrome. Trophic disorders in hand and fingers may be impressive.

The *plexus lumbalis* (L1–L3) (see Fig. 1.25) is seldom injured, because of its well-protected location. Signs of damage to this plexus result from lesions such as an abscess of the psoas muscle, pelvic tumor, trauma, or inflammation. The obturator and femoral nerves are particularly vulnerable.

Among the nerves that derive from the *sacral plexus* (see Fig.1.25) are the peroneal and tibial nerves, which together form the sciatic nerve. These two nerves separate near

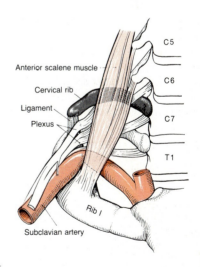

Fig. 2.15 Scalenus syndrome caused by narrowing of the scalenus hiatus by a cervical rib.

the knee and follow their own courses. *Peroneal paralysis* produces palsy of the dorsiflexors of the foot, making it impossible to lift the foot upward (steppage gait). Interruption of *tibial nerve* function causes paralysis of plantiflexors, making it impossible to walk on toes. In its course, the tibial nerve is more protected than the peroneal nerve; therefore, tibial paralysis is less common than peroneal paralysis. Peroneal palsy is associated with sensory disorder over the lateral aspect of the lower leg and over the dorsum of the foot. In paralysis of the tibial nerve, the sensory disorder involves the sole of the foot.

Functional muscle deficits caused by involvement of individual peripheral nerves are listed in Table 2.1. For the patterns of sensory disorders caused by peripheral nerve damage, see Fig. 1.**29**. Damage to a single peripheral nerve can usually be attributed to a mechanical injury such as chronic pressure or trauma. Depending on whether the nerve is solely sensory or motor or is a mixed nerve, the deficits are correspondingly sensory, motor, or autonomic.

Each time the continuity of an axon is interrupted, a distally progressing breakdown of axon and myelin sheath begins within hours or days and is usually completed after 15 to 20 days (*secondary or wallerian degeneration*). Injured axons do not regenerate within the central nervous system but can do so in peripheral nerves, provided that the nerve sheaths remain intact and can serve as guide rails for the sprouting axons. Even if the nerve is completely severed, approximation of its endings by suture may lead to a complete regeneration. The electromyogram is an important tool for determining the extent of damage to peripheral nerves.

If injury to numerous peripheral nerves produces a syndrome characterized by widespread sensory, motor, and autonomic alterations, a polyneuritis or a polyneuropathy exists. It may appear in various forms, for example, as a multiplex condition affecting various parts of the body at once.

This generalized disease is characterized more often by degenerative than by inflammatory changes in multiple peripheral nerves. The neurologic deficits are most often bilateral and involve predominantly the distal portions of the extremities. Complaints concern paresthesias and pain. The findings consist of sensory deficits of glove or stocking-like distribution, flaccid paralysis of muscles associated with atrophy, and trophic disorders of the skin. If nerve roots are also damaged, the condition is called *polyneuroradiculitis*. In rare cases the disease spreads to the spinal cord; in those instances, it is referred to as polyneuroradiculomyelitis. Cranial nerves also may become involved. The term Landry's paralysis (*Guillain-Barré syndrome*) signifies a generalized radiculoneuritis, possibly of infectious or immunological origin.

Polyneuropathy has many causes, among them *intoxicants* (lead, arsenic, thallium, isoniazid, and others), *dietary deficiencies* (from alcohol intake, cachexia, carcinoma, and other conditions), *infections* (diphtheria, spotted fever, typhus, and others), and *metabolic disorders* (diabetes mellitus, porphyria, pellagra, uremia, and others). Quite often no definite cause can be established, in which case the condition is referred to as *idiopathic polyneuropathy*.

Frequent Syndromes of Peripheral Nerve Damage

Scalenus syndrome (Naffziger's syndrome, cervical rib syndrome). As is illustrated in Fig. 2.**15**, the nerve cords of the brachial plexus proceed through a hiatus or gap formed by the anterior and medial scalenus muscles and the first rib. Under normal conditions, the scalenus gap is large enough to accomodate the cords of the plexus as well as the subclavian artery. Under abnormal conditions, as, for example, in the presence of a cervical rib, the gap may become too small. The cords of the plexus and the artery must pass the tendon connecting the tip of the cervical rib with the first thoracic rib and may easily be damaged at this point. The first sign of plexus involvement is pain radiating into the arm. The intensity of pain changes, depending on the position of the arm. In addition, there are often paresthesias and hypesthesias, predominantly involving the ulnar supply area of the hand. Muscle pareses of the type of Klumpke's paralysis follow. Damage to the sympathetic fiber network surrounding the subclavian artery often causes vasomotor disorders in the arm.

Carpal tunnel syndrome (Fig. 2.16). This syndrome is caused by damage to the median nerve where it passes through the narrow carpal tunnel underneath the transverse carpal ligament. Characteristically, it produces pain and paresthesias in the hand which are most annoying at night (brachialgia paraesthetica nocturna) and the sensation of swelling of the hand and wrist. Trophic disorders and atrophy of the lateral thenar eminence of the thumb follow. The median nerve carries many autonomic fibers. If they become damaged, the paralysis of the median nerve may be accompanied by *Sudeck-Leriche syndrome* (posttraumatic osteoporosis associated with vasospasm) or with *causalgia* (burning pain).

Syndrome of ulnar nerve damage (Fig. 2.17). Of all the peripheral nerves, the ulnar nerve is most often paretic. The nerve is easily damaged by pressure at the extensor side of the elbow joint. The trauma may be acute or chronic; it occurs if the arm is leaned on a hard support. This is unavoidable in certain trades, such as glass-blowing. The same damage may occur if the ulnar nerve jumps out of its sulcus (luxation). The results are paresthesias and hypesthesias in the ulnar region of the hand. Chronic damage leads to atrophy of the hypothenar eminence of the little finger and of the adductor pollicis muscle (ulnar paralysis with claw hand).

Syndrome of Spinal Cord and Peripheral Nerve Damage

Syndrome of the spinal ganglion (Fig 2.18). A viral infection is one of the diseases that may

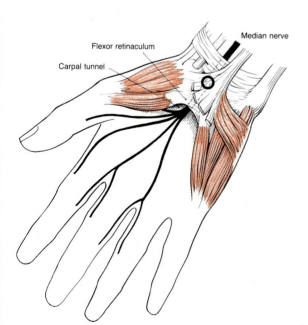

Fig. 2.16 Carpal tunnel syndrome.

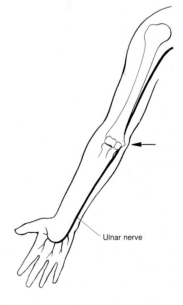

Fig. 2.17 Location of pressure lesion or of luxation of ulnar nerve.

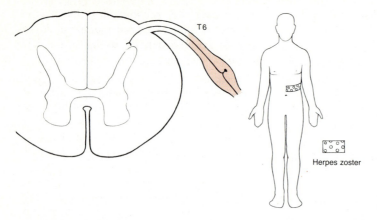

Fig 2.18 Syndrome of spinal ganglion.

involve one or several spinal ganglia, particularly those of the thoracic area. The corresponding dermatome develops a painful reddening and, thereafter, small blisters varying in number. The syndrome is called *herpes zoster*. There are paresthesias in the diseased dermatome, and pain is annoying and lancinating. The inflammation may invade the spinal cord but usually remains localized. A flaccid paralysis from involvement of the anterior horns is rare, and still rarer is the syndrome of hemi-transection or even complete transection of the cord. Occasionally, herpes zoster is grafted on already existing disease (carcinoma metastases of vertebrae, tuberculous spondylitis, leukemia, etc.).

The actual mechanism leading to the inflammatory skin alterations with formation of vesicles is not fully understood. Presumably, certain substances (histamine? acetylcholine?) are set free at the nerve endings of the involved dermatome and produce the vasodilatation and exudation (antidromic impulses).

Syndrome of the posterior roots (Fig. 2.19). Complete transection of neighboring posterior roots abolishes sensitivity in the corresponding dermatomes. If the damage is not complete, however, there is a difference in the involvement of the various sensory qualities, pain sensation being particularly vulnerable to involvement (Achilles tendon, testicles). In addition, the interruption of the peripheral reflex arc produces hypotonia as well as hypo- or areflexia (*tabes dorsalis*). Lancinating pain is a posterior root sign. In all cases,

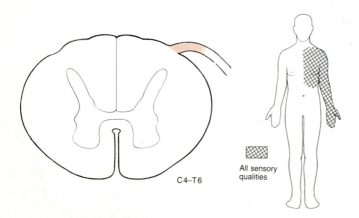

Fig. 2.19 Syndrome of posterior roots.

the development of typical deficits indicates that several adjacent roots are involved.

Syndrome of the posterior tracts (Fig. 2.20). Damage to posterior roots produces secondary alterations in the posterior tracts. Typical deficits attributable to posterior tract damage are astereognosis and the loss of sensation for position, vibration, and discrimination. In addition, Romberg's sign is present, and ataxia occurs when the eyes are closed. There is often also a hypersensitivity to pain. The most frequent causes of posterior tract damage are tabes dorsalis, subacute combined degeneration of the spinal cord, Friedreich's ataxia, trauma, and extramedullary tumors.

Syndrome of the posterior horns (Fig. 2.21). The posterior horn syndrome is seen in conditions such as syringomyelia, hematomyelia, and, occasionally, intramedullary tumors. The sensory deficit shows a segmental distribution pattern identical to that in the deficit caused by damage to the posterior roots. The sensory loss, however, essentially is of pain and temperature sensation in the ipsilateral segment; epicritical and proprioceptive sensations transmitted via the posterior tracts remain intact. In the area insensitive to pain, spontaneous attacks of pain may occur. The loss of pain and temperature sensation in the presence of preservation of the other sensory qualities is a *dissociated sensory disorder*. The fibers transmitting pain and temperature stimuli connect in the posterior horn with the "second neuron" that gives rise to the lateral and anterior spinothalamic tracts. Both cross through the anterior commissure to the opposite side. Because posterior funiculi remain

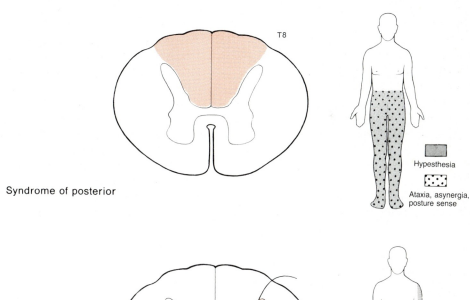

Fig. 2.20 Syndrome of posterior tracts.

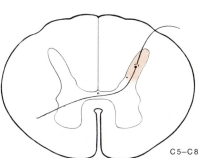

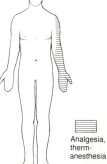

Fig. 2.21 Syndrome of posterior horn.

intact, the sensation of touch is not diminished, in spite of the involvement of the anterior spinothalamic tract. The preservation of unaltered pain and temperature sensation below the level of damage indicates that the spinothalamic tracts have not been damaged while ascending in the anterolateral funiculi.

Syndrome of the gray matter (Fig. 2.22). Diseases damaging the central gray matter, such as *syringomyelia, hematomyelia*, and *intramedullary tumors*, interrupt all pathways that cross through the anterior gray substance in front of the central canal. This interruption produces a bilateral dissociated sensory disorder. Syringomyelia most often involves the cervical cord and produces loss of pain and temperature sensation in shoulders and arms. The central cavitation characteristic of syringomyelia usually involves several segments. The tissue surrounding the syrinx often shows degenerative changes, which are probably caused in part by pressure exerted by the fluid filling the cavity. If both anterior horns are damaged, there will be a flaccid paralysis of the arms associated with muscular atrophy. If the lateral horns are involved, the arms may develop trophic disorders, possibly of such degree that the fingers become crippled. Occasionally, the pyramidal tracts degenerate, and this degeneration may be the cause of a spastic paresis of the legs. Extension of the syringomyelia into the medulla oblongata is not rare and may cause damage to motor nuclei of muscles subserving speech and swallowing (syringobulbia).

Syndrome of combined degeneration of posterior funiculi and corticospinal tracts (subacute combined degeneration of spinal cord) (Fig. 2.23). This disease is usually related to *pernicious anemia*, but it may be caused also by *other anemias* and various *dietary deficiencies*. It involves, progressively, the posterior funiculi and the pyramidal tracts; the gray substance is not involved. The damage to the posterior funiculi causes loss of position sensation in the lower extremities and, for example, the inability to feel vibrations in the feet. In addition, there will be ataxia and a positive Romberg's sign. The involvement of the pyramidal tracts simultaneously produces a spastic paraparesis of the legs with increased tendon reflexes and bilateral positive Babinski's sign.

Syndrome of the anterior horns (Fig. 2.24). The neurons of the anterior horns are selective victims in acute *poliomyelitis* and in chronic *progressive spinal muscular atrophy*. The neurons in the areas of the cervical and lumbar swelling of the cord appear to be particularly vulnerable.

In *poliomyelitis* so many anterior horn cells may die that a flaccid paralysis of the corresponding muscles ensues. The lack of innervation produces an atrophy of the muscle tissue which may be so severe that the tissue vanishes and is replaced by connective tissue

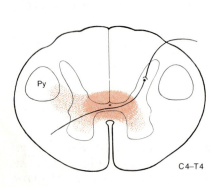

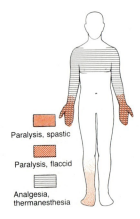

Fig. 2.22 Syndrome of gray matter.

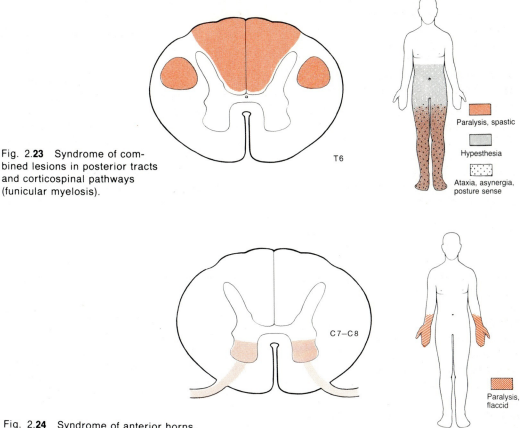

Fig. 2.**23** Syndrome of combined lesions in posterior tracts and corticospinal pathways (funicular myelosis).

Fig. 2.**24** Syndrome of anterior horns.

and fat. The degree of muscular involvement varies, depending on the degree of spinal cord damage. It is rare for all muscles of an extremity to be involved, mainly because the anterior horn cells of the various muscles are grouped in columns that extend for some distance within the anterior horns (see Fig. 2.**10**).

In *progressive spinal muscular atrophy* and also in *amyotrophic lateral sclerosis*, the anterior horn cells die slowly. In between areas of total degeneration, there are always neurons that are less severely damaged or remain intact. They are probably responsible for the fasciculation of muscles involved. Because the innervation of the musculature is plurisegmental, it is necessary that several adjacent segments be damaged for a paralysis to be complete. In addition to flaccid paralysis, secondary contractures develop as time passes. Involvement of sympathetic fibers coming from the lateral horns may be responsible for vasomotor disorders in the paralyzed areas and also for a transient sweating disorder.

Aside from poliomyelitis, progressive spinal muscular atrophy, and amyotrophic lateral sclerosis, the anterior horns may be involved in syringomyelia, hematomyelia, myelitis, and disorders of circulation of the cord.

Syndrome of combined anterior horn and pyramidal tract damage (Fig. 2.**25**). This combination of alterations is called *amyotrophic lateral sclerosis*. It leads to muscular

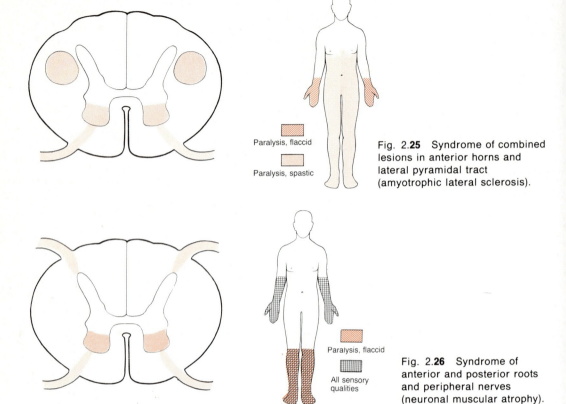

Fig. 2.25 Syndrome of combined lesions in anterior horns and lateral pyramidal tract (amyotrophic lateral sclerosis).

Fig. 2.26 Syndrome of anterior and posterior roots and peripheral nerves (neuronal muscular atrophy).

atrophy as a result of the disease of the anterior horns and to pareses of other muscles because of the degenerative disease of the pyramidal tract. The damage to the anterior horn cells produces a flaccid paresis, and that to the pyramidal tracts a spastic paresis. Consequently, in examining the patient, one will find a combination of flaccid and spastic paresis. For example, the muscles of arms and hands may show atrophy and decrease in tone; nevertheless, it may be possible to elicit signs of spasticity in these muscles. Although atrophy is present and reflexes should be absent, it is not rare to find normal reflexes, suggesting that some fibers of the pyramidal tracts and some anterior horn cells are still functioning. If the nuclei of cranial motor nerves are involved, there will be a disorder of swallowing and speech (*progressive bulbar paralysis*).

Syndrome of anterior and posterior roots and peripheral nerves (Fig. 2.26). This syndrome is also called *neural muscular atrophy*. It consists of a combination of sensory disorders and flaccid pareses. There are also paresthesias and occasionally pain. The peripheral nerves appear upon touch to be thickened and are often sensitive to pressure. The neural muscular atrophy is hereditary and occurs predominantly in young men. It is a chronic disease, with its progression being interrupted by remissions of longer duration. Atrophy predominantly of the lower legs (stork's legs) with steppage gait is characteristic of the disease.

Syndrome of the corticospinal tracts (Fig. 2.27). This condition is called *progressive spastic spinal paralysis*. A degenerative disappearance of neurons in the motor cortex

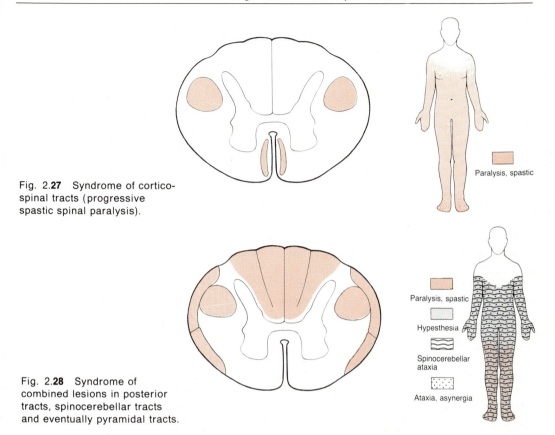

Fig. 2.27 Syndrome of corticospinal tracts (progressive spastic spinal paralysis).

Fig. 2.28 Syndrome of combined lesions in posterior tracts, spinocerebellar tracts and eventually pyramidal tracts.

leads to a degeneration of the corticospinal tracts. This rare condition is probably hereditary. The disease commences in early childhood and progresses extremely slowly. At first the patient complains about extreme heaviness of the legs. This symptom is followed by an increasing weakness. Gradually a spastic paraparesis of the legs develops, with a spastic gait disorder. The muscle tone is spastically elevated, and the reflexes are brisk and increased. Spastic paresis of the arms develops rather late. *Spastic paraparesis of the legs* is not infrequent. This syndrome is usually caused by multiple sclerosis or by a tumor. Amyotrophic lateral sclerosis as well may produce an early spastic paraparesis of the legs.

Syndrome of combined disease of posterior funiculi, spinocerebellar pathways, and possibly pyramidal tracts (Fig. 2.28). Involvement of these systems is the basis of the disease called *Friedreich's ataxia*. The symptomatology reflects the deterioration of the various systems. The disease commences with degeneration of the neurons of the spinal ganglia, which leads to a degeneration of the posterior funiculi. Consequently, there will be loss of position sense, discrimination, and stereognosis. Pain and temperature sensations are involved to a small extent if at all. Because of the posterior funicular disease, there will be a positive Romberg's sign and ataxia. Ataxia is often the leading sign because of the degeneration of the spinocerebellar tracts. The ataxia can be noticed while the patient is walking, standing, or sitting and is clearly revealed by the finger-to-nose and heel-to-knee tests. Walking is broad based and proceeds in a zigzag fashion. Later, a spastic component can be detected, indicating a degeneration of the pyramidal tracts. The development of a pes cavus, a so-called *Friedreich foot*, is characteristic of the disease. It is seen in 75% of the cases. Quite often, it is present already in childhood, but may develop later in life. Occasionally, it may be an isolated sign among family members. Eighty percent of the patients have a kyphosis or scoliosis. In general, the proprioceptive reflexes disappear. They may return as the pyramidal tracts degenerate and the toe reflexes become abnormal. *Marie's hereditary ataxia* combined with spastic paraparesis and the *Strümpell–Lorrain syndrome* with atrophy of the peroneal muscles are variants of the syndrome.

Syndrome of hemisection of the spinal cord (Fig. 2.**29**). This condition is also known as *Brown-Séquard syndrome*. A true hemisection of the spinal cord is extremely rare and may be the result of a stab wound. Usually the lesion involves only parts of the injured side of the cord. Briefly, the symptomatology is as follows: on the side of the lesion the descending motor pathways are interrupted, and after the initial spinal shock has dissipated, this interruption causes an *ipsilateral spastic paralysis* below the level of the lesion with hyperreflexia and abnormal reflexes of the toes. Injury to the posterior funiculus abolishes sensation for position, vibration, and tactile discrimination below the level of the injury. Ataxia should be present but cannot be demonstrated because of the paralysis. Pain and temperature sensations are not diminished below the level of the injury, because here the fibers of the lateral spinothalamic tract have already crossed to the opposite "healthy" side. In contrast, pain and temperature sensations are abolished on this contralateral healthy side up to the level of the lesion, because the crossing fibers are interrupted at the level of the hemisection. Simple tactile sensations are not decreased, because fibers transmitting these sensations use two pathways: the posterior funiculi and the anterior spinothalamic tract. In addition to the interruption of descending pathways, anterior horn cells are lost at the level of the injury. This loss causes a flaccid paresis in the corresponding myotome above the level of the lesion, where paresthesias and sometimes radicular pain also exist because of irritation of the posterior roots.

Syndrome of complete transection of the spinal cord (Fig. 2.**30**). A complete transection of the spinal cord may be produced by a myelitis (*transverse myelitis*) but is in most instances traumatic. The sudden interruption of the cord produces a so-called *spinal shock*. Below the lesion there is a complete flaccid paralysis and loss of all sensory qualities. Voluntary control of bladder and rectum and sexual potency are abolished. Below the lesion there are trophic disorders of the skin, particularly involving sweat secretion. Also, there is a malfunction of temperature regulation and a great tendency to develop decubital ulcers. The rostral border of sensory

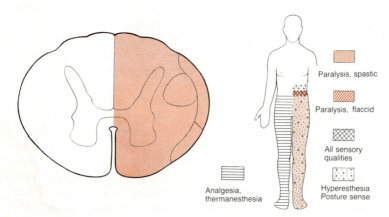

Fig. 2.**29** Syndrome of hemisection of spinal cord (Brown–Séquard syndrome).

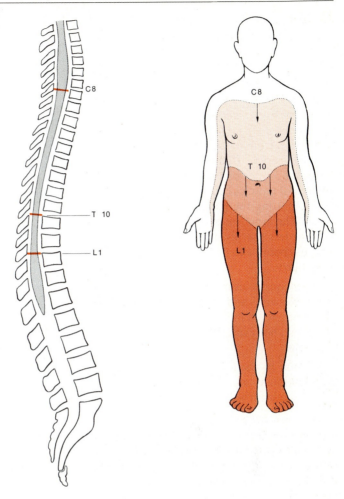

Fig. 2.**30** Paraplegia from transection of spinal cord at three different levels.

loss is usually characterized by a zone of hyperalgia.

How *spinal shock* develops is still unknown. It is assumed that it is caused in part by the sudden absence of the central stimulating impulses which continuously enter and tonicize the intrinsic neuronal apparatus of the spinal cord. It takes days or weeks for the spinal neurons gradually to regain their function, if only in part. At this time *spinal automatisms* appear. A painful stimulus below the level of the lesion may produce a sudden flexing in hip, knee, and foot joints (flexor reflex). If the transverse paralysis is partial, the legs are flexed at the beginning but later return to their original position. Gradually, bowel movements and bladder contractions return; they are automatic and involuntary, however. The automatic bladder contractions occur because a certain filling pressure produces a spontaneous reflex contraction. As time passes, muscle reflexes and tone may return. The reflexes are now often hyperreactive. Sexual potency remains abolished.

A spinal shock does not develop if the transverse paralysis develops slowly, as in the case of a growing tumor. Usually, transverse paralysis is incomplete in such situations. As a result, and increasing spastic paralysis below the level of the lesion is associated with disorders of bladder and rectum control and with impotence and automatic abnormalities such as vasomotor paralysis, sweating disorders, and a tendency to develop decubital ulcers. Certain sensory qualities remain more or less intact.

All *transverse injuries above the third cervical vertebra* are fatal because of cessation of respiration from paralysis of phrenic and intercostal nerves. If the transverse lesion involves the *lower cervical cord*, paralysis of the intercostal muscles causes respiratory insufficiency, putting the patient in a critical condition. The arms are partially paralyzed. The more or less sharply outlined border of sensory loss permits to determine the level of the cord injury.

A transverse lesion in the *upper thoracic cord* leaves arms and respiration undisturbed. There may be an involvement of the splanchnic nerves, however, that may lead to a paralytic ileus.

A lesion in the *lower thoracic cord* leaves the abdominal musculature intact. Respiration is undisturbed.

A transverse lesion in the *lumbar cord* may be very destructive, because it is most likely to involve the main artery of the lumbosacral cord, the *A. radicularis magna* (see Fig. 2.**38**). If this artery is obstructed or transected, the entire lumbar and sacral cord will be destroyed by infarction.

As long as the lower lumbar and sacral cord remains intact, any lesions involving the corticospinal pathways or even the motor portion of the cortex of the paracentral lobule produce a spastic paralysis of bladder and rectum. The bladder will be automatic, that is, will empty automatically by reflex action when it becomes filled to a certain level. Also, stimulating the perineum or its vicinity often produces a reflex contraction of the bladder. Voluntary control is no longer possible.

Syndrome of the epiconus (L4 to S2). The area called the *epiconus* is illustrated in Fig. 2.**31**. The epiconus syndrome is rela-

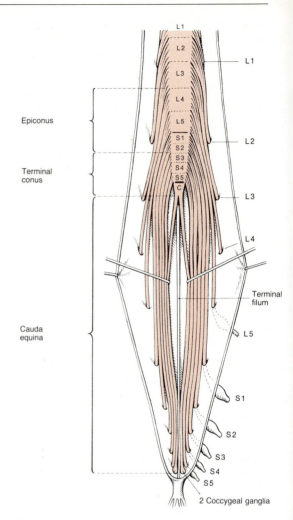

Fig. 2.**31** Syndromes of epiconus, conus, and cauda equina.

tively rare. In contrast to the conus syndrome, the altitude of the lesion in this syndrome determines whether it produces a paresis or a flaccid paralysis. Outward rotation (L4 to S1) and dorsal flexion in the hip joints (L4, L5), and possibly flexion in the knee joint (L4 to S2) and flexion and extension in the joints of the foot and toes (L4 to S2), are reduced or abolished. The Achilles tendon reflexes are absent; the knee tendon reflexes are preserved. There are sensory disorders in the dermatomes L4 to S5. The bladder and rectum empty only by reflex. Occasionally there is priapism, although potency is absent. There may be transient paralysis of vasomotors and absence of sweat secretion.

Syndrome of the conus (S3 to C). The cord segment called the conus terminalis is illustrated in Fig. 2.**31**. This syndrome is also rather rare and may be caused by alterations such as an intramedullary tumor, a carcinoma metastasis, or a deficiency in blood supply. Signs and symptoms of isolated conus damage are as follows:

1. flaccid paralysis of bladder associated with incontinence (continuous drip of urine)
2. incontinence of rectum
3. impotence
4. anesthesia of the saddle region (S3–S5)
5. absence of anal reflexes
6. absence of paralysis in the lower extremities and presence of Achilles tendon reflexes (L5–S2)

A tumor, at first restricted to the conus, will eventually involve adjacent lumbar and sacral roots (see Figs. 2.**31** to 2.**34**). Therefore, signs of involvement of the cauda equina consisting of paresis and more extensive sensory disorders will be superimposed on the originally pure conus syndrome.

Syndrome of the cauda (Fig. 2.**31**). Signs and symptoms indicative of involvement of the long nerve roots forming the cauda equina are most often caused by tumors such as ependymomas and lipomas. At first there is radicular pain in the territory of the sciatic nerve and severe pain in the bladder which is exacerbated by coughing and sneezing. Later, sensory disorders for all qualities develop to various degrees, showing a radicular pattern that extends downward from the level of L4. If the alteration involves the rostral cauda, the sensory disorder involving the saddle region extends down to the lower legs. With a more caudal location of the lesion, only the saddle area is involved (S3–S5). A rostral lesion may also produce flaccid paralysis of the lower extremities with loss of reflexes, incontinence of bladder and rectum, and potency disorders (see also pp. 212, 216).

In contrast to tumors of the conus, those of the cauda equina produce symptoms slowly and irregularly, because the roots can tolerate some displacement before dysfunction sets in.

Aside from tumors, the most frequent cause of conus or cauda syndrome, or both, is a prolapsing intervertebral disk. This disease is the most frequent cause of spinal radicular syndromes and deserves some specific comments.

Spinal Radicular Syndromes Caused by Diseases of the Disk (Osteochondrosis, Disk Protrusion, Prolapse, or Herniation)

The center of a disk is occupied by the jelly-like *nucleus pulposus,* which is regarded as the persistent remains of the embryonic notochord. It is surrounded and contained by the *anulus fibrosus,* composed of fibrocartilage and fibrous tissue. With the end of spinal column development, the disks lose their blood vessels. During life they become gradually less elastic and less effective as mechanical shock absorbers. This change may lead to disorders in the most flexible portions of the spinal column, its cervical and lumbar segments. As the disks lose their thickness, the bodies of adjacent vertebrae move closer to each other. Consequently, the intervertebral foramina become smaller, endangering the soft tissues they contain (Fig. 2.**32b**; see Fig. 2.**37b**). The progressing atrophy of the disks and approximation of the vertebrae is called *osteochondrosis.*

The *cervical radicular syndrome* is almost always caused by osteochondrosis. The superior compact bone layers of the bodies of the cervical vertebrae are raised laterally to form the *uncinate processes,* saddle-shaped structures (see Fig. 2.**32d**). As the disks shrink, each preceding vertebral body presses wedge-like into the saddle-shaped cavity of the lower body and exerts pressure on the lateral uncinate processes. These processes undergo structural change and become dis-

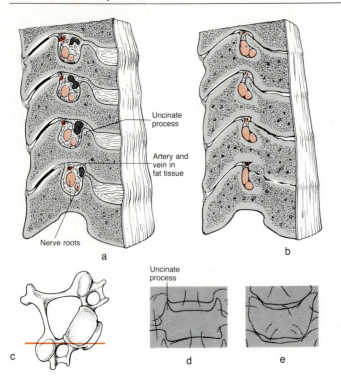

Fig. 2.**32** Intervertebral foramina of cervical column between 3rd and 7th cervical vertebrae.
a Normal foramina;
b narrowing of foramina due to atrophy of intervertebral disks (drawn from specimen); **c** plane of cut section; **d** normal uncinate processes;
e unicate processes deformed by atrophy of intervertebral disks.

placed laterally and dorsally, compromising the intervertebral foramina (see Fig. 2.**32b**).

The osteochondrosis of the cervical column involves the cervical vertebrae from C3 downward and the first thoracic vertebra. The spaces between the fifth and sixth, as well as the sixth and seventh cervical vertebrae are most often involved in the narrowing process. The narrowing may be restricted to individual foramina or may involve several of them unilaterally or bilaterally to different degrees. This is the reason one may encounter monosegmental as well as plurisegmental radicular syndromes. These syndromes usually consist of radicular irritation producing paresthesias and pain in segmental distribution patterns. More severe damage may lead to radicular sensory and motor losses associated with abnormal reflexes.

Syndromes of lesions limited to individual cervical nerve roots (see Fig. 2.**11**).

C3, C4: pain in neck and shoulder; rarely, partial paresis of diaphragm.

C5: pain, potentially hypalgesia in dermatome C5; disorder in innervation of deltoid and brachial biceps muscles.

C6: pain, potentially hypalgesia in dermatome C6; paresis in brachial biceps and brachioradial muscles; decreased biceps reflex.

C7: pain, potentially paresthesia or hypalgesia in dermatome C7; paresis of brachial triceps and pronator teres muscles and possibly atrophy of thenar muscles of thumb; decreased triceps reflex.

C8: pain, possibly paresthesias and hypalgesia in dermatome C8; paresis and possibly atrophy of hypothenar muscles of little finger; triceps reflex decreased.

If several adjacent foramina become very narrow, there is the rare possibility that a radicular artery feeding into the anterior spinal artery will become compressed (Fig. 2.**33**). The circulatory deficiency of the cord may be so severe that it produces spinal

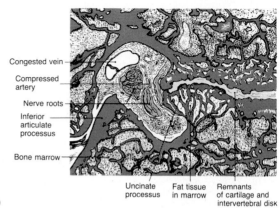

Fig. 2.**33** Histologic preparation of a severely narrowed foramen showing the narrowing as well as the expanding alterations of the uncinate and articulate processes (bone marrow). (Drawn from microscopic preparation.)

cord signs overriding the syndrome of root compression.

The degenerative process of the disk is often combined with *spondylosis deformans*, gradually reducing the mobility in the respective segment of the cervical spine. This quasi-fixation of the spinal column, together with a process that widens the foramen, may be the reason no radicular syndrome develops. The situation is usually labile, however. A slackening of the vertebral joints, whatever its cause, may immediately provoke complaints (Duus, 1948, 1951, 1974).

The *lumbar disks* are rather thick, and the adjacent vertebral surfaces are flat. As degeneration takes place, there may be *disk protrusion* or even *disk prolapse* directly compromising spinal roots and ganglia. An osteochondrosis narrowing the intervertebral spaces will also reduce the lumina of the intervertebral foramina and thereby trigger radicular pain (see Fig. 2.37).

The caudal disks between L4 and L5, and L5 and S1, are more often abnormal than is the disk between L3 and L4.

Fig. 2.**34** illustrates the close topographical relationship between lumbar and sacral vertebrae, disks, and nerve roots. The roots leave the spinal canal at the level of the superior third of each vertebra. In a ventrocaudal course toward the spinal ganglia they pass through a pouch of the dura that terminates at the exit of the foramen. Because of their ventrocaudal direction, a dorsolateral protrusion of a disk is more likely to press on the roots of the subsequent segment than on those of its own level. For example, if the disk between L4 and L5 protrudes dorsolaterally, it does not impinge on the L4 but on the L5 root as it passes in a caudal direction behind the protrusion of the disk, as illustrated in Fig. 2.**35**. The root of the same segment can be directly damaged only if the disk does not protrude but prolapses and does so rather laterally.

The disk between L5 and S1 is often smaller dorsally than the other disks, because of the more pronounced lordosis. This is the reason a prolapse of this disk may involve the roots of S1 as well as of L5, producing a combined L5–S1 syndrome.

As with cervical disks, those in the lumbar area cause irritation to the nerve roots, felt as pain and paresthesias in the corresponding segments (lumbago, sciatica). More severe damage to the roots produces segmental sensory and motor deficits.

Syndromes of lesions limited to individual lumbar roots (see Fig. 2.12).

L3: pain, possibly paresthesias in dermatome L3; paresis of femoral quadriceps muscle; decreased or missing quadriceps tendon reflex (patellar reflex).

L4: pain, possibly paresthesias or hypalgesia in dermatome L4; paresis of femoral

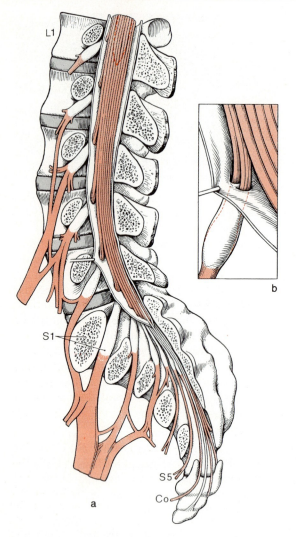

Fig. 2.**34 a** Conus terminalis and cauda equina in spinal canal. Lateral view after removal of half of vertebral arches and opening of dural sac, showing topography of spinal column, vertebral disks and nerve roots.
b Funnel-like widening of dura with two openings for anterior root (ventral) and posterior root (dorsal).

quadriceps and anterior tibial muscles; reduced patellar reflex.

L5: pain, possibly paresthesias or hypalgesia in dermatome L5; paresis and possibly atrophy of extensor hallucis longus as well as extensor digitorum brevis muscles; absence of posterior tibial reflex.

S1: pain, possibly paresthesias or hypalgesia in dermatome S1; paresis of peroneal and triceps surae muscles; loss of triceps surae reflex (Achilles tendon reflex).

Should sciatic pains from radicular irritation suddenly disappear and be replaced by a motor paresis or a sensory loss, it signifies that the radicular fibers can no longer conduct. Immediate surgical relief of the involved roots is indicated.

In rare instances, a disk that prolapses medially through the posterior longitudinal ligament into the spinal canal may be the cause of a cauda syndrome (Fig. 2.**36**).

Acute lumbago is often caused by entrapment of articular capsule tissue in the verte-

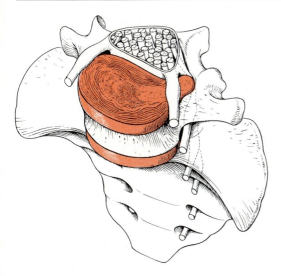
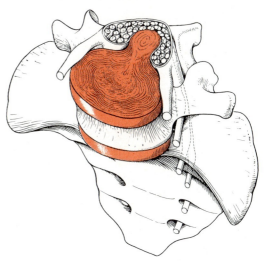

Fig. 2.**35** Posterolateral protrusion of vertebral disk between 4th and 5th lumbar vertebrae. The 4th lumbar root is intact, but the 5th lumbar root passing behind the 4th lumbar disk is damaged.

Fig. 2.**36** Medial protrusion of vertebral disk in area between 4th and 5th lumbar vertebrae with pressure on cauda equina.

bral joint. This entrapment occurs if the atrophy of the disk causes a rostral shifting of the articular process into the foramen (Fig. 2.**37**). As the articular capsule slackens it may become caught in the joint during an awkward movement. These cases explain why chiropractic manipulations are sometimes blessed with instant success.

Blood Supply of the Spinal Cord

Arterial Supply

Before the vertebral arteries join to form the basilar artery, they give off branches that run toward the uppermost portion of the cervical cord and become the rostral feeders of the *one anterior* and the *two posterior spinal arteries*. These longitudinal anastomotic arteries receive blood at various intervals and distribute it among the arteries proper of the spinal cord. The anterior spinal artery runs as a continuous single artery over the ventral median sulcus (fissure) of the cord down to the conus terminalis (Figs. 2.**38** and 2.**39a**). Here it loops to the posterior aspect of the lumbosacral cord and connects with the posterior spinal arteries. These arteries descend in the dorsolateral sulci of the cord next to the posterior roots. They are not continuous

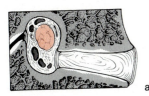
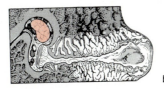

Fig. 2.**37 a** Normal width of intervertebral foramen between 5th lumbar and 1st sacral vertebrae with spinal ganglion in center. **b** Narrowed foramen with deformation of spinal ganglion by upward displacement of inferior articulate process. (Drawn from microscopic preparation.)

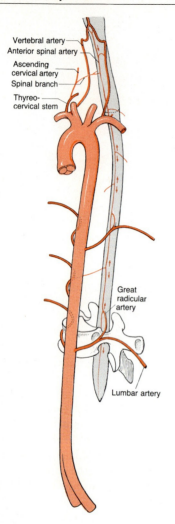

Fig. 2.**38** Arterial feeders of spinal arteries.

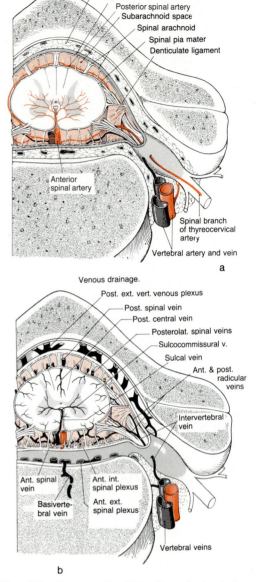

Fig. 2.**39** Cross-section through cervical vertebra showing **a** arterial supply to spinal arteries and **b** venous drainage.

individual vessels but represent anastomosing chains of small arteries in which the blood may flow in opposite directions.

Occasionally, the posterior inferior cerebellar arteries are the rostral feeders of the posterior spinal arteries. Aside from the rostral feeder arteries, the anterior as well as the posterior spinal arteries receive blood from radicular arteries coming from one or both vertebral arteries in the neck, from the thyreocostocervical trunk of a subclavian artery, and, below T3, from the segmental intercostal and lumbar arteries. Originally, each segment of the cord has its pair of radicular arteries. Later, only five to eight arteries accompany the ventral roots to the anterior spinal artery and four to eight arteries the dorsal roots to the posterior spinal arteries, at irregular intervals. The ventral radicular arteries are larger than the dorsal; the largest among them is called the *A. radicularis magna* (Adamkiewicz). It usually accompanies the right or the left root at L2 on its way to the anterior spinal artery. The segmental spinal arteries that regressed after early development do not disappear; they supply the roots, the spinal ganglia, and the dura. The anterior spinal arteries give off *sulcocommissural* and *circumferential branches* at close intervals. The approximately 200 sulcocommissural branches run horizontally through the ventral median sulcus and fan out in front of the anterior commissure to both sides, supplying almost the entire gray matter and the surrounding rim of white matter, including part of the anterior funiculi (see Figs. 2.**39a** and 2.**40**). The circumferential branches anastomose with like branches of the posterior spinal arteries, forming a *vasocorona*. Twigs of the anterior vasocorona supply the anterolateral and the lateral funiculi, including much of the lateral pyramidal tracts (see Fig. 2.**40**). The main structures supplied by the posterior spinal arteries are the posterior funiculi and the tips of the posterior horns.

Venous Drainage (Fig. 2.39b)

The intraspinal capillaries, which in the gray matter form clusters corresponding to the columns of neurons, drain into the intraspinal veins. Most of these veins run radially to the periphery of the cord. More centrally located veins extend first longitudinally parallel to the central canal before leaving the cord in the depth of the ventral or dorsal median sulci. Outside the cord the veins form plexuses draining into meandering longitudinal collecting veins, the *ventral and dorsal spinal veins*. The dorsal collecting vein is the larger and increases in size toward the caudal portion of the cord. The blood in the collecting veins drains via central and dorsal radicular veins (5 to 11 on each side) into the *internal vertebral venous plexus*. Surrounded by loose connective tissue and fat tissue, the plexus is located in the extradural space. The plexus is analogous to the cranial dural sinuses. In fact, it communicates through the foramen magnum with these sinuses at the

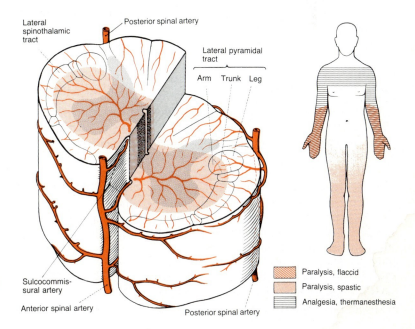

Fig. 2.**40** Syndrome of thrombosis of anterior spinal artery.

base of the skull. The blood drains only in part through these connections; most of it leaves by intervertebral veins through the intervertebral foramina and enters the *external vertebral venous plexus*. This plexus, among others, drains into the azygos vein, which on the right side of the spinal column connects the superior and inferior venae cavae.

Syndromes Caused by Spinal Vascular Lesions

Anterior spinal artery occlusion. A sudden, usually thrombotic obstruction of the cervical portion of the anterior spinal artery produces paresthesias and severe pain, soon followed by flaccid paralysis of the arms and spastic paraparesis of the legs from involvement of the pyramidal tracts; disorders of bladder and rectum function; and decreased sensation for pain and temperature at the segmental level of the arterial obstruction. Sensations of proprioception and touch are usually preserved (Fig. 2.**40**). Anhidrosis in the paralyzed portions of the body may raise the body temperature, particularly if the ambient temperature is high, simulating fever from infection.

Posterior spinal artery obstruction. An occlusion of one or both posterior spinal arteries is very rare. The resulting infarction involves the posterior tracts and horns and, in part, the lateral pyramidal tracts. Below the level of the lesion, deficits such as anesthesia and analgesia, spastic paresis, and reflex disorders are found.

Angiodysgenetic necrotizing myelopathy. This condition, also called *Foix-Alajouanine's disease* (*myélite nécrotique subaigue*), consists of lesions of circulatory atrophy combined with infarction, most often in the lower thoracic and lumbar cord. The alterations are caused by progressive changes (vascular ectasia, hypertrophy of vessel walls, symptomatic inflammation) in originally abnormal intra- and extraspinal arteries and veins. The clinical subacute or chronic course is dominated by paraplegia of the lower extremities, first mild and spastic, later flaccid and associated with muscular atrophy. Initial disorders of pain and temperature sensation are followed by loss of all sensory qualities.

Intraspinal hematoma. Bleeding in such cases may be caused by spontaneous rupture of an intrinsic vascular malformation such as a telangiectasia in the gray matter. Most often it is the result of trauma. If the bleeding originates centrally, it usually extends up and down the axis of the cord for several segments and is generally referred to as *hematomyelia*. It produces an acute syndrome which may be very similar to the chronic syndrome characteristic of syringomyelia.

Spinal epidural bleeding. This bleeding is rare. It is usually not traumatic but caused by the rupture of a vascular malformation, usually a small-vessel angioma in the epidural space or next to it in the vertebral bone. (Roentgenography will show vertical strands of spongiosa in the vertebral bone characteristic of angioma.) The blood does not always collect at the site of the angioma. The hematoma usually develops over the dorsal portion of the midthoracic cord. It may produce acute radicular pain at the level of the bleeding. Thereafter, the syndrome of a transverse myelopathy begins, with paresthesias followed by sensory deficits. Motor paresis starts in toes and feet and ascends to the level of the cord compression. Immediate neurosurgical consultation is a necessity.

Spinal Tumors

These tumors may be classified according to their locations as *extramedullary* or *intramedullary*. Extramedullary tumors may be *extradural* (sarcoma or carcinoma of the vertebrae, fibroma, lipoma, angiolipoma, neurinoma) or *intradural* (meningioma, neurinoma, ectopic ependymoma). Most of the intramedullary tumors are gliomas, ependymomas, or angiomas.

Extramedullary Tumors

These tumors may originate in the area of posterior roots (Fig. 2.**41**) and produce early

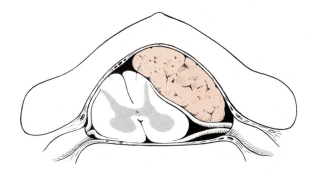

Fig. 2.41 Syndrome of dorsally located extramedullary tumor.

radicular pain and dysesthesias. As they grow, they exert more and more pressure on the posterior roots and on the spinal cord.

In *dorsomedial locations* the tumor may press first on the posterior roots and posterior tracts and involve the lateral pyramidal tracts later. This pattern produces a growing ipsilateral spastic paresis of the leg, as well as paresthesias, particularly for cold, in both legs, and a disorder of epicritical and proprioceptive sensations ipsilaterally and later bilaterally. The sensory disorder has a tendency to ascend in a caudocranial direction until it becomes stationary at the segment involved. At this segment the vertebrae are sensitive to tapping. Coughing and sneezing exacerbate the pain. The pain related to involvement of the posterior tracts is similar to rheumatic pain and is felt first in the distal portions of the extremities. In the dermatome of the damaged roots, there is often a zone of hyperesthesia helpful in diagnosing the altitudinal location of the lesion. Finally, paralysis of bladder and rectum sphincters develops as a result of spinal cord compression.

In *ventral locations* tumors may press first on one or both anterior roots (Fig. 2.42). Cervical tumors in this position cause flaccid paresis of one or both hands. Later, pyramidal tract involvement leads to a spastic paresis, first of the ipsilateral leg and later of both legs. Damage to the pyramidal tracts may be caused in part by mechanical stress resulting from stretching of the denticulate ligament. Pressure on one ventrolateral funiculus may produce hypesthesias for pain and temperature contralaterally. Ultimately bladder and rectum control will be lost.

If the symptomatology defies satisfactory analysis, one must suspect a *subarachnoid angioma*. Such a tumor often extends over several segments and prefers the dorsal aspect of the cord. It may affect the cord by pressure, by bleeding, or by producing a local oligemia because of an arteriovenous shunt.

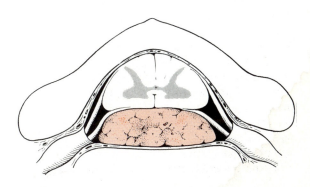

Fig. 2.42 Syndrome of ventrally located extramedullary tumor.

A subarachnoid angioma may easily be misdiagnosed, particularly as multiple sclerosis.

Intramedullary Tumors

These tumors (Fig. 2.**43**) differ from extramedullary tumors in the following features:

1. Radicular pain is rare.
2. Dissociated sensory disorders start early.
3. Disorders in bladder and rectum control appear early.
4. Because of *longitudinal* growth the upper border of sensory disorders may migrate rostrally, in contrast to the situation in extramedullary tumors. Their rostral border finally becomes stationary because of *transverse* growth of the neoplasm.
5. Atrophy of muscles stemming from involvement of anterior horns is more frequent than with extramedullary tumors.
6. Spasticity is rarely as severe as it is with extramedullary neoplasms.

If the tumor involves the upper cervical cord, the symptomatology may include signs of bulbar involvement. Also, fasciculations and fibrillations in the muscles of the corresponding extremity are not rare with such a high-level tumor. Statistically, extramedullary tumors are considerably more frequent than those within the spinal cord.

A tumor in the area of the foramen magnum (meningioma, neurinoma) often indicates its presence by pain as well as by paresthesia and hypesthesia in the area of C2 (great auricular nerve, occipital nerve) and paresis of the sternocleidomastoid and trapezius muscles (accessory nerve).

Hourglass tumor

This tumor (Fig. 2.**44**) is invariably a neurinoma originating within the intervertebral foramen growing to the outside as well as into the spinal canal. It produces signs and symptoms of root compression. It may also gradually lead to Brown-Séquard syndrome when

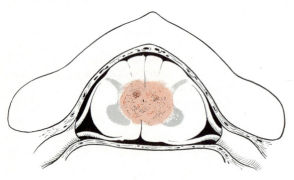

Fig. 2.**43** Syndrome of intramedullary tumor.

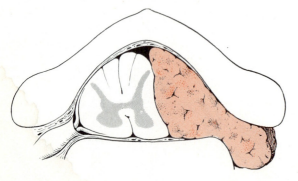

Fig. 2.**44** Syndrome of hour-glass tumor.

it presses on the lateral aspect of the spinal cord. The diagnosis can be made easily by the presence of an enlargement of the intervertebral foramen on oblique roentgenograms.

Disorders of Neuromuscular Junctions and Muscles

Myopathies

The word *myopathy* is used for a variety of diseases caused by anatomic and biochemical alterations in and around the motor endplates, in muscle fibers, or in the connective tissue of the muscles, and not by lesions in the nervous system.

These diseases include:

1. progressive muscular dystrophy (Erb-Goldflam disease)
2. myotonia congenita (Thomsen's disease)
3. dystrophia myotonica (Curschmann-Steinert syndrome)
4. paroxysmal paralysis (hyper- and hypokalaemic type)
5. amyotonia congenita (Oppenheim's disease)
6. dermatomyositis
7. acute, subacute, and chronic polymyositis
8. scleroderma

The myopathies have several features in common. The disease of the muscles is almost always bilateral and often even symmetric in distribution. Except in myotonia congenita the musculature and, therefore, the strength of the muscles slowly dwindles. Neurologic signs such as sensory disorders, fasciculations, fibrillations, reaction of degeneration, and spastic phenomena are missing. Reflexes attenuate corresponding to the decrease in muscle tissue. Muscle atrophy may be masked by proliferation of intramuscular connective tissue and fat tissue, as is the case in progressive muscular dystrophy. The proliferation of these tissues may lead one to assume that there is a hypertrophy of the musculature. Electromyography and muscle biopsy will show that the atrophy is myogenic and not neurogenic. Some myopathies, such as the first four listed, are hereditary. In myotonia congenita the muscles remain strong and do not become atrophic. The abnormality consists in a prolongation of muscle contracture after innervation. For example, the handshake is firm, but subsequent opening of the hand is very slow and halting. Dermatomyositis and polymyositis are not causally distinct. Some myopathies fall into the category of collagen diseases. The causes of others include viral and bacterial infection, toxoplasmosis, trichinosis, malignant growth, and sarcoidosis. In contrast to the degeneration muscular diseases, the polymyositides are often accompanied by pain. Sensitivity of the muscles to pressure is common. The course of these conditions can be acute, subacute, or chronic.

Myasthenia gravis pseudoparalytica is not hereditary. The muscles do not become atrophic but suffer from great, abnormal fatigability. This is an autoimmune disease, in which circulating antibodies act on the acetylcholine receptors of the postsynaptic membrane of the neuromuscular junction. Acetycholine needed for the transmission of nerval impulses to the musculature is not available in sufficient amount or is too rapidly degraded by cholinesterase. The diagnosis of myasthenia can be made if after injection of an inhibitor of cholinesterase the myasthenic signs rapidly and temporarily disappear (Tensilon test).

3 Brainstem and Cranial Nerves

External Structure

In general, *brainstem* is used as the collective term for the *medulla oblongata (myelencephalon), pons (metencephalon),* and *midbrain (mesencephalon)*. Pons and medulla oblongata together are also referred to as *hindbrain (rhombencephalon)*.

As can be seen in Fig. 3.1a, the brainstem extends from the crossing of the pyramidal tracts – that is, from the level of the origin of the roots of C1 – upward to the level of the optic tracts, which, on their way from the chiasm to the lateral geniculate bodies, embrace the *crura cerebri* of the midbrain. On ventral and lateral views, the three components of the brainstem are rather well delineated (Fig. 3.1a and c). A horizontal groove marks the pontocerebellar junction. A similar groove is present where the peduncles of the midbrain meet the rostral margin of the pons. The dorsal aspect of the brainstem can be seen only after removal of the cerebellum (derivative of the metencephalon). Fig. 3.1b shows the two rather large stumps of the fiber masses that connected brainstem and cerebellum. They are subdivided into three groups. The *superior cerebellar peduncle* (brachium conjunctivum) connects cerebellum and midbrain. Most of its fibers leave the dentate nucleus and other cerebellar nuclei, cross the midline at the junction of pons and midbrain, and connect predominantly with the contralateral red nucleus. The *middle cerebellar peduncle* (brachium pontis) carries pontocerebellar fibers from neurons in the contralateral portion of the base of the pons.

These neurons are the recipients of impulses from corticopontine fiber bundles descending through the internal capsules. Thus, they are the second neurons of the connections between cerebral and cerebellar cortex. The *inferior cerebellar peduncle* (corpus restiforme) carries ascending fibers going to the cerebellar cortex.

Medulla Oblongata

The medulla oblongata is best seen by looking at the ventral aspect of the brainstem (see Fig. 3.1a). The structure is approximately 2.5 to 3 cm long, the distance from the pontomedullary junction to the roots of C1. The longitudinal, elevated, clublike structures on either side of the median sulcus are the pyramids. They are made up of the descending corticospinal tracts; thus, these motor pathways are also called *pyramidal tracts*. In the midbrain these tracts pass through the middle of the peduncles together with corticopontine fiber bundles. In the pons they pass through the base and are hidden from external view by surrounding pontine nuclei and crossing fibers. In the medulla oblongata, however, as pyramids, they are superficial, rendering them vulnerable under certain conditions. For example, a pathologically enlarged vertebral artery may deeply depress the pyramid that it crosses on its way to the midline. Also, the lower pyramids face the margin of the foramen magnum and may be pressed against it as result of a space-occupying alteration in or around the cerebellum. The *inferior olivary nuclei* are the

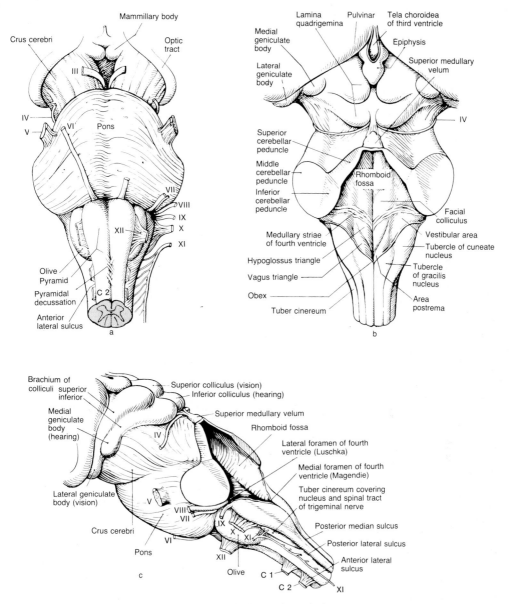

Fig. 3.1 Brainstem. **a** ventral view; **b** dorsal view; **c** lateral view.

natural neighbors of the pyramids. They are separated from the pyramids by the anterior lateral or ventrolateral sulci. The hypoglossal nerves emerge from these sulci with multiple rootlets along the surface of the inferior olives. The *hypoglossal nerve* (XII) and the *abducens* (VI), *trochlear* (IV) and *oculomotor* (III) *nerves* are close relatives of the anterior motor roots of the spinal cord. Their nuclei develop from the basal plate from which the anterior horns of the spinal cord also were derived. These nuclei are characteristically located on either side of the midline near the fourth ventricle and aqueduct (see Figs. 3.2 and 3.3).

Several cranial nerves are visible at the lateral aspect of the medulla oblongata (Fig. 3.1c). The most caudal is the *accessory nerve (XI)*, which is formed by a number of small rootlets. Some of these originate in the cervical cord, so that the cervical portion of the nerve has to ascend through the foramen magnum in order to pick up the medullary rootlets. Next follow the *vagus (X)* and *glossopharyngeal (IX)* nerves. In the corner of the pontomedullary junction, also referred to as the *cerebellopontine angle*, the vestibulocochlear nerve (VIII) enters the brainstem.

The dorsal aspect of the medulla oblongata shows three symmetrically located protuberances on either side of the midline (see Fig. 3.1b). The most lateral is called the *tuberculum cinereum*. It is produced by the underlying spinal nucleus and tract of the trigeminal nerve. The eminences caused by the cuneate and gracilis nuclei immediately follow. These structures form the caudal border of the floor of the fourth ventricle, which, because of its shape, is also referred to as the rhomboid fossa (hence the term *rhombencephalon* for pons and medulla oblongata). Here, the border between medulla oblongata and pons is roughly indicated by the *medullary striae* running across the floor of the fourth ventricle. These myelinated fibers are axons of the arcuate nuclei. These caudal extensions of the nuclei of the base of the pons form a half shell around the periphery of the pyramidal tracts. The fibers pass dorsally close to the midline and, after reaching the fourth ventricle, enter the inferior cerebellar peduncles. Below these striae and to either side of the midline are the trigones of the hypoglossal and vagus nerves. More laterally, slight bulgings are produced by the vestibular nuclei (area vestibularis). Near the caudal tip of the fourth ventricle, the area postrema forms a small bilateral elevation. This is the level of the *foramen of Magendie* (apertura mediana ventriculi quarti). The *foramina of Luschka* (aperturae laterales ventriculi quarti) are located in the pontomedullary angle, just beneath the vestibulocochlear nerves.

Pons

The *pons* (bridge) was thus named by Varolio (1543–1575) because it ventrally connects the two cerebellar hemispheres and bridges the fourth ventricle. A belly-like protrusion is produced by the base of the pons. Here, corticopontine fibers terminate ipsilaterally at the neurons of pontine nuclei (second neurons), the axons of which cross the midline and proceed to the contralateral cerebellar cortex. The base also contains, on either side of the midline, the pyramidal tracts. A shallow, longitudinal grooving divides the base of the pons into symmetrical halves (see Fig. 3.1a). This grooving is not caused by the basilar artery; rather, the elevations on either side of the midline are caused by the pyramidal tracts. If the cerebral portion of a pyramidal tract is interrupted by a lesion, such as an infarct that destroys the internal capsule, the distal portion of the tract becomes atrophic and the ipsilateral elevation of the pons disappears. In the medulla oblongata the ipsilateral pyramid becomes small and atrophic.

Laterally, the transverse fibers of the base of the pons form the pontine peduncles. The stumps of the trigeminal nerves (V) are located in the rostral portions of the peduncles where they emerge from the base of the pons. Most of the nerve fibers are sensory and come from neurons of Gasser's trigeminal ganglia (*ganglion semilunare Gasseri*). The small bundle of motor fibers attached to the dorsal portion of the nerve stumps and supplying the muscles of mastication originate in the tegmentum of the pons, as do the abducens nerves (VI) and the facial nerves (VII). These nerves emerge from the pontomedullary junction: the abducens nerves near the midline and between pons and pyramids, the facial nerves laterally in front of the vestibuloauditory nerves (see Fig. 3.1a). When viewed from behind (see Fig. 3.1b), the territory of the pons extends from the level of the medullary striae to that of the trochlear nerves (IV). Above the medullary striae and on either side of the midline is a circumscribed elevation of the floor of the fourth ventricle caused by the *internal knee* of the fibers of the *facial nerve*. Fig. 3.1b shows this facial colliculus and also a portion of the rostral roof or tectum of the fourth ventricle, the *velum medullare superius*, which is fastened to the upper vermis of the cerebellum (see Fig. 4.2).

Midbrain

At its ventral aspect, the midbrain is characterized by its *cerebral peduncles* (crura cerebri), which consist of the corticopontine and corticospinal fiber tracts as they leave the internal capsule on either side posterior to the level of the mamillary bodies (see Fig. 3.1a). Between the peduncles is the *interpeduncular fossa*. The *oculomotor nerves (III)* emerge from the midbrain on either side of the midline of the caudal portion of the fossa. The *trochlear nerves (IV)* differ from all cranial nerves in two respects: (1) they emerge from the dorsal aspect of the midbrain, and (2) they cross in the rostral portion of the superior medullary velum just before they leave the midbrain. As can be seen in Fig. 3.1b, the nerves swing around the dorsal and lateral aspects of the pontomesencephalic junction and proceed laterally from the cerebral peduncles on their way to the cavernous sinuses. They run below the level of the margin of the tentorium (see Fig. 3.16). The *tectum*, or roof, of the midbrain is formed by the *quadrigeminal plate*, which is subdivided into

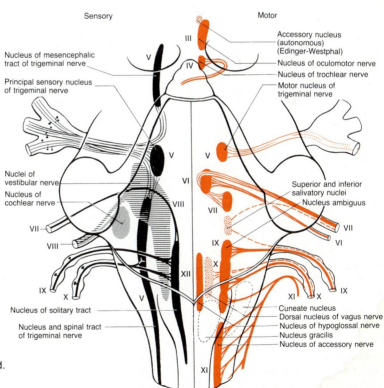

Fig. 3.2 Nuclei of cranial nerves viewed from behind. Sensory nuclei are black; motor nuclei, red.

two *superior* and two *inferior colliculi*. The former receive optic and the latter acoustic stimuli.

Cranial Nerves

Origin, Components and Function

Fig. 3.2 shows the brainstem as viewed from the rear. On the right, the motor nuclei of III through XII and their nerves are shown in red. On the left, the sensory nerves and the nuclei at which they terminate appear in black. Figs. 3.3 and 3.4 demonstrate the topographical distribution of the motor and sensory nerves and their nuclei as seen from the side of the brainstem. Fig. 3.3 shows the motor nerves and their nuclei in red, and Fig. 3.4 the sensory nerves and respective nuclei in black.

The components of the cranial nerves, along with their origins and functions, are listed in Table 3.1. Fig. 3.5 shows all cranial nerves, including olfactory tract and optic nerves, in their topographical arrangement at the base of the brain and, in a semicircle, the organs they supply (red lines) or from which their impulses originate (black lines).

It was mentioned earlier that spinal nerves are classified as somatic afferent, somatic efferent, autonomic afferent, or autonomic efferent. The functional classification of cranial nerves is more complicated, because some of them are connected with highly specialized sensory organs and subserve such functions as vision, hearing, smell and taste. Other cranial nerves are branchiomeric (V, VI, IX, X, and XI), and their efferent fibers innervate the muscles derived from branchial arches.

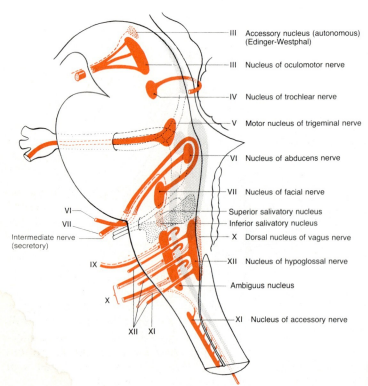

Fig. 3.3 Motor nuclei of cranial nerves (lateral view).

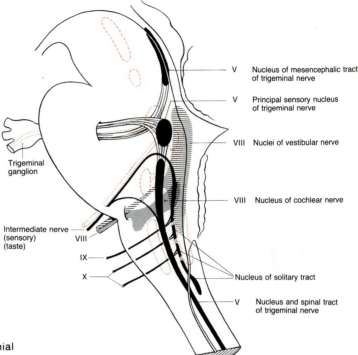

Fig. 3.4 Sensory nuclei of cranial nerves (lateral view).

The following types of fibers are encountered in cranial nerves:

1. somatic afferent fibers (transmitting pain, temperature, touch, pressure, and proprioceptive sensations via receptors in skin, joints, tendons, etc.)
2. autonomic (visceral) afferent fibers, transmitting impulses (pain) from the viscera
3. a) special somatic afferent fibers, transmitting impulses from special receptors (eye, ear)
   b) special afferent visceral fibers, conducting taste and smell impulses
4. general somatic efferent fibers, innervating the skeletal muscles (III, IV, VI, XII)
5. visceral efferent fibers, innervating smooth muscles, heart muscles, and glands parasympathetically as well as sympathetically
6. special branchiomeric efferent fibers, innervating the muscles that are derived from branchial arches (V for musculature of first arch, VII for musculature of second arch, IX for musculature of third arch, X and XI for musculature of fourth and subsequent arches).

Fig. 3.6 shows, on the right, the distribution of the cranial nerves at the base of the skull, which is still covered with dura. On the left, the dura has been removed, and the various foramina through which the nerves enter or leave the skull are identified.

3 Brainstem

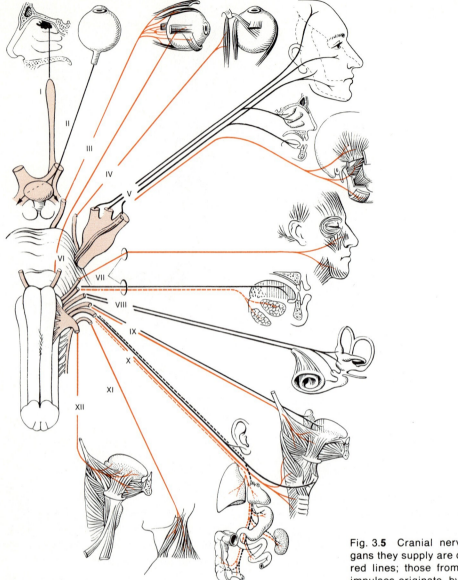

Fig. 3.5 Cranial nerves. The organs they supply are connected by red lines; those from which their impulses originate, by black lines.

Olfactory System (I)

The olfactory system is illustrated in Figs. 3.7 and 3.8. Starting with the site of reception of olfactory stimuli, the system consists of the following subdivisions: olfactory mucosa in the upper part of the nasal cavity; fila olfactoria; bulbus olfactorius; tractus olfactorius; cortex (paleocortex) in the temporal lobe uncus and the subcallosal area at the medial aspect of the orbital lobe.

The *olfactory mucosa* covers an area of approximately 2 cm² at the roof of each nasal cavity and extends toward the superior nasal concha and the nasal septum. Small sensory

Cranial Nerves

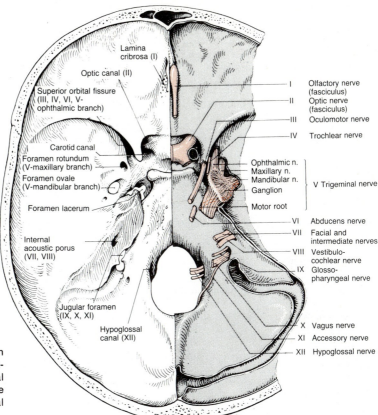

Fig. 3.6 Base of skull. On the left the foramina of exiting and entering cranial nerves are identified; on the right, the stumps of cranial nerves are shown.

cells and their supporting cells are scattered in the highly specialized olfactory epithelium. Also located here are the Bowman's glands, which produce the serous fluid, also called olfactory mucus, in which aromatic substances probably go into solution. The sensory cells (olfactory receptors) are bipolar neurons. Their peripheral processes terminate at the surface of the epithelium in the form of short olfactory hairs. The central processes are more delicate. Hundreds of them join to form unmyelinated fascicles, the *fila olfactoria*. On each side are approximately 20 such fila, which pass through foramina in the cribriform plate of the ethmoid bone (lamina cribrosa) and connect with the olfactory bulb. These fila are the olfactory nerves proper and are believed to have the slowest conduction rate of any nerves.

The *olfactory bulbs* are protruding portions of the brain (telencephalon). They are the site of complicated synapses or dendrites of mitral cells, tufted cells, and granular cells. Thus, the bipolar olfactory cells are the first neurons in the smelling system, the mitral and tufted cells of the olfactory bulbs representing the second neurons. The axons of these neurons make up the *olfactory tracts*, which on either side lie laterally from the gyri recti on top of the olfactory sulci.

In front of the anterior perforated substances, through which the blood vessels of striate bodies and pallida enter and leave, the tracts form the *olfactory trigones*, where each tract splits into lateral and medial striae. The fibers of the lateral stria proceed over the limen of the insula (junction of insular and orbital cortex) to the *semilunar* and *ambient gyri* (*area prepiriformis*) into the amygdala. Here the third neuron starts, which extends to the anterior portion of the parahippocampal gyrus (*area entorhinalis*), representing

Table 3.1 Cranial Nerves.

Number and Name	Components	Origin	Function
I: Olfactory nerve (fasciculus olfactorius)	Special visceral afferent	Bipolar olfactory neurons in olfactory mucosa	Smell
II: Optic nerve (fasciculus opticus)	Special somatic afferent	Ganglion cell layer of the retina	Vision
III: Oculomotor nerve	Somatic efferent	Oculomotor nucleus (midbrain)	Mm. rectus superior, inferior, medialis; M. obliquus inferior; M. levator palpebrae
	Visceral efferent (parasympathetic)	Westphal-Edinger nuclei	M. sphincter pupillae; M. ciliaris
	Somatic afferent	Proprioceptors of eye muscles	Proprioception
IV: Trochlear nerve	Somatic efferent	Trochlear nucleus (midbrain)	M. obliquus superior
	Somatic afferent	Proprioceptors	Proprioceptors
V: Trigeminal nerve	Somatic afferent	Bipolar cells in ganglion semilunare	Sensibility of skin of face and mucosa of nose & mouth
1st branchial arch	Branchial efferent	Motor nucleus of V	Masticatory muscles
	Somatic afferent	Proprioceptors in masticatory muscles	Proprioception
VI: Abducens nerve	Somatic efferent	Abducens nucleus	M. rectus lateralis
	Somatic afferent	Proprioceptors	Proprioceptors
VII: Facial nerve	Branchial efferent	Facial nucleus	Muscles of facial expression; platysma; M. stylohyoideus; M. digastricus
2nd branchial arch	Visceral efferent	Superior salivatory nucleus	Nasal, lacrimal, salivary glands (sublingual and submandibular)
Intermediate nerve	Special visceral afferent	Ganglion geniculi	Taste, anterior two-thirds of tongue
	Somatic afferent	Ganglion geniculi	External ear, parts of the auditory canal, external surface of membrane tympani (sensibility)
VIII: Vestibulocochlear nerve	Special somatic afferent	Ganglion vestibulare	Equilibrium; cristae canalis semilunaris; macula utriculi and sacculi
		Ganglion spirale	Hearing; organ of Corti
IX: Glossopharyngeal nerve	Branchial efferent	Nucleus ambiguus	M. stylopharyngeus; pharynx muscle
	Visceral efferent (parasympathetic)	Inferior salivatory nucleus	Salivation; glandula parotis

Table 3.1 (continued)

Number and Name	Components	Origin	Function
3rd branchial arch	Special visceral afferent	Ganglion inferius	Taste (posterior third of tongue)
	Visceral afferent	Ganglion superius	Sensibility; posterior third of tongue & pharynx (retching reflex)
	Somatic afferent	Ganglion superius	Middle ear; eustachian canal (sensibility)
X: Vagus nerve	Branchial efferent	Nucleus ambiguus	Pharynx & larynx musculature
	Visceral efferent (parasympathetic)	Dorsal nucleus of vagus nerve	Viscera of chest & abdominal cavity (motor)
4th branchial arch	Visceral afferent	Ganglion inferius (nodosum)	Abdominal cavity (sensibility)
	Special visceral afferent	Ganglion inferius (nodosum)	Taste; epiglottis
	Somatic afferent	Ganglion superius (jugulare)	Auditory canal; dura (sensibility)
XI: Accessory nerve	Branchial efferent	Nucleus ambiguus (cranial root)	Pharynx & larynx musculature
	Somatic efferent	Anterior horn cells (spinal root)	M. sternocleidomastoideus; M. trapezius
XII: Hypoglossal nerve	Somatic efferent	Hypoglossal nucleus	Musculature of the tongue

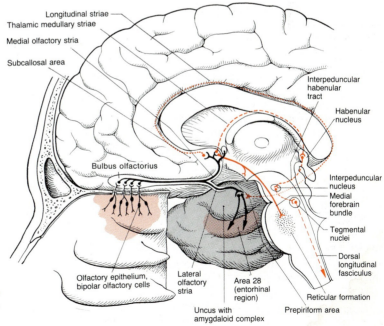

Fig. 3.7 Olfactory nerve (tract) and its cortical terminals.

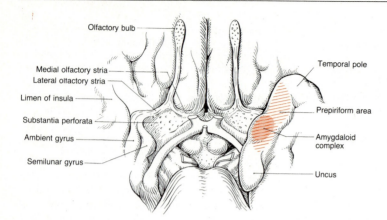

Fig. 3.8 Olfactory nerves (tract) viewed from below.

Brodmann's area 28. This is the cortical region of projection fields and an association area of the olfactory system.

The axons of the stria medialis become continuous with the area beneath the rostrum of the corpus callosum (*area subcallosa*) and with the septal area in front of the *anterior commissure*. This is the commissure of the paleocortex, which connects both olfactory areas and carries fibers communicating with the *limbic system*. It also connects the middle and, in part, the inferior temporal gyri of those hemispheres. The olfactory system is the only sensory system in which the impulses reach the cortex without first being relayed to the thalamus. Its central interconnections are complex, and some are not fully understood.

An odor that provokes an appetite induces reflex salivation, whereas a foul odor triggers nausea, retching, and vomiting. These reactions are associated with emotion. Smells can be pleasant or offensive. The main fiber connections with autonomic areas are the medial forebrain bundles and the medullary striae of the thalamus.

The *medial forebrain bundle* is composed of fibers arising from the basal olfactory region, the periamygdaloid region, and the septal nuclei. On their way through the hypothalamus, some fibers terminate at hypothalamic nuclei. Most fibers proceed into the brainstem and connect with autonomic areas in the reticular formation and with the salivatory nuclei and the dorsal nucleus of the vagus nerve.

The *thalamic medullary striae* synapse in the habenular nuclei. The *habenulopeduncular tract* (tractus retroflexus) extends from these nuclei to the *interpeduncular nucleus* (Ganser's ganglion) and to tegmental nuclei and, further down, to the autonomic centers of the reticular formation of the brainstem (See Fig. 3.51).

The emotions accompanying olfactory stimuli are probably related to fiber connections with thalamus, hypothalamus, and limbic system. The septal area is in contact with, among other areas, the cingulate gyrus through association fibers.

Disorders of olfaction may be caused by:

1. Agenesis of olfactory tracts, which occurs as the sole malformation of the brain.
2. Diseases of the olfactory mucosa (rhinitis, nasal tumor).
3. Tearing of fila olfactoria caused by fracture of the lamina cribrosa.
4. Destruction of olfactory bulbs and tracts by contrecoup contusions, usually caused by a fall on the back of the head. Unilateral or bilateral anosmia may be the only neurologic evidence of orbital region trauma.
5. Ethmoidal sinusitis, osteitis of ethmoid bone, and inflammation of adjacent meninges and their spaces.

6. Tumors of the midline of the anterior cranial fossa, particularly olfactory groove (ethmoid fossa) meningiomas, which may produce the triad of anosmia, Foster Kennedy syndrome, and orbital lobe type of personality disorder (lack of inhibitions, as in general paresis and orbital lobe Pick's disease). A rostrally extending pituitary adenoma may also damage olfaction.

7. Diseases involving the anterior temporal lobe and its base (intrinsic or extrinsic tumors), which may produce uncinate fits in the form of unpleasant or, occasionally, pleasing *olfactory hallucinations*. Temporal lobe seizures may start with an *olfactory aura*. The prepiriform and parahippocampal gyri (Brodmann's area 28) are probably involved in the perception and recognition of odors, in comparing them with former olfactory impressions, and in associating such impressions with distinct situational experiences.

A patient may not be aware of his olfactory loss. Instead he may complain about having lost taste sensation, because his ability to perceive aroma, an important adjuvant to taste, is missing.

Optic System (II, III, IV, VI)

The Visual Pathway (II)

The retina is the receptor for visual impulses. It represents a forward extension of the brain and essentially is made up of three layers of neurons (Fig. 3.**9a**).

The first neurons are called *rods* and *cones*. When light enters the eye, a photochemical reaction in these elements produces impulses which are transmitted to the visual cortex (area striata or area 17). It had been assumed that the rods react to brightness and serve twilight (scotopic) vision, and that the cones are sensitive to color and serve daylight vision. This theory has been called into question. Recent studies have shown that the events taking place in the retina are much more complicated, and too complicated to be discussed here.

Except in the fovea centralis of the macula, rods and cones are mixed, the rods being more than ten times as numerous as the cones. In the area of the fovea that subserves the highest visual acuity, only cones are present, and each cone connects with only one of the *bipolar cells* representing the second neuron. The bipolar cells transmit the impulses to the third neuorn, the *ganglion cells* of the inner layer of the retina. The approximately 1 million axons of these ganglion cells run in the retinal fiber layer to the papilla or head of the optic nerve, pass through the lamina cribrosa of the sclera of the eye, and finally reach the lateral geniculate bodies of the thalamus.

The lens of the eye functions like the lens of a camera: it causes altitudinal and lateral inversion of the visual object projected on the retina.

The fiber tracts extending from the eye to the *chiasm* are called *optic nerves* (fasciculi optici). As the nerve arrives at the *chiasm*, the one half of its fibers that originate in the nasal half of the retina cross through the chiasm to the opposite side. The other half, coming from the temporal half of the retina, continue ipsilaterally. Behind the chiasm, they join the crossed fibers from the contralateral eye and form the *optic tract*. Each tract terminates at its *lateral geniculate body* (Fig. 3.**9b**). In the optic nerve and tract and also in the *optic radiation*, which originates from a new neuron in the lateral geniculate body, the fibers are arranged in a strict retinotopic order, also found in the *calcarine* or *visual cortex* (Fig. 3.**10**).

Fig. 3.**11** illustrates how the nerve fibers originating in the four quadrants of macula and peripheral retina converge to the head (papilla, disk) of the optic nerve and how these fibers are arranged in optic nerve, chiasm, and optic tracts.

The macular fibers for central vision enter the temporal nerve head. They soon reach a

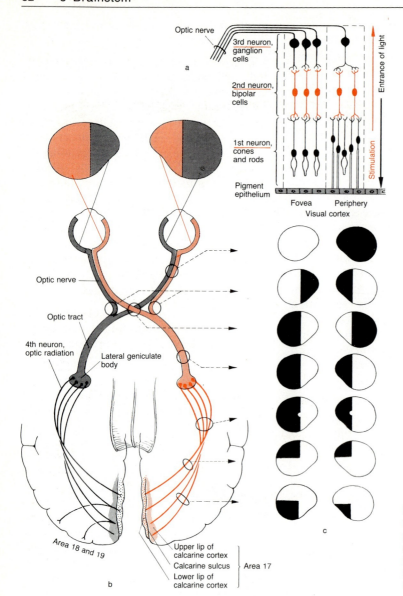

Fig. 3.9 Optic nerve (fasciculus) and optic pathway. a Microscopic structure of retina; b visual pathway interrupted by lesions; c corresponding defects of visual fields.

central position in the orbital portion of the nerve. Atrophy of the macular fiber bundles produces a characteristic paleness of the temporal portion of the nerve head, which may be associated with impairment of central vision; peripheral vision remains intact. If the peripheral fibers of the optic nerves are damaged (periaxial nerve injury), visual acuity remains intact, but peripheral vision is constricted. Damage to the entire nerve leading to atrophy is followed by paleness of the entire papilla. One speaks of *primary optic atrophy* if the nerve was damaged directly, as, for example, by the pressure exerted on the nerve by a tumor. Such atrophy and central scotoma on the side of the tumor and papill-

Cranial Nerves 83

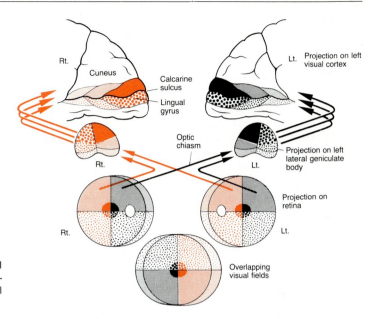

Fig. 3.10 Projection of visual fields on retina, in lateral geniculate body, and in visual cortex.

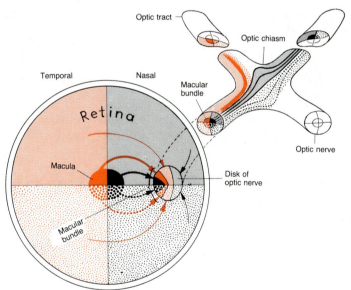

Fig. 3.11 Arrangement of macular bundles in retina, optic nerve, and optic chiasm.

edema on the other side is known as *Foster Kennedy Syndrome. Secondary optic atrophy* occurs following papilledema.

In the absence of intraocular disease, impairment of vision in one eye always suggests a lesion in the orbital, foraminal, or cranial portion of the optic nerve (Figs. 3.9b and c).

If the center of the chiasm is damaged to such an extent that the crossing fibers become interrupted (by pituitary tumor, craniopharyngioma, meningioma of tuberculum sellae), the result is a *bitemporal hemianopia*. Usually, the fibers coming from the lower halves of the retinas and occupying the ventral portion of the chiasm are damaged first; which explains why the hemianopia begins in the upper bitemporal quadrants of the visual fields. It first involves color vision. In rare cases the heteronymous *hemianopia may be binasal.* Such a finding indicates that the lateral portions of the intracranial optic nerves, chiasm, or postchiasmatic tracts are damaged (by abnormal arteries, unusual growth of a tumor, basal meningitis).

In contrast to the heteronymity of the chiasm lesions, those injuring the optic tract produce *homonymous hemianopias.* For example, a lesion in the right optic tract interrupts the impulses that originate in the right halves of both retinas. Consequently, visual impairment involves the left halves of the visual fields (see Figs. 3.**9b** and **c**).

Just before the optic tract arrives at the lateral geniculate body, a small contingent of fibers, the *medial pupillosensory bundle,* proceeds to the superior colliculi and the nuclei in the pretectal area (see Fig. 3.**25**). These are afferent fibers for several optic reflexes, particularly the important pupillary reflex to light, to be discussed later. If interruption of the optic tracts includes these fibers, the light falling on the involved homonymous halves of the retinas produces no pupillary reaction. Unfortunately, the test for a hemianopic light reflex has little diagnostic use because of the difficulty of concentrating the light on only half of the retina.

The bulk of the fibers of the optic tract enters the *lateral geniculate body* by joining thin sheets of white matter that separate the neurons into six, partially interconnected layers. The first layer runs parallel to the base of the body. Layers 2, 3, and 5 receive the uncrossed fibers from the ipsilateral eye and layers 1, 4, and 6 the crossed fibers of the contralateral eye. The axons of the neurons form the *optic radiation* (radiation of Gratiolet).

The radiation projects into the visual or *calcarine cortex,* which extends with an upper and a lower lip along the calcarine fissure (Brodmann's area 17). The cortex of this area is well marked by *Gennari's stripe,* a thicker-than-usual layer of horizontal myelinated fibers dividing the fourth layer of small nerve cells. The fibers of the optic radiation are close together only where they emerge from the lateral geniculate body. After passing through the so-called *isthmus of the temporal lobe,* they fan out in the deep white matter of the temporal lobe near the lateral wall of the inferior and posterior horns of the lateral ventricle (see Figs. 3.**9b** and 3.**12**).

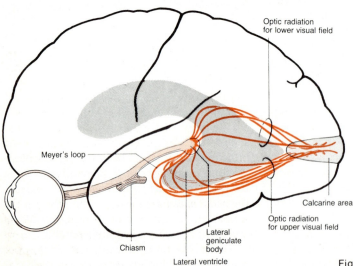

Fig. 3.**12** Gratiolet's optic radiation.

The *retinotopic order* of the cells in the lateral geniculate body illustrated in Fig. 3.10 is maintained also in their *axons* and in the points of termination of the axons in the calcarine cortex. The fibers representing the homonymous halves of the axons of both eyes form the central core of the radiation. They proceed in a fairly straight course to the caudal half of the visual cortex at the medial aspect of the occipital lobe and at the convexity of its pole. The dorsal quadrants of the macular and peripheral retinal halves project into the upper (dorsal) lip, and their ventral quadrants into the lower (ventral) lip, of the visual cortex (see Figs. 3.10 and 3.12).

As can be seen in Fig. 3.12, some of the ventral fibers of the radiation first take a rostral course toward the temporal pole. Thereafter, each fiber forms a loop before turning toward the lower lip of the visual cortex. The most rostral fibers of *Meyer's loop* (Adolf Meyer, 1907) may reach the level of the tip of the inferior ventricular horn. The looping fibers represent the lower quadrants of the peripheral portion of the homonymous halves of the retinae.

This anatomic situation explains why an interruption of fibers of an optic radiation also produces a homonymous hemianopic defect contralateral to the lesion. The hemianopia may be complete, but it is often incomplete because of the wide spreading of the fibers. A homonymous hemianopia limited to the two upper quadrants and ending sharply at the vertical midline ("pie-in-the-sky" defect) always indicates a temporal lobe lesion involving Meyer's loop (see Figs. 3.9b and c).

Brodmann's area 17, the primary recipient of the visual impulses, is surrounded by areas 18 and 19, which extend from the medial aspect of the occipital lobe over its convexity (see Figs. 8.23 and 8.24). Experimental studies and clinical experiences suggest that these two cortical areas represent secondary and tertiary optical fields—in other words, association areas for visual imprints (*fields of optical memories*). Electrical stimulation in areas 18 and 19 produces an optical aura in the form of flashing lights, color, and simple forms and lines. Visual impressions arriving at area 17 probably become conscious experiences in the adjacent association areas and may be compared with former experiences and interpreted. It is likely that other cortical territories participate in this activity. Destruction of areas 18 and 19 reduces ability to recognize objects by their form, size, and outlines and to be aware of their significance (*optical agnosia, alexia*). The disorder is particularly evident if commissural fibers of the splenium of the corpus callosum interconnecting both visual areas are interrupted. Areas 18 and 19 participate also in several important optical reflexes that will be discussed later.

Oculomotion (III, IV, VI)

The muscles of each eye are innervated by oculomotor (III), trochlear (IV), and abducens (VI) nerves (Figs. 3.13 and 3.14). The nuclei of these three pairs of nerves are located on either side of the midline of the tegmentum of midbrain and lower pons, near the aqueduct and the fourth ventricle (see Figs. 3.2, 3.13, and 3.21).

Oculomotor nerve (III)

The nuclei of the oculomotor nerves are located in part in front of the periaqueductal gray matter (motor nuclei) and in part within the gray matter (autonomic nuclei). The *motor* nuclei are responsible for the innervation of the medial, superior, and inferior rectus muscles, the inferior oblique muscles, and the levator muscles of the superior eyelids. In each nucleus the neurons responsible for each muscle form columns. The topographical arrangement of these columns is illustrated in Fig. 3.15, representing Warwick's scheme (monkey). The *autonomic* or *Edinger-Westphal nuclei* are located within the poorly myelinated periaqueductal gray matter. Their small neurons give off parasympathetic fibers for the innervation of the internal eye muscles (sphincter pupillae, ciliary muscle). The *para-*

sympathetic Perlia's nuclei are located between the Edinger-Westphal nuclei.

Some of the axons of the motor neurons responsible for the external muscles cross at the level of the nuclei. Together with the uncrossed axons and the parasympathetic fibers, they swing around and through the red nuclei on their way to the lower lateral wall of the interpeduncular fossa, where they join and emerge as oculomotor nerves. Both nerves pass between the posterior cerebral and superior cerebellar arteries (Fig. 3.**16**). On their way to the orbit, they pass first through the subarachnoid space of the basal cistern and then through the subdural space. Where each crosses the sphenopetrosal ligament before entering the cavernous sinus, it is vulnerable to pressure caused by a herniating uncus. After passing through the sinus (see Fig. 3.**17a**), the nerve enters the orbit through the superior orbital fissure (see Fig. 3.**13**). Thereafter, the parasympathetic fibers leave the nerve and join the *ciliary ganglion*, where the preganglionic fibers are relayed to short, postganglionic fibers that innervate the internal eye muscles.

Upon entering the orbit, the somatic fibers of the oculomotor nerve divide into two branches, of which the upper or dorsal branch proceeds to the levator of the upper lid and the superior rectus muscle. The lower or ventral branch innervates the medial and inferior rectus and the inferior oblique muscles (see Fig. 3.**13**).

If all fibers of the oculomotor nerve are interrupted, paralysis occurs of all extraocular muscles except the lateral rectus muscle, supplied by the abducens nerve (VI), and the superior oblique muscle, supplied by the trochlear nerve (IV). In addition, there is paralysis of the parasympathetic innervation of the internal eye muscles, with loss of pupillary light reflex, mydriasis, and disorders of convergence and accommodation.

Trochlear nerve (IV)

The nuclei of the trochlear nerves are located at the level of the inferior colliculi in front of the periaqueductal gray matter and immediately below the nuclei of the oculomotor nerves. The internal roots circle around the lateral portions of the central gray matter and cross behind the aqueduct within the *velum medullare superius*, the thin membrane that forms the tectum of the rostral fourth ventricle. After crossing, the nerves leave the midbrain beneath the inferior colliculi (see Figs. 3.**1** and 3.**13**). They are the only cranial nerves that exit from the dorsal aspect of the brainstem. In their ventral course to the cavernous sinus, the nerves first pass through the *rostral pontocerebellar fissure* and then proceed beneath the margin of the tentorium

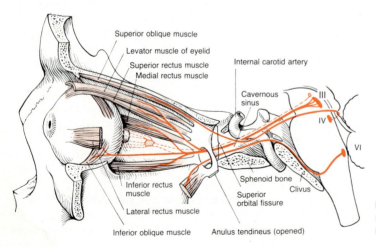

Fig. 3.**13** Course of oculomotor, trochlear and abducens nerves (lateral view).

Cranial Nerves

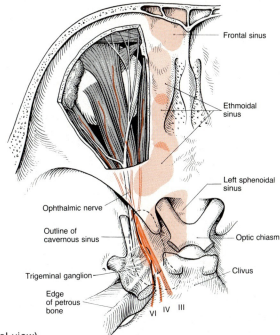

Fig. 3.14 Course of ocular motor nerves (dorsal view).

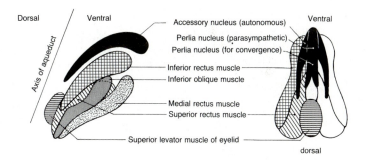

Fig. 3.15 Oculomotor nucleus complex (according to Warwick).

to the cavernous sinus and from there into the orbit in the company of the oculomotor nerve.

The trochlear nerve supplies the *superior oblique muscle*, which lowers the eye, turns it inward, and abducts it to a small extent. Paralysis of the muscle produces a deviation of the diseased eye upward and slightly inward toward the healthy side. This deviation is particularly noticeable if the involved eye looks downward and inward in the direction of the normal eye.

Abducens nerve (VI)

The nuclei of the abducens nerves are situated on either side of the midline of the tegmentum of the lower pons near the medulla oblongata and immediately beneath the floor of the IVth ventricle. The internal knee of the facial nerve (VII) passes between the nucleus of VI and the fourth ventricle. The root fibers of the abducens proceed through the base of the pons on either side of the midline and emerge as nerves from the pontomedullary junction just above the pyramids.

From here, both nerves run upward through the subarachnoid space on either side of the basilar artery. Then they proceed through the subdural space in front of the clivus, perforate the dura, and adjoin the other two motor nerves in the cavernous sinus. Here they are in close contact with the first and second branches of the trigeminal nerves and with the internal carotid artery, which also passes through the cavernous sinus (Fig. 3.17, see Fig. 3.16). The nerves are also not far away from the upper and lateral portions of the sphenoid sinus and the ethmoidal sinus (see Fig. 3.14).

If the abducens nerve is paralyzed, the eye cannot move laterally. Because the medial rectus muscle no longer has an antagonist, the eye is slightly deviated nasally. This condition is referred to as *convergent strabismus* or *esotropia*.

Damage to any of the ocular motor nerves produces double vision, because the image of objects on the retina does not cover corresponding areas. It is the combined action of the six muscles on either side that permits eye movements in all directions (Table 3.2). The movements are always delicately atuned and conjugate, assuring that the image is projected precisely on the two foveas. A rather complicated central mechanism controls the fine synergism of the various eye muscles and their nerves, as will be discussed later. No eye muscle can be innervated independently.

All of the eye muscles function in precise coordination with one another in such a way that, as they act together, the desired direction is encouraged, while any distracting side effects are suppressed. For example, the lifting

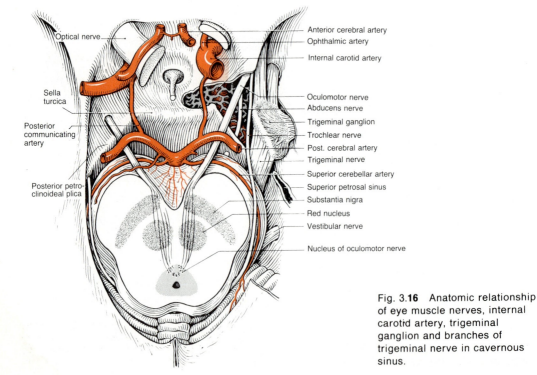

Fig. 3.16 Anatomic relationship of eye muscle nerves, internal carotid artery, trigeminal ganglion and branches of trigeminal nerve in cavernous sinus.

Table 3.2 Innervation and Action of the Extraocular Muscles.

Nerves	Muscles	Actions	
		Primary	Secondary
Oculomotor	Superior rectus	Moves eye up	Adducts; rotates inwards
	Inferior rectus	Moves eye down	Adducts; rotates outwards
	Medial rectus	Adducts	None
	Inferior oblique	Moves eye up	Abducts; rotates outwards
Trochlear	Superior oblique	Moves eye down	Abducts; rotates inwards
Abducens	Lateral rectus	Moves eye out	None

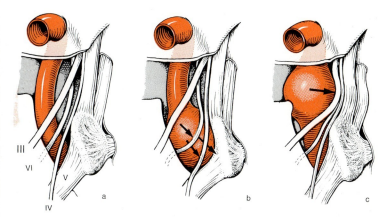

Fig. 3.17 Encroachment of eye muscle nerves and trigeminal nerve by an intracavernous aneurysm of the internal carotid artery. **a** Normal conditions; **b** caudal aneurysm; **c** rostal aneurysm.

effect of the superior rectus muscle is supported by the inferior oblique muscle, while the horizontal and rotational component is inhibited. Similarly, abduction by the lateral rectus muscle is supported by the two oblique muscles as a result of simultaneous inhibition of their vertical and rotational components.

To better understand the functioning of the individual eye muscles, it is important to bear in mind the divergence of the orbital axis from the optic axis (Fig. 3.**18**a).

Fig. 3.**18**b shows schematically the cooperation among individual eye muscles necessary to perform the most *basic conjugate eye movements*. Figs. 3.**19** and 3.**20** illustrate the influence of the paralysis of individual eye

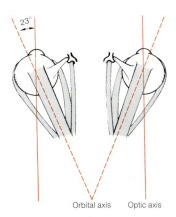

Fig. 3.**18a** View from above of the orbit, eyeball, superior rectus muscle, and superior oblique muscle. The optic axis diverges from the orbital axis by 23°.

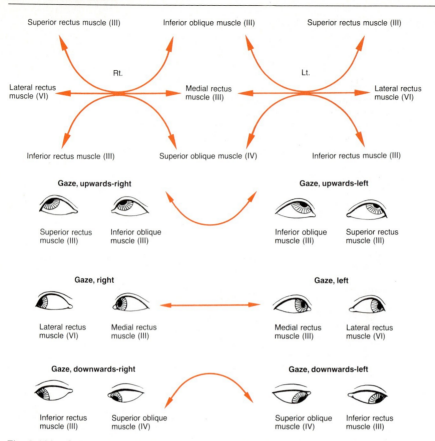

Fig. 3.18b Schematic illustration of eye positions in six diagnostic directions of gaze revealing most clearly a paralysis of the leading eye muscles.

muscles on the position of the eye and on the resulting double vision.

When one checks the diplopia with red-green glasses and a hand light, the double image of an object appears in the paralyzed eye if the patient tries to look in the direction in which the paralyzed muscle normally would pull the eye. When the patient looks in this direction, the distance between the double images is the largest. The most outward image is from the paralyzed eye (see Figs. 3.**19** and 3.**20**).

Paralysis of Eye Muscles

Only if the paralysis of a single muscle is acute, is it possible to determine with the method described in the last paragraph which of the muscles is paralyzed. Diagnostic procedures become rather difficult and require particular instrumentation (such as Maddox rods, Hess screen, etc.) and experience, if the paralysis is old or if several eye muscles are paralyzed. A longer lasting paralysis of an eye muscle may lead to contraction or hyperfunction of the ipsilateral antagonist, to a hyperactivity of the contralateral synergist, and to paralysis from inhibition of the contralateral antagonist.

Regardless of whether a disorder involves the nuclear territory of a nerve or the peripheral fiber bundle, the consequences for the eye muscles are the same. A nuclear lesion usually also produces signs and symptoms

Cranial Nerves

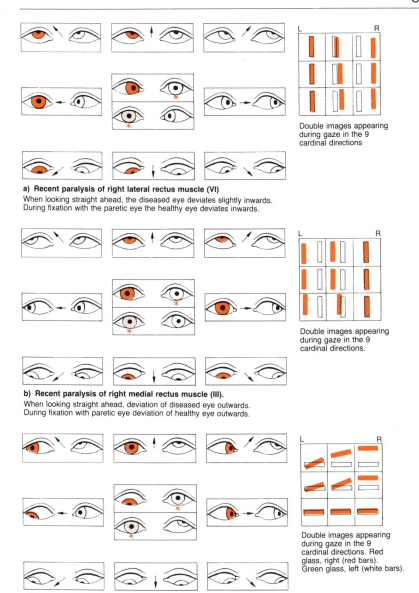

Double images appearing during gaze in the 9 cardinal directions

a) Recent paralysis of right lateral rectus muscle (VI)
When looking straight ahead, the diseased eye deviates slightly inwards. During fixation with the paretic eye the healthy eye deviates inwards.

Double images appearing during gaze in the 9 cardinal directions.

b) Recent paralysis of right medial rectus muscle (III).
When looking straight ahead, deviation of diseased eye outwards. During fixation with paretic eye deviation of healthy eye outwards.

Double images appearing during gaze in the 9 cardinal directions. Red glass, right (red bars). Green glass, left (white bars).

c) Recent paralysis of right superior rectus muscle (III).
When looking straight ahead, deviation of diseased eye downwards and outwards. During fixation with paretic eye deviation of the healthy eye upwards and outwards.

Fig. 3.**19** Deviation of eyes in recent paralysis of **a** lateral, **b** medial, and **c** superior rectus muscles (right).

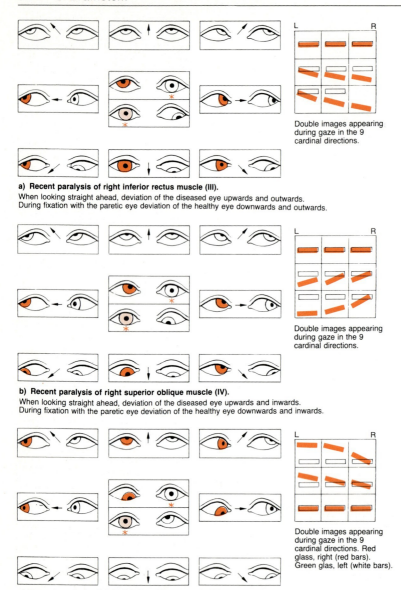

a) **Recent paralysis of right inferior rectus muscle (III).**
When looking straight ahead, deviation of the diseased eye upwards and outwards.
During fixation with the paretic eye deviation of the healthy eye downwards and outwards.

Double images appearing during gaze in the 9 cardinal directions.

b) **Recent paralysis of right superior oblique muscle (IV).**
When looking straight ahead, deviation of the diseased eye upwards and inwards.
During fixation with the paretic eye deviation of the healthy eye downwards and inwards.

Double images appearing during gaze in the 9 cardinal directions.

c) **Recent paralysis of right inferior oblique muscle (III).**
When looking straight ahead, deviation of the diseased eye downwards and inwards.
During fixation with the paretic eye deviation of the healthy eye upwards and inwards.

Double images appearing during gaze in the 9 cardinal directions. Red glass, right (red bars). Green glas, left (white bars).

Fig. 3.20 Deviation of eyes in recent paralysis of **a** inferior rectus muscle, **b** superior and **c** inferior oblique muscles (right).

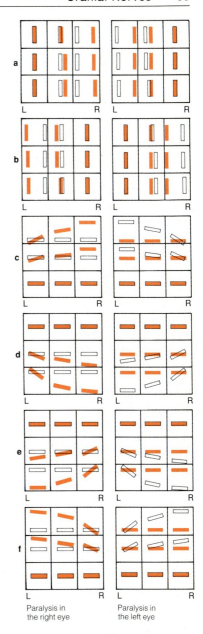

Fig. 3.20 A Contrast between the double images of paralysis in the individual muscles of the right eye (left) and left eye (right). **a** Lateral rectus muscle, **b** medial rectus muscle, **c** superior rectus muscle, **d** inferior rectus muscle, **e** superior oblique muscle, **f** inferior oblique muscle.

stemming from involvement of neighboring structures.

Paralysis of the oculomotor nerve

A complete oculomotor palsy produces the following syndrome:

1. ptosis caused by paralysis of the levator palpebrae muscle and the unopposed action of the orbicularis oculi innervated by the facial nerve
2. fixed position of the eye, with pupil directed downward and laterally because of

unopposed action of the lateral rectus (VI) and superior oblique (IV) muscles

3. dilated pupil not reacting to light and accommodation.

Partial paralysis may produce only part of the syndrome, for example, *ophthalmoplegia interna or externa*. If all the muscles are acutely paralyzed, the damage is usually peripheral. On the other hand, paralysis of a single muscle suggests that the damage involves the oculomotor nucleus.

Paralysis of the trochlear nerve

When the patient is looking straight ahead, the axis of the diseased eye is higher than that of the other eye. When the patient looks downward and inward, the eye rotates. Diplopia occurs with every direction of gaze except upward. In order to avoid diplopia the patient tilts his head to the healthy side, lowers the chin, and turns the head toward the contralateral shoulder. A paralysis limited to the trochlear nerve is rare and is often caused by trauma, usually by a fall on forehead or vertex.

Paralysis of the abducens nerve

When the patient is looking straight ahead, the diseased eye is adducted and cannot be moved laterally. When the patient looks nasally, the paralyzed eye turns inward and up because of the predominance of the inferior oblique muscle.

If all three motor nerves of one eye are interrupted, the eye looks straight ahead and cannot be moved in any direction, and its pupil is wide and does not react to light (*ophthalmoplegia totalis*). Bilateral paralysis of the eye muscles is usually the result of the nuclear damage.

The most frequent causes of *nuclear paralysis* are encephalitis, neurosyphilis, multiple sclerosis, circulatory conditions, hemorrhages, and tumors. The most frequent causes of *peripheral eye muscle palsies* are meningitis, sinusitis, cavernous sinus thrombosis, aneurysm of internal carotid artery (see Fig. 3.17) or posterior communicating artery, fractures, tumors of the cranial base as well as of the orbit, diphtheria, and botulism. One should be aware, however, that ptosis and diplopia are often caused by myasthenia.

Voluntary and Reflex Innervation of the Eye Muscles

The extremely precise cooperation among the individual ocular muscles that move the eyes in various directions requires a close interrelationship among all nuclei of the nerves in charge of ocular movements. Such intimate connections are provided by the *medial longitudinal fasciculus*, which runs bilaterally parallel to the midline from the tegmentum of the midbrain down to the cervical cord. It interconnects the nuclei of the motor nerves of the eye muscles. It also receives impulses from the cervical cord (serving anterior and posterior neck muscles), from the nuclei of the vestibular nerves, from the reticular formation controlling pontine and mesencephalic "centers of vision," and from cerebral cortex and basal ganglia.

The eyes can be moved both *voluntarily* and *by reflex*. They can, however, move only jointly–in other words, conjugately (Fig. 3.21). In whatever direction the eyes move, all eye muscles participate in the action, in part by increasing muscular tension (agonists), in part by relaxation (antagonists).

When looking voluntarily at an object, the eyes perform extremely fast jerking and most precise movements (*saccades*). Most eye movements take place by reflex, however, and are not voluntary. Any object entering the field of vision attracts attention, and vision is involuntarily directed to it. As the object moves, the eye follows involuntarily in an attempt to keep the image of the object continuously in the area of most acute vision, the fovea of both maculae. If we voluntarily focus on an object of interest, the eye is automatically kept on it, even if we as well as the object of interest are moving. Thus, all volun-

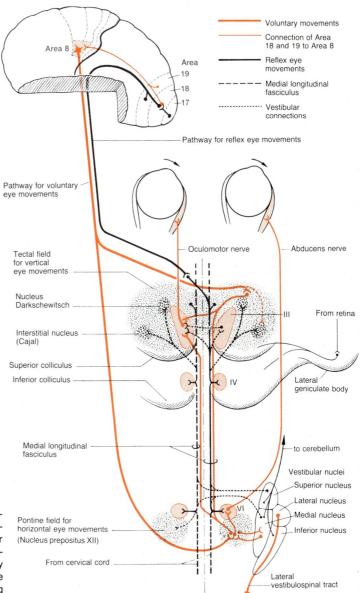

Fig. 3.21 Nuclei of eye muscles, medial longitudinal fasciculus and complex of vestibular nucleus with supra- and infranuclear pathways for voluntary and reflexive conjugate eye movements (in part according to Hassler).

tary eye movements are appended by involuntary reflex movements. This reflex – holding the image of the object of interest in the retinal area of most acute vision – is called the *fixation reflex*.

The afferent portion of this reflex runs from the retina over the visual pathway to the visual cortex (area 17). From here the impulses are transmitted to areas 18 and 19. The efferent fibers probably originate in these areas and temporarily join the optic radiation on their course to contralateral mesencephalic and pontine centers of oculomotion (see Fig. 3.21). From there they join the corresponding nuclei of the ocular motor nerves. It is likely that some of the efferent fibers go directly to the ocular motor centers and the rest do so indirectly, making a detour over Brodmann's area 8.

Special components of the reticular formation contained in the anterior portion of the midbrain regulate individual directions of vision. According to Hassler (1967), the *prestitial nucleus* in the posterior wall of the third ventricle regulates upward movements; the nucleus of the posterior commissure, downward movements; and the interstitial Cajal's nucleus and Darkschewitsch's nucleus, rotatory movements of the eyes.

Segments of the superior colliculi can also produce eye movements in certain directions. Upward movements are represented at the anterior margin of the superior colliculi. Destruction of this area produces paralysis of upward gaze (Parinaud's syndrome discussed on page 156).

Impulses originating at the convexity of the occipital lobes also travel to contralateral pontine centers for eye movement and produce conjugate lateral movements of the eyes.

Experimental stimulation of areas 18 and 19 results in conjugate lateral as well as downward and upward gaze. The movements of lateral gaze undoubtedly are the most prominent in man and the most frequent of these occipitally initiated movements.

Voluntary eye movements are triggered in the frontal eye field of Brodmann's area 8, located in front of the precentral gyrus, and perhaps also in parts of areas 6 and 9. A conjugate movement of the eyes (déviation conjuguée) toward the opposite side (the patient looks away from the side of irritation) is the most frequent response to stimulation in this territory. The movement of the eyes is sometimes accompanied by a movement of the head toward the opposite side. Unilateral destruction of area 8 creates a predominance of the contralateral area, producing a conjugate movement toward the side of the lesion (the patient looks towards the paralyzing focus). This deviation abates with time. The situation is reversed with pontine lesions (Fig. 3.22), because the corticopontine pathways cross. A pontine paralysis of gaze is seldom followed by full recovery.

It is not quite clear how the frontal eye fields are connected with the nuclei for ocular motion. The fibers accompany the corticonuclear tract on its way to the internal capsule and cerebral peduncle. They do not terminate directly in the nuclei of the cranial nerves, however. It appears that their impulses arrive at the nuclei via intercalated neurons in the reticular formation and via the medial longitudinal fasciculus (see Fig. 3.21).

All voluntary movements of the eyes are under the influence of reflex arcs. Some of these arcs belong to the optical and others to the acoustic, vestibular, and proprioceptive reflex arcs (originating in ventral and dorsal muscles of the neck and transmitted via the spinotectal tract and the medial longitudinal fasciculus).

After unilateral destruction of the *frontal eye field*, the eyes for a time cannot be turned voluntarily to the opposite side, but such movement is still possible by reflex action. The patient is able to pursue with his eyes an object that moves slowly through his field of vision even if he is not able to follow its direction voluntarily (*pursuit reflex*).

In contrast, if the *occipital fields* are destroyed, the reflex movements of the eyes are abolished. The patient can move his eyes voluntarily in every direction, but he cannot pursue an object. It immediately escapes from the area of highest acuity and must be searched for again by voluntary eye movements.

If attention is paid to a visual object, its images are fused in both eyes in the area of greatest acuity. Regardless of whether the object moves up or down, left or right or approaches or recedes, its image is always kept in both foveas by finely tuned sequences of movements called *smooth pursuit movements*. As the images leave the foveas, messages are sent by the retinas via the visual

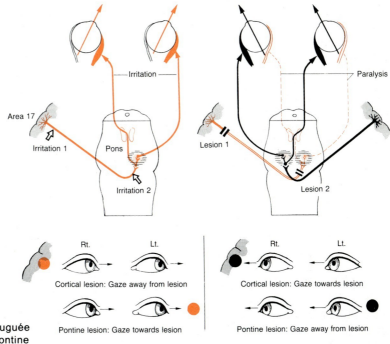

Fig. 3.22 Déviation conjuguée caused by cortical and pontine lesions (irritation or paralysis).

pathways to the calcarine cortices and from here via occipitotectal fibers to the nuclei of the ocular motor nerves. The result is that the images are brought back into the foveas by the *optokinetic process*. In this process the eyes perform a jerking movement (*optokinetic nystagmus*). Such nystagmus occurs when one is looking out of a moving train or reading or, experimentally, when one focuses on a slowly turning cylinder displaying alternating black and white stripes. The jerks of the eyes occur in a direction opposite to the movement of the gaze. The optokinetic nystagmus is abolished if this reflex arc is interrupted at any point.

Convergence and Accommodation

Different reflexes are triggered if an object caught in the center of vision comes closer and closer. These are the reflexes of convergence and accommodation (Fig. 3.23). Three different events take place:

1. *Convergence:* Both medial rectus muscles become innervated simultaneously, so that the axes of both eyes are directed toward the object. This process places the images of the object precisely on corresponding portions of the retinas, that is, on the areas of greatest visual acuity.

2. *Accommodation:* Because of contraction of the ciliary muscle, the lens relaxes and becomes more rounded. By this mechanism the retinal image of an approaching object is continuously kept in focus. (Looking into the distance relaxes the ciliary muscle, and this produces a flattening of the lens.)

3. *Constriction of the pupils:* Narrowing of the pupil permits the retinal image of the object to remain sharply outlined, just as a narrowing of the aperture in a photographic camera increases the sharpness of the object image.

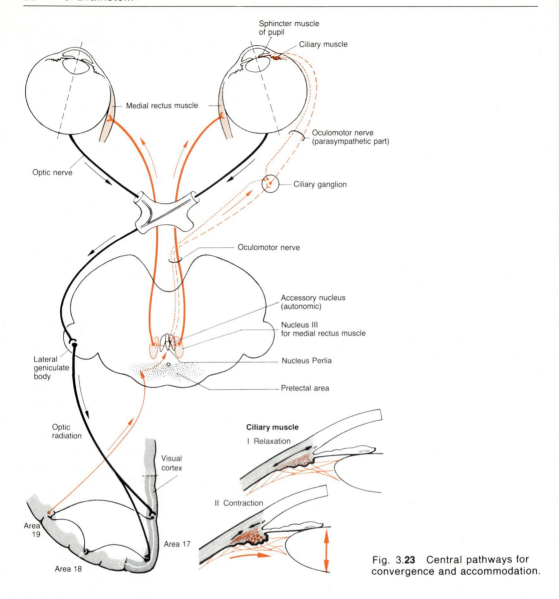

Fig. 3.23 Central pathways for convergence and accommodation.

All three reactions can be triggered by *voluntary fixation* on a nearby object. They also take place by *reflex* if a distant object suddenly approaches. The afferent impulses travel from the retina to the calcarine cortex. From here the efferent impulses proceed over the area pretectalis to a parasympathetic nuclear area called *Perlia's nuclei* located at the midline ventral to the *Edinger-Westphal nuclei*. Impulses from these nuclear groups go to the neurons innervating both medial rectus muscles (for convergence of the eyes), to the Edinger-Westphal nuclei, and from there to the ciliary muscle via the ciliary ganglion (accommodation) as well as to the sphincter pupillae (narrowing of the pupils). The fiber connections to the ciliary muscle and to the sphincter muscle of the pupils are probably not the same, because the pupillary reflex for accommodation and that to light can be lost individually. In syphilis, for example, the pupillary reaction to light can be abolished but the reactions for convergence and accommodation preserved (*Argyll Robertson pupil*).

It is still not known how this condition occurs. Furthermore, the pupil is very narrow and irregular for a very long time, and this myosis continues after death. For this reason one can assume that the pupillary disorder is caused by local alterations in the iris. *Adie's syndrome*, which consists of an abnormally slow, myotonic reaction of the pupil to brightness and darkness and to accommodation, is also not fully understood. (Transmitter disturbance in the ciliary ganglion?)

Internuclear ophthalmoplegia

If the medial longitudinal bundle is damaged unilaterally, the patient can no longer innervate the ipsilateral medial rectus muscle. In Fig. 3.**24** the left bundle is damaged, and the left medial rectus muscle is paralyzed. This paralysis occurs although there is no damage to the nucleus or peripheral portion of the nerve responsible for the muscle. Reflex contraction of the muscle as it occurs, for example, in response to convergence remains intact. When the patient attempts to look to the right, the left eye cannot follow; the right eye, innervated by the abducens, exhibits *mono-ocular nystagmus*.

Because of their proximity, there may be involvement of both medial longitudinal fasciculi by the same lesion. In such instances neither eye can adduct in direct horizontal gaze. The leading eye shows *monoocular nystagmus*. All other eye movements are unrestrained, and the reaction of the pupils is undisturbed.

Unilateral internuclear ophthalmoplegia suggests a vascular cause, particularly in an elderly person. Bilateral ophthalmoplegia is usually the result of multiple sclerosis.

Light Reflex

When light falls on the retina, the diameter of the pupil changes. This pupillary light reflex has the same effect as an automatic adjustment of the diaphragm of a photographic camera: it protects the retina and its photoreceptors against exposure to an overdose of

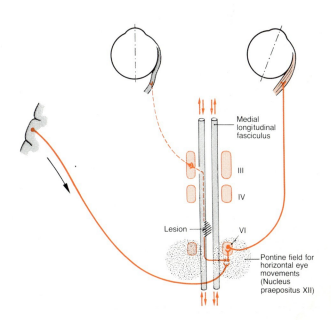

Fig. 3.**24** Internuclear opthalmophlegia caused by lesion of medial longitudinal fasciculus.

light and sharpens the image of a visual object projected on the retina. The reflex arc does not involve cortex. Therefore, the pupillary reactions do not enter the level of consciousness.

The afferent fibers of the reflex arc accompany the optic nerve and tract and leave the tract near the lateral geniculate body as its medial bundle, which proceeds toward the superior colliculi and terminates in *nuclei of the pretectal area*. Intercalated neurons connect with the parasympathetic *Edinger-Westphal* or *autonomic accessory nuclei* of both sides (Fig. 3.25), causing the *light reflex to be consensual*; that is, light falling into one eye causes narrowing of the pupil also in the contralateral, unilluminated eye. The topography of the fibers subserving the light reflex also explains why destruction of optic radiation or visual cortex has no effect on the reflex.

The fiber connections leading to the Edinger-Westphal nuclei have not been fully determined. It has been shown, however, that destruction of the superior colliculi has no effect on the light reflex but that injury to the pretectal area abolishes the reflex, suggesting that the afferent fibers of the reflex arc must pass through the latter region.

The efferent motor fibers originate in the Edinger-Westphal nuclei and accompany the oculomotor nerve into the orbit. Here the parasympathetic preganglionic fibers become independent and enter the ciliary ganglion, where the impulses are transmitted to short, postganglionic fibers. These fibers enter the eye and innervate the sphincter muscle of the pupil (see Fig. 3.25).

The sphincter muscle is paralyzed if the ipsilateral oculomotor nerve, preganglionic fibers, or ciliary ganglion is damaged. As a result, the light reflex is extinguished, and the pupil is dilated because it is now solely under the influence of the sympathetic innervation. Interruption of the afferent fibers along the course of the optic nerve abolishes the light reflex in both the ipsilateral and the contralateral eye, because the consensual reaction is interrupted. If in such a case the con-

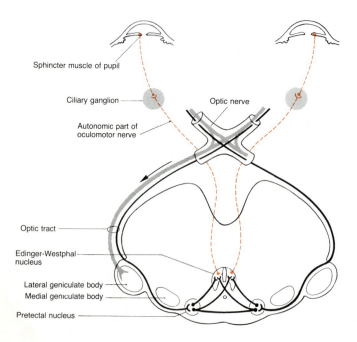

Fig. 3.25 Circuit controlling light reflex.

tralateral eye is exposed to light, however, the light reflex functions bilaterally.

The width of the pupil is not controlled only by light reflex; extraocular stimuli may have an influence. Severe pain, particularly pain involving the musculature in the neck, and strong emotional reactions may produce a widening of the pupils. So far it has been assumed that this kind of mydriasis results from a predominance of sympathetic impulses that cause contraction of the *dilator muscle of the pupil*. A different explanation is offered on page 102.

Sympathetic Innervation of the Eye

The area of the sympathetic nuclei, also called the *ciliospinal center*, is located in the lateral horn of the spinal gray matter of C8 to T2. From here, preganglionic fibers ascend to the superior cervical ganglion, from which postganglionic fibers emerge. The postganglionic fibers adjoin the internal carotid artery and accompany it up to the level of the orbit. Here, the fibers proceed to the dilator muscle of the pupil (Fig. 3.26; see Fig. 3.27). How the ciliospinal center receives afferent

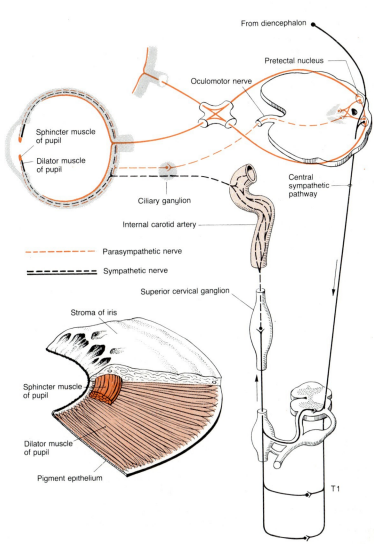

Fig. 3.26 Parasympathetic and sympathetic innervation of inner eye muscles.

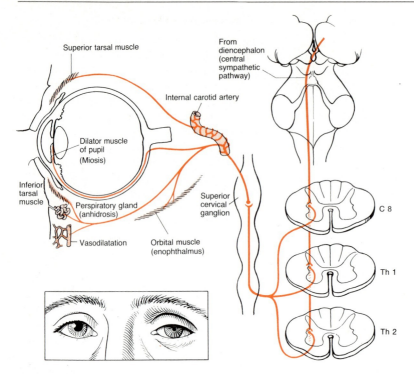

Fig. 3.27 Horner's syndrome. Sympathetic innervation of various structures. Anhidrosis and vasodilatation caused by paralysis.

impulses is not fully understood. The optic tract probably has indirect connections with the hypothalamus. The central sympathetic tract originates here, descends to the midbrain, where it crosses, and continues through brainstem and cervical cord to the ciliospinal center.

An interruption of impulses in the central sympathetic tract, in the ciliospinal center, in the superior cervical ganglion, or in the area of the postganglionic fibers on their way to the eye produces *Horner's syndrome* (Fig. 3.27). The sympathetic nerve innervates the smooth fibers of the pupillary dilator, the superior and inferior tarsal, and the orbital muscles and, in addition, the sweat glands and the blood vessels of the corresponding half of the face. Consequently, if the ciliospinal center or its efferent fibers on their way to the eye are damaged, the following conditions occur:

1. narrowing of the palpebral fissure (paralysis of superior and inferior tarsal muscles)
2. miosis (paralysis of pupillary dilator; predominance of parasympathetic innervation of pupillary sphincter)
3. enophthalmus (paralysis of orbital muscle)
4. anhidrosis
5. vasodilatation in the corresponding half of the face

Although the dilator of the pupil influences the width of the pupil, more recent studies suggest that pupillary dilatation accompanying pain and emotional reactions is predominantly caused by inhibition of the parasympathetic innervation and that sympathetic innervation of the dilator of the pupil plays only a minor role.

As was mentioned earlier, paralysis of the pupillary sphincter muscle caused by interruption of its parasympathetic innervation from damage to either the Edinger-Westphal nuclei, their fibers, or the ciliary ganglia is followed by mydriasis because of the action of the sympathetically innervated dilator muscles of the pupils. Inequality in the diameter of the pupils is called *anisocoria*.

Protective blink reflex

An object suddenly appearing in front of the eyes causes an immediate reflex closure of the lids, or *blink reflex*. The afferent impulses of this reflex extend from the retina directly to the tectum of the midbrain and proceed from there via the tectonuclear tract to the nuclei of the facial nerves that innervate the orbicularis oculi muscles. If the impulses reach the anterior horn cells of the cervical spinal cord via the tectospinal fibers, they produce a turning away of the head.

Trigeminal Nerve (V)

The trigeminal nerve is mixed: its major portion carries sensory fibers from the face, and a smaller portion carries the motor fibers for the muscles of mastication. The sensory portion originates in the *trigeminal ganglion* (*ganglion semilunare Gasseri*), which corresponds to the spinal ganglia and contains pseudounipolar ganglion cells. The peripheral axons of these cells are in contact with the receptors for touch, discrimination, pressure, pain, and temperature. Their central processes enter the pons and terminate in the principal sensory nucleus (touch, discrimination) and spinal nucleus (pain, temperature) of the nerve. One aspect of the *nucleus of the trigeminal mesencephalic tract* points out a special feature of the nerve. The neurons of this nucleus correspond to those of the spinal ganglia. Thus, the nucleus may be considered as a ganglion that became displaced, so to speak, into the brainstem. The axons of its cells connect with the peripheral receptors in the muscle spindles of the chewing muscles and with receptors that respond to pressure.

The three nuclei cover a large territory which, as is shown in Fig. 3.**29**, extends from the cervical cord upward to the midbrain.

The *gasserian ganglion* rests in a shallow groove (impressio trigemini) of the rostral apex of the petrous bone outside the posterolateral portion of the cavernous sinus. The peripheral axons of the ganglionic neurons form three major divisions:

1. the *ophthalmic nerve*, which passes through the *superior orbital fissure*
2. the *maxillary nerve*, which goes through the *foramen rotundum*
3. the *mandibular nerve*, which extends through the *foramen ovale* (see Fig. 3.**6**).

The peripheral branches of these nerves are illustrated in Fig. 3.**28**. Their sensory territory includes delineated areas of the skin of forehead and face (Fig. 3.**29**); the mucosa of mouth, nose, and sinuses; the mandibular and maxillary teeth; and large areas of the dura in anterior and middle cranial fossae. For the ear, the Vth nerve reports only from anterior portions of the outer ear and the auditory canal and from parts of the tympanic membrane. The earlobe and the remaining portions of the auditory canal receive sensory innervation from the intermediate (pars intermedia of facial nerve), glossopharyngeal, and vagus nerves. The mandibular nerve carries, among other impulses, the proprioceptive impulses from masticatory muscles and from the roof of the mouth for the control of biting strength.

The skin areas supplied by the trigeminal nerve border on the dermatomes of the C2 and C3 spinal nerves. The roots of C1 are purely motor and innervate the individual neck muscles between skull and upper cervical vertebrae.

Within the pons the nerve fibers carrying pain and temperature sensations proceed in a caudal direction as the *spinal trigeminal tract*. This tract terminates at the *spinal nucleus* of the nerve, which extends downward as far as the upper cervical cord. Here the tract rep-

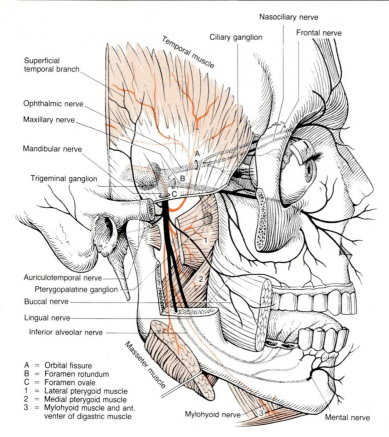

Fig. 3.28 Trigeminal nerve.

resents the cranial extension of Lissauer's zone and of the substantia gelatinosa of the posterior horns, which receive pain sensations from the uppermost cervical segments.

The caudal portion of the spinal nucleus shows some somatotopic patterning. The lowest portion receives pain fibers from the ophthalmic nerve. More cranially, fibers from the maxillary nerve arrive. They are followed by fibers from the mandibular nerve. Fibers of VII (intermediate nerve) and of IX and X, transmitting pain impulses from ear, posterior third of tongue, pharynx, and larynx, join the spinal tract of the trigeminal nerve (see Figs. 3.**41** and 3.**42**). The midsegment (pars interpolaris) and the cranial segment (pars rostralis) of the spinal nucleus probably receive afferent fibers transmitting pressure and touch impulses. It is assumed that the midsegment receives pain fibers originating in the pulp of the teeth. The function of these areas of the nucleus needs further clarification, however.

Fibers of second neurons in the spinal nucleus fan out while crossing to the opposite side, where they proceed through the tegmentum of the pons to the thalamus together with the lateral spinothalamic tract. The fibers terminate in the ventral posteromedial nucleus of the thalamus (see Fig. 3.**29**).

The *principal sensory nucleus of V* occupies a circumscribed area of the dorsolateral tegmentum of the pons. It receives the afferent impulses of touch, discrimination, and

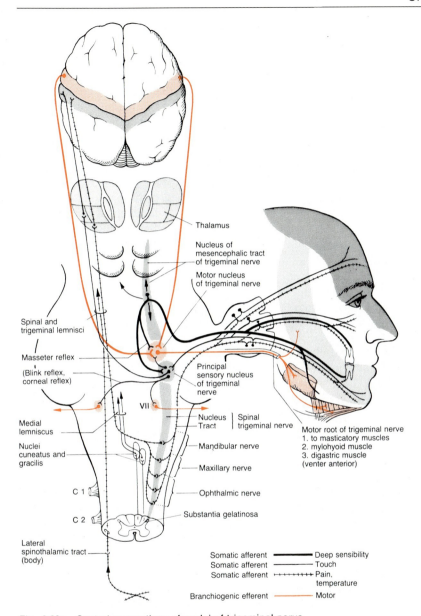

Fig. 3.29a Central connections of nuclei of trigeminal nerve.

pressure, which, in the spinal cord, are transmitted by the posterior funiculi. The fibers of the second neurons in this nucleus also cross to the other side and proceed with the medial lemniscus to the ventral posteromedial nucleus of the thalamus.

The third neurons of the trigeminal pathway, located in the thalamus, send their axons through the posterior limb of the internal capsule to the lower third of the postcentral gyrus (see Figs. 3.29a and 1.20).

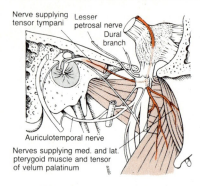

Fig. 3.29b Medial aspect of motor portion of V.

The *motor*, or, *minor portion of the trigeminal nerve* has its nucleus in the pontine tegmentum, located medially from the principal sensory nucleus. The motor nerve leaves the skull together with the mandibular nerve. It innervates the masseter, the temporal, lateral, and medial pterygoid, the mylohyoid, the anterior digastric, and the tensor veli palatini muscles (Fig. 3.29b).

The motor nuclei receive their central stimuli via the *corticonuclear tract*. This supranuclear pathway originates in the large pyramidal cells of the lower third of the precentral gyrus (see Figs. 3.29a, 2.2, and 8.20). The impulses come predominantly from the opposite side. Because some are of ipsilateral origin, a unilateral interruption of the supranuclear trigeminal pathway produces no noteworthy weakness of the chewing muscles.

In contrast, a lesion damaging the nucleus or the peripheral portion of the motor nerve results in a flaccid paralysis of the corresponding chewing muscles, which is followed by atrophy. Such unilateral paralysis can easily be diagnosed by feeling the absence of chewing muscle contraction when the patient bites down. If the patient is asked to open his mouth and to push his chin forward, the chin will deviate to the side of the paralysis because of the predominance of the pterygoid muscle of the other side. Also, the reflex of the masseter muscles (*masseter reflex*) will be absent on the paralyzed side. Normally, the masseter muscle contracts when tapped with the reflex hammer while the mouth is open.

Sensory stimuli originating in the mucous membranes of the eye are carried via the ophthalmic nerve to the principal sensory nucleus. There they are transmitted to other neurons that represent the afferent portion of the *corneal reflex* and connect with the nucleus of the facial nerve of the same side. The efferent portion of the reflex is represented by the peripheral neuron of the facial nerve. This reflex arc may be interrupted in its afferent (trigeminal) or its efferent (facial) portion. In either case the result will be an extinction of the reflex.

Sensory fibers that carry impulses from the mucosa of the nose to the nuclear area of the trigeminal nerve represent the afferent portion of the *sneezing reflex*. Several nerves participate in the efferent part of this reflex: nerves V, VII, IX, and X, and the nerves responsible for expiration.

A traumatic tear in one of the branches of the trigeminal nerve produces loss of sensitivity in the corresponding area of supply but is not usually followed by pain.

Facial Pain

Trigeminal neuralgia

The facial pain called trigeminal neuralgia (*tic douloureux*) is of particular importance. It characteristically occurs in paroxysmal attacks of sharp, lancinating, agonizing pain limited to a territory supplied by one or more branches of the trigeminal nerve and is usually accompanied by vasomotor and secretory disturbances. The shooting pain occurs suddenly with great severity and lasts for several seconds. Often it is triggered when a certain area is touched, for example, when the patient is washing or shaving his face or brushing his teeth (trigger zone). Usually no signs of organic alteration of the nerves can be found. No definite cause of this traumatizing affliction has been identified. It is assumed that there may be pathological alterations in the area of the trigeminal ganglion and perhaps also in the spinal nucleus of the trigeminal nerve. It is also believed that there are causative mechanical factors related to movement of the jaw.

What has been described by Janetta (1981), is probably the most frequent cause of the typical tic douloureux. He found that it was triggered by a blood vessel, most often the superior cerebellar artery, looping around the most proximal, still unmyelinated root of the nerve (Fig. 3.**29c**). A microsurgical displacement of the vessel stopped the tic from reoccurring. Ever since, this method has been employed world-wide with great success. In a few cases, veins have been the triggering blood vessels. All this suggests that the tic douloureux actually constitutes one of the symptomatic trigeminal neuralgias to be discussed now.

Symptomatic trigeminal pain

Symptomatic pain in the territory of one of the branches of the trigeminal nerve may be produced by diseased teeth, sinusitis, fractures or tumors in the area of nose or mouth, an inflammation of the eyes, multiple sclerosis, herpes zoster, and other conditions. This pain does not have the paroxysmal, lancinating character of true trigeminal neuralgia. *Glaucoma* or *iritis* may be the cause of pain in eyes and forehead. A paroxysmal attack of glaucoma may produce pain as sudden and severe as that in idiopathic trigeminal neuralgia.

Charlin's syndrome of neuralgia consists of severe pain in the inner corner of an eye disproportionate to the degree of ocular inflammation. There is pain also in the root of the nose, with secretion of tears and discharge of watery fluid from the side of the nose ipsilateral to the painful eye. It is suggested that an irritation of the ciliary ganglion may be the cause of this syndrome.

Gradenigo's syndrome refers to pain in the area of the frontal branch of the trigeminal nerve, associated with paresis of the abducens nerve. It is related to an inflammation of the pneumatic cells of the apex of the petrous bone.

Bing-Horton syndrome is also called *erythroprosopalgia* because the attacks of facial pain are associated with marked reddening of the ipsilateral half of the face. In contrast to the symptoms in trigeminal neuralgia, the pain in erythroprosopalgia occurs during sleep and is of brief duration. There is tearing and a watery discharge from the nose, and it is not rare to find a concurrent Horner's

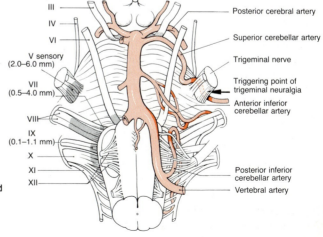

Fig. 3.**29c** Ventral aspect of pons and medulla oblongata showing roots of cranial nerves. On the left side of the figure, the proximal, nonmyelinated portions of the roots are indicated by gray color. On the right, branches of vertebral and basilar arteries are looping around corresponding portions and are in close contact. (With kind permission by Prof. J. Lang. From Lang J. and W. Wachsmuth: Praktische Anatomie. Springer Berlin-Heidelberg, 1985.)

syndrome. An irritative condition in the area of the greater petrosal nerve has been suspected as causative.

An *aneurysm of the internal carotid artery* within the cavernous sinus may irritate the first and possibly the second branch of the trigeminal nerve and thus be responsible for pain in the territory supplied by these nerves (see Fig. 3.**17**).

Among painful conditions involving the face, one must also consider pain that radiates from the temporomandibular joint (*Costen's syndrome*), pain caused by *rheumatic temporal arteritis*, and pain related to *neuralgia of the auriculotemporal nerve*.

Other diseases involving V

Within the cranium, nerve damage may occur from conditions such as meningitis, tumor (pontocerebellar angle tumor), and various types of otitis.

The nuclei or the central pathways may be involved in, among other conditions, circulatory or degenerative processes (progressive bulbar paralysis, syringobulbia). Diseases such as these produce loss of sensation but, in general, no pain.

The word *trismus* stands for a tonic spasm of the masticatory muscles caused by acute encephalitic lesions in the pons, by rabies, by tetanus, or by other conditions. Because of the strong abnormal tension in these muscles, the patient is not able to open his mouth.

Facial and Intermediate Nerves (VII)

The facial nerve has two subdivisions. The larger of the two is purely motor and innervates the expressive musculature of the face (Fig. 3.**30**). It is the facial nerve proper and is accompanied by a much thinner nerve,

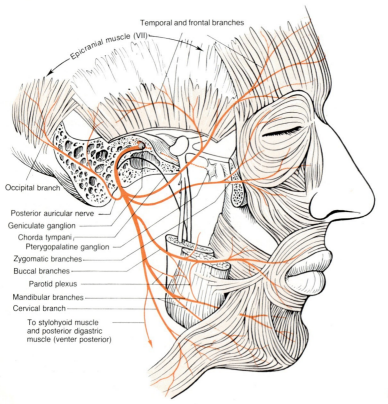

Fig. 3.**30** Facial nerve.

the *intermediate*, which carries autonomic and somatic afferent as well as autonomic efferent fibers (see Table 3.1).

Facial Nerve Proper

The motor nuclei are located in the ventrolateral portion of the lower pontine tegmentum near the medulla oblongata (Fig. 3.31; see Figs. 3.2 and 3.3). While still in the tegmentum of the pons, the axons of the neurons first proceed toward the floor of the fourth ventricle near the midline, then loop around the nuclei of the abducens nerves (*inner knees*) and proceed toward the pontocerebellar angles, where they emerge at the pontomedullary junction just in front of cranial nerves VIII. As shown in Fig. 3.1b, the knee of the facial nerve produces a colliculus facialis in the floor of the fourth ventricle just above the horizontal medullary striae. The intermediate nerve emerges between facial and acoustic nerves, and all three (facial, intermediate, and vestibulocochlear) proceed laterally into the *internal acoustic canal*. Within the canal the facial and inter-

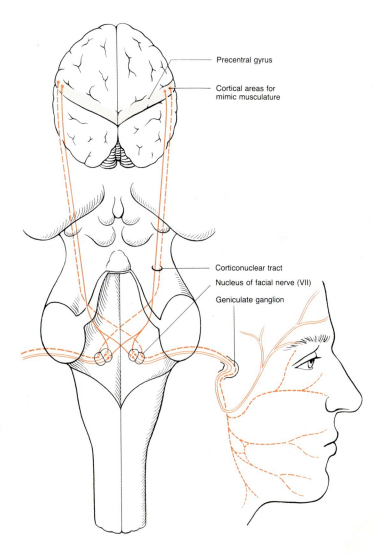

Fig. 3.31 Central pathways of facial nerves. Fibers for the forehead (solid lines) cross incompletely in lower pons explaining preservation of frontal muscle function in paralysis due to cerebral and upper brainstem lesions. (See Fig. 3.32a.)

mediate nerves separate from cranial nerve VIII and continue somewhat laterally in the *facial canal* up to the level of the geniculate ganglion.

Here the facial canal makes a sharp turn in a caudal direction. Because the facial nerve follows the canal, it also makes such a turn, which is called the *outer or external knee of the facial nerve*. At the end of the canal the facial nerve leaves the cranium through the stylomastoid foramen. From this point the motor fibers spread over the face (see Fig. 3.30). In doing so, some perforate the parotid gland. The muscles innervated by VII serve facial expression and are derivatives of the second branchial arch. The orbiculares oris and oculi, buccinator, occipital, frontal, stapedius, stylohyoid, and posterior digastric muscles and the platysma constitute this group.

The motor nucleus of the facial nerve is part of several reflex arcs. The *corneal reflex* has already been mentioned. Optical impulses also arrive at the nucleus from the superior colliculi via the tectobulbar tract, causing the lids to close in the presence of a sufficiently bright light (*blink reflex*). Acoustic impulses reach the nucleus via the dorsal nucleus of the trapezoid body. Depending on the intensity of the noise, this reflex arc produces either relaxation or tension of the stapedius muscle.

The supranuclear innervation of the forehead musculature is located in both cerebral hemispheres, whereas the remaining facial musculature is innervated only from the contralateral precentral gyrus. Consequently, a unilateral interruption of the corticonuclear tract by a lesion, such as an infarct, leaves the innervation of the frontal muscles intact (central paralysis) (Fig. 3.**32a**). If, however, a lesion involves the nucleus or the peripheral nerve, the entire ipsilateral facial musculature is paralyzed (peripheral paralysis) (Fig. 3.**32b**).

The facial nuclei also receive impulses from the thalamus that direct the emotionally expressive movements of the facial musculature. There are also connections with the basal ganglia. If these or other parts of the extrapyramidal system are diseased, there may be a decrease in or absence of facial expression (*hypomimia or amimia*) as in Parkinson's disease, or a hyperkinetic reaction causing a *mimetic facial spasm* or *blepharospasm* (see page 228). The connections with thalamus and basal ganglia are not known in detail.

The mimetic facial spasm has been found to be due to an irritation of the proximal, unmyelinated portion of the root of the nerve by a looping blood vessel. A microsurgical relocation of such a vessel has resulted in improvement of the condition as it has done in trigeminal neuralgia (Janetta, 1967; Samii, 1983).

Intermediate Nerve

The intermediate nerve has several afferent and efferent components (see Table 3.**1**). The

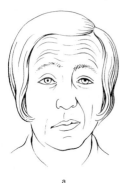
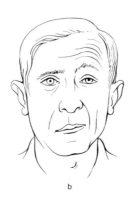

Fig. 3.**32** Facial paralysis. **a** Central paralysis (musculature of forehead not involved); **b** peripheral paralysis (musculature of forehead also paralyzed).

Cranial Nerves 111

afferent fibers belong to the neurons of the *geniculate ganglion*. These cells, like those of the spinal ganglia, are pseudounipolar. Some of these afferent fibers report stimuli from taste buds in the anterior two-thirds of the tongue (Fig. 3.33). These taste fibers at first accompany the lingual nerve (mandibular branch of V). Thereafter they follow the *chorda tympani* to the geniculate ganglion and then the intermediate nerve to the nucleus of the solitary tract, where taste fibers of the glossopharyngeal nerve (posterior third of tongue, papillae vallatae) and of the vagus nerve (epiglottis) also terminate.

The *nucleus of the solitary tract* is a relay station for the *taste fibers* of the nerves mentioned. From there the taste impulses go to the contralateral thalamus (the exact pathway is not known) and terminate in the most medial portion of the posteromedial ventral nucleus (see Fig. 8.22). From the thalamus

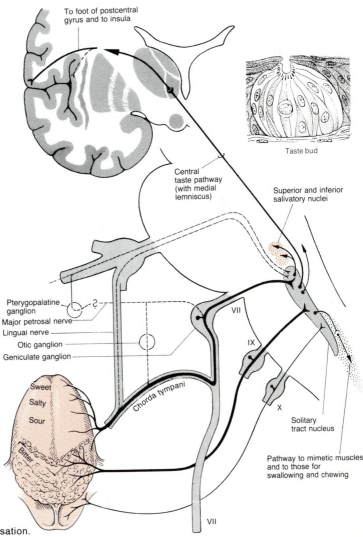

Fig. 3.33 Pathways of taste sensation.

another neuron runs to the foot of the opercular portion of the posterior central convolution near the insula (see Fig. 3.33). Because the centrally transmitted taste sensations are collected by three different nerves (VII, IX, and X), a complete loss of taste sensation (*ageusia*) is rare.

Some somatic afferent fibers from a small area of the external ear, auditory canal, and external surface of the tympanic membrane join the facial nerve. They travel via the geniculate ganglion to the groups of trigeminal nuclei in the brainstem. The skin eruptions of *herpes zoster oticus* indicate the presence of this contingent of fibers.

Efferent parasympathetic fibers are also part of the intermediate nerve. The *superior salivatory nucleus* (Fig. 3.34) is the site of origin of these fibers. This nucleus is located caudally and medially from the facial nucleus just at the border between pons and medulla oblongata near the floor of the fourth ventricle. One group of the axons of this nucleus separates from the stem of the facial nerve at the level of the geniculate ganglion. These fibers turn and go to the *pterygopalatine ganglion* and from there to the lacrimal gland and the glands of the nasal mucosa. Another group of axons continues caudally and accompanies the chorda tympani and the lingual nerve to the submandibular ganglion. From there the impulses travel to the sublingual and submandibular glands, where they stimulate salivation (see Fig. 3.34). We have already mentioned that the superior salivatory nucleus receives impulses from the olfactory system via the *dorsal longitudinal*

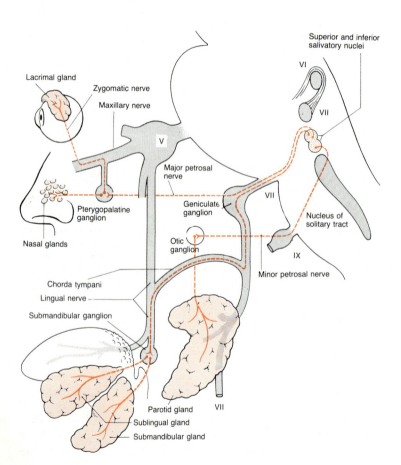

Fig. 3.**34** Innervations of glands in the area of the face.

bundle (see Fig. 3.7). Appetite-stimulating odors cause reflex salivation. Tearing is related to central stimuli from the hypothalamus (emotions) via the reticular formation and over the spinal nucleus of the trigeminal nerve (irritation of conjunctiva).

The rare attacks of neuralgia that occur in connection with the intermediate nerve are of the following types:

1. *Sluder's neuralgia* is caused by involvement of the pterygopalatine ganglion stemming from a spreading inflammation of the paranasal sinuses. Symptoms are pain in the eye, nasal root, maxilla, and palate radiating into neck and shoulders. Tearing and salivation are disturbed.

2. *Hunt's neuralgia* is caused by a pathologic condition of the geniculate ganglion. Signs are *herpes zoster oticus*, with pain and formation of vesicles in the auditory canal as well as behind the auricle (posterior auricular nerve), associated with peripheral facial paralysis, tinnitus, impairment of hearing, and disorders of taste, tearing, and salivation.

Frequent Types of Damage to VII

Peripheral paralysis

Peripheral paralysis is the most common type of loss of facial nerve function. It is usually caused by a viral infection along the course of the nerve through the facial or fallopian canal (Leibowitz, 1969; Esslen, 1970; and Edwards, 1973). A vascular disorder has also been considered as cause, because edema and hemorrhagic infarction have been observed where the nerve enters the canal (Esslen, and others). The result is a peripheral flaccid paralysis of all muscles subserving facial expression, including the musculature of the forehead. This basic finding is accompanied by other signs, which vary depending on the segment of the nerve involved within the canal. The various syndromes connected with alterations in each topographical location within the nerve are listed and illustrated in Fig. 3.**35**.

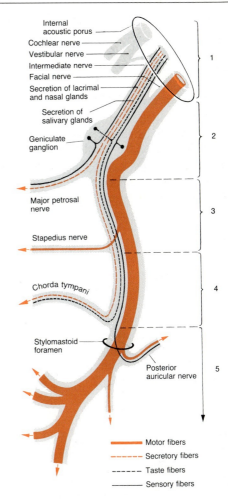

Fig. 3.**35** Fiber components of the facial and intermediate nerve and signs from damage to its individual segments. 1 = Peripheral motor paralysis of the muscle supplied by the facial nerve as well as impairment of hearing or deafness and decrease in vestibular excitability. 2 = Peripheral motor paralysis and impairment of taste sensation and lacrimal and salivary secretion. 3 = Peripheral motor paralysis and impairment of taste sensation and salivary secretion; hyperacusis. 4 = Peripheral motor paralysis and impairment of taste sensation and salivary secretion. 5 = Peripheral motor paralysis.

Intracranially, the facial and intermediate nerves accompany the vestibulocochlear nerve (VIII) as it passes through the internal auditory meatus. There, the two nerves may be damaged by a neurinoma in VIII. Other types of tumors and a large aneurysm of a vertebral artery may have the same effect on the nerves.

Some additional causes of peripheral facial palsy are otitis media, mastoiditis, fracture of the petrous bone, inflammation of the parotid gland, and iatrogenic damage during surgery in the area of the parotid gland.

After a peripheral facial palsy, regeneration of damaged fibers, particularly autonomic fibers, may be partial or misdirected. Preserved fibers may send new axonal sprouts into the damaged portion of the nerve. Such abnormal reinnervation may explain contracture or synkineses (associated movements) in the mimetic musculature of the face. The syndrome of *crocodile tears* (*paradoxical gustolacrimal reflex*) appears to be based on faulty reinnervation. One assumes that secretory fibers for the salivary glands grew into the sheaths of Schwann of degenerated injured fibers that originally were responsible for the lacrimal gland.

Nuclear paralysis

The nuclei may suffer damage from degenerative diseases (progressive bulbar paralysis, syringobulbia), circulatory and inflammatory processes (polioencephalitis), tumors of the pons, or pontine bleeding. Because of the close topographical relationship of the facial nucleus and internal knee of the facial fibers to the nucleus and fibers of the abducens nerve (VI), it is not unusual for a single disease process to damage both nerves.

Supranuclear paralysis

The supranuclear pathway can be interrupted anywhere but is most often interrupted in its course through the internal capsule. One possible cause is infarction caused by obstruction of the internal carotid artery or, more often, the middle cerebral artery; by massive bleeding from an angioma or other vascular changes, such as hypertensive vascular disease; or by tumors. An isolated supranuclear facial palsy can be brought about by a small cortical lesion in the portion of the precentral gyrus that represents the face. Such isolated palsy may be accompanied by Jacksonian attacks in facial muscles. Despite supranuclear palsy the facial musculature may still perform involuntary movements in the form of *clonic tics* or *tonic facial spasms*, because the facial nerve is still connected with the extrapyramidal system.

Auditory System (VIII)

The vestibulocochlear organ develops bilaterally in the petrous bone from a common primordium. The vestibular system arises from the utricle, with the three semicircular ducts, and the auditory organ develops out of the sacculus, with the cochlear duct.

Vibrations in the air, or sound waves (tones, speech, singing, music, sounds, noise, etc.) enter via the external auditory canal and pass to the eardrum (tympanic membrane), which separates the external auditory canal from the middle ear (*tympanic cavity*) (Fig. 3.35 A). The tympanic cavity contains air and is connected to the nasopharyngeal space (exterior) via the auditory tube (eustachian tube). It consists of a bony space covered with mucosa, the *vestibulum*. In the medial wall, there are two openings sealed by collagenous tissue: the oval window (fenestra vestibuli, or fenestra ovalis) and the round window (fenestra cochleae, or fenestra rotunda). These two openings separate the *tympanic cavity* from the *inner ear*, which is filled with perilymph. Within the tympanic cavity, there are also two small muscles: the tensor tympani muscle (V) and the stapedius muscle (VII), which can influence the motion of the ossicles by tensing, protecting the organ of Corti against excessive shock due to strong acoustic effects. Sound waves are conducted by the eardrum via the three small auditory ossicles (the malleus, incus, and stapes) to the oval window, causing it to vibrate. The auditory part of the inner ear consists of bony and membranous elements. The bony cochlea, with its tube winding in two and a half spiral turns, resem-

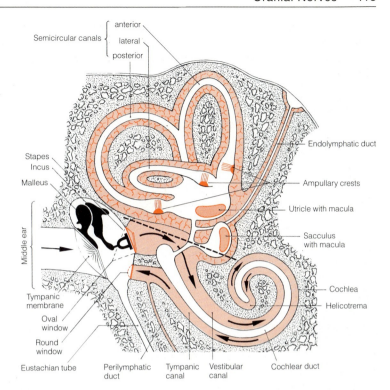

Fig. 3.35 A Schematic diagram of the hearing and vestibular apparatus.

bles a garden snail. It is depicted here in an abbreviated form for learning purposes. It consists of the vestibule and the bony tube covered in epithelium, which winds round the columella (modiolus), a wedge-shaped bony axis that contains the spiral ganglion of the cochlea. A section through the cochlear duct shows that it consists of three parts: the vestibular canal (scala vestibuli), the tympanic canal (scala tympani), and the cochlear duct (scala media), which contains the organ of Corti (Fig. 3.35 B). The vestibular canal and the tympanic canal are filled with perilymph, while the cochlear duct contains endolymph produced by the vestibular stria. The cochlear duct begins blindly at the vestibular cecum and ends blindly at the cupular cecum. The upper wall of the cochlear duct is formed by Reissner's membrane, the very thin vestibular membrane. Reissner's membrane separates the endolymph from the perilymph in the vestibular canal but nevertheless transmits pressure waves in the vestibular canal without obstruction, causing the basilar membrane to vibrate. The pressure waves traverse the perilymph from the oval window through the vestibular canal up to the apex of the cochlea, where they communicate with the tympanic canal through a small opening, the helicotrema, and back to the round window, which is separated from the middle ear by a membrane. Along its entire length, the organ of Corti (spiral organ) lies on the basilar membrane, from the vestibule to the apex (Fig. 3.35 C). It consists of hair cells and supporting cells (Figs. 3.35 B c, d). The hair cells are the receptors for the auditory organ and are able to transform mechanical energy into electrochemical potentials. A distinction is made between inner hair cells and outer hair cells. The inner hair cells (3500) form a single row, while the outer hair cells (12000–19000) are arranged in three or more rows. Each of them carries some 100 stereocilia, some of which reach into the tectorial membrane of the cochlear duct. When the basilar

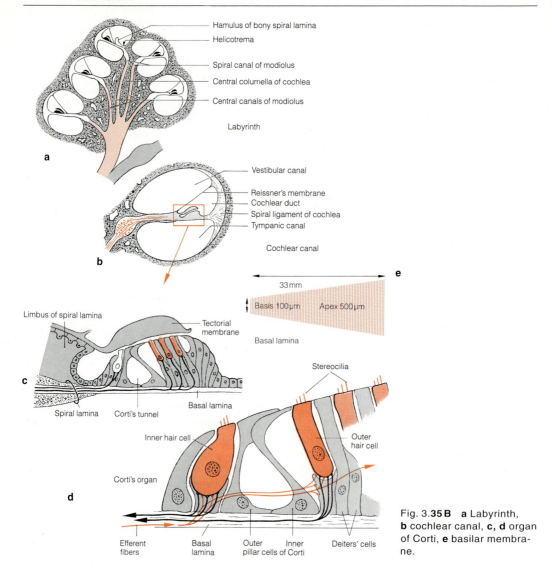

Fig. 3.35B a Labyrinth, b cochlear canal, c, d organ of Corti, e basilar membrane.

membrane oscillates, the stereocilia are bent by the tectorial membrane, which does not oscillate, and this probably represents the appropriate stimulus for the auditory receptor cells. In addition to the sensory cells, the organ of Corti contains various supporting cells, e.g., Deiters' cells and hollow spaces (tunnels), which are not discussed here in detail (see Fig. 3.35 B d, however). Inward movements of the footplate of the stapes in the oval window produce a "wandering wave" along the strands of the basilar membrane, which lie at right angles to the direction of the wave. Any given tone has its own special position with maximum shift (amplitude maximum) in the basilar membrane (tonotopic order, or spatial arrangement). High frequencies have a more basal position, while lower frequencies have increasingly apical positions. The basilar membrane is broader in the area of the apex than in its basal part (Fig. 3.35 B e).

The spiral ganglion (cochlear ganglion) (Fig. 3.35 D) contains some 25 000 bipolar nerve cells, and ca. 5000 unipolar ones. These cells have central and peripheral processes. The peripheral processes enter into contact with the inner hair cells, while the central processes form the cochlear nerve.

The central processes form the cochlear nerve, which together with the vestibular nerve passes through the internal acoustic meatus and enters the brainstem at the cerebellopontine angle, behind the inferior cerebellar peduncle. In the ventral cochlear nucleus, the fibers of the cochlear nerve separate in a T shape, and switch—partly in the ventral cochlear nucleus and partly in the dorsal cochlear nucleus—to a secondary neuron. The secondary neuron transmits the impulses along various paths in a central direction, sometimes in interrupted form, as far as the inferior colliculi and the medial geniculate bodies (Fig. 3.36).

The axons deriving from the *ventral cochlear nucleus* cross the midline as "trapezoid" fibers. Some of these fibers at this point transmit the impulses to neurons of nuclei of the trapezoid body; others transmit them to neurons in the superior olivary nucleus, in the nucleus of the *lateral lemniscus,* or in the reticular formation. Thereafter the acoustic

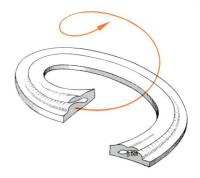

Fig. 3.35 C Course of the basal lamina with the organ of Corti.

impulses travel via the lateral lemniscus rostrally to the inferior colliculi, and some of them probably travel directly to the medial geniculate bodies.

The axons of the *dorsal cochlear nucleus* run dorsally from the inferior cerebellar peduncle to the opposite side, in part as striae medullares, in part via the reticular formation. Finally, they join the fibers coming from the ventral cochlear nucleus in the lateral lemniscus and accompany them to the inferior colliculi.

One group of these fibers runs ipsilaterally; therefore, interruption of one lateral lem-

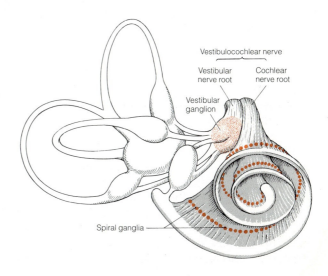

Fig. 3.35 D Spiral ganglion.

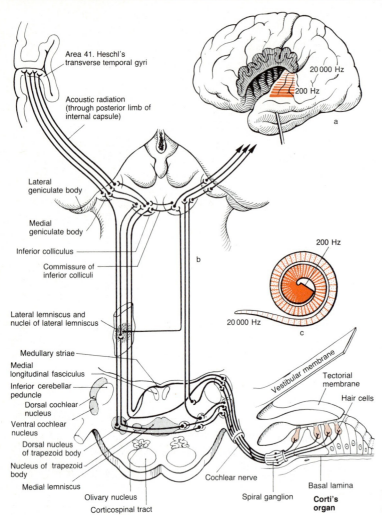

Fig. 3.36 Central pathways of cochlear nerve.

niscus does not cause unilateral deafness. Rather, there will be some reduction in hearing on the opposite side (hypacusis) and some impairment in the recognition of the direction of sound.

Starting in the inferior colliculi, new neurons connect with the medial geniculate bodies of the thalamus. From there the acoustic impulses travel via the *acoustic radiation* through the ventral posterior limb of the internal capsule to the primary cortical fields (Brodmann's area 41) in *Heschl's transverse temporal convolutions* (see Fig. 8.6).

Similar to the retinotopic arrangement of fibers in the visual system, there is an arrangement of fibers in the auditory system according to sound frequencies, called *tonotopic order*. This order exists from the organ of Corti rostrally to the auditory cortex (see Figs. 3.**36a** and **c**).

The primary cortical field of area 41 is partially surrounded by area 42, which is followed laterally by area 22, occupying the external surface of the first temporal convolution (see Fig. 8.**9a**). In these secondary areas the auditory stimuli are analyzed, identified, and compared with former acoustic memories. They are also interpreted and recognized as noises, tones, melodies, vowels and consonants, words and sentences, in other words, as symbols of speech. If these cortical areas are damaged in the dominant hemisphere, the ability to recognize noises and to understand speech is lost (*sensory aphasia*).

On their way from the organ of Corti to the cortex, the fibers of the *auditory pathway* pass through four to six relay stations (superior olivary nucleus, neurons of the reticular formation, nucleus of the lateral lemniscus, inferior colliculi, medial geniculate bodies). At these points they give off collaterals that are part of reflex arcs. Some collaterals connect with the cerebellum. Others travel along the *medial longitudinal bundle* to nuclei of the eye muscles and are instrumental in conjugate eye movements in the direction of a noise. Still other fibers run via the inferior and superior colliculi to the pretectal nucleus and via the tectobulbar tract to nuclei of various cranial nerves, among them the nucleus of the facial nerve (for adjustment of the tone of the stapedius muscle) and the anterior horn motor cells in the cervical cord. The latter connections are responsible for turning the head toward or away from the source of a noise. Collaterals feeding impulses into the ascending activating system of the reticular formation subserve awakening. Some impulses descend via the lateral lemniscus to intercalated neurons that have a regulatory influence, supposedly in part inhibitory, on the tension of the basilar membrane. It is assumed that these neurons enable the ear to focus on certain frequencies of sound by simultaneously inhibiting neighboring frequencies.

Impairments of Hearing

Clinically, there are two basic types of hearing difficulties: *middle ear* or *conduction deafness and inner ear* or *nerve deafness*.

Conduction deafness is caused by disease processes involving the external auditory meatus or, more frequently, the middle ear. None or only some of the sound waves are transmitted to the inner ear and, therefore, to the organ of Corti. Some causes of conduction deafness are otitis media, otosclerosis, and tumors such as glomus tumor. These conditions produce noises in the ear (tinnitus), reduced hearing acuity, and even deafness. Obstruction of the external auditory canal by cerumen should always be considered as a cause.

Nerve or inner ear deafness is the result of a pathologic alteration involving the organ of Corti, the cochlear nerve, or its central pathways.

Should hearing impairment be caused by a disease process in the middle ear that impedes or interrupts the transmission of sound waves, the patient is still able to hear sound waves transmitted by the cranial bone to the organ of Corti. Therefore, it is possible to test with a tuning fork whether the middle ear or the inner ear is afflicted.

The *Schwabach test* is used if the hearing deficit involves both ears. Its purpose is to determine how long the patient can hear the sound of a tuning fork held against the bone, for example, against the mastoid process. If the inner ear is diseased, the period of bone conduction is shortened or absent. It is prolonged if the middle ear is involved.

The *Rinne test* provides information on whether the sound is conducted better through air or through bone. The vibrating tuning fork is held against the mastoid process. When the tone can no longer be heard, the tuning fork is held in front of the ear to determine whether the patient can still hear the tone in this position. He is able to do so if his ear is normal. If the middle ear is damaged, however, he hears the tone longer through bone than through air.

In *Weber's test* the vibrating tuning fork is held on top of the patient's head. If the hearing impairment is caused by conduction failure, he will hear the fork better on the damaged side. With inner ear impairment the tone is heard better on the healthy side.

In testing with an audiometer, loss of low frequencies points to a middle ear affliction, and loss of high frequencies (*senile hypacusis*) suggests a nervous origin for the hearing difficulty.

Middle ear diseases belong to the domain of otolaryngology. Signs and symptoms of involvement of the cochlear nerve and its pathways should be evaluated by a neurologist.

As stated earlier, unilateral interruption of hearing pathways in the brainstem is of little importance because the pathways ascend bilaterally to the primary hearing centers. Signs and symptoms related to damage of the cochlear nerve itself, however, are of practical importance. They may be produced, for example, by a neurinoma of VIII, that is, an *acoustic schwannoma*. Initial irritation of the cochlear fibers may produce *tinnitus* as a first symptom. Further damage proceeds very slowly, so that the increasing deafness and impairment in perceiving the direction of sound often escape the attention of the patient. Only if he specifically uses the diseased ear, for example, by holding the telephone receiver to it instead of to the ear he commonly uses, will he detect the deafness. Otherwise he will find no reason to see his physician until the tumor becomes so large that it damages neighboring structures (vestibular nerve, cerebellum, facial nerve, trigeminal nerve) and produces increased intracranial pressure, headaches, nausea, and vomiting.

If hearing loss is acute (*apoplectiform deafness*), it will be noticed immediately, as will be the inability to determine the direction of sound (caused in such cases by viral infection or circulatory disorders such as vertebrobasilar insufficiency).

Other causes of involvement of the organ of Corti and the cochlear nerve are meningitis, aneurysm, perilymphatic fistula, overdose of certain drugs (streptomycin, quinine, aspirin), and overwhelming, sudden noises (detonation).

The central pathways within the brainstem are subject to circulatory deficiencies from vascular disease, inflammation, and tumors. The result is a *hypacusis*. Only bilateral interruption of the auditory pathways leads to bilateral deafness. In temporal lobe epilepsy the seizure may commence with an acoustic aura. Diseases of the temporal lobes are responsible for auditory agnosia and aphasic disorders, as is discussed in Chapter 8 (Telencephalon).

Vestibular or Equilibrium System (VIII)

Three system subserve the maintenance of the equilibrium: the vestibular system, the system of proprioception from muscles and joints, and the optical system.

The *vestibular system* consists of the labyrinth, the vestibular nerve, and the central vestibular pathways (Fig. 3.37). The *labyrinth* is situated in the petrous bone and consists of the *utriculus*, the *sacculus*, and *three semicircular canals*. The labyrinth is a membranous organ separated from the bony labyrinth by a thin space filled with *perilymph*. The organ itself is filled with *endolymph*.

On each side, the three semicircular canals extend in different planes. The anterior canals are perpendicular, the posterior canals parallel, and the lateral canals horizontal to the axis of the petrous bone. The petrous bone tilts 45° anteriorly, so the anterior canal of one side lies in the same plane as the posterior canal of the other side and vice versa. The horizontal canals of both sides are located in the same plane.

Receptor organs maintain the equilibrium of the body and are located in the utriculus, in the sacculus, and in the ampullae of the semicircular canals. In both utriculi and sacculi the receptor organs are the *maculae staticae* (Fig. 3.38). The macula of the utriculus occupies the floor of the utriculus, parallel to the base of the cranium. The macula of the sacculus occupies the medial wall of the sacculus in a vertical position. The hair cells

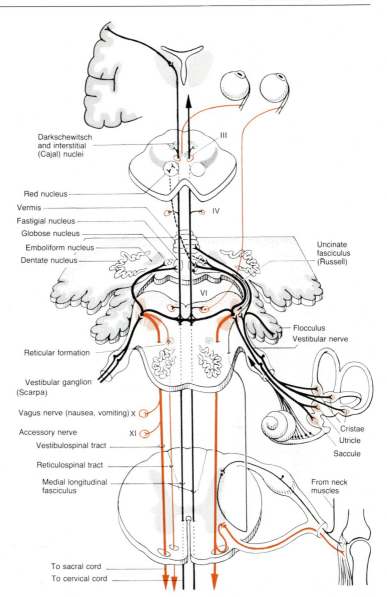

Fig. 3.37 Central pathways of vestibular nerve.

of each macula are embedded in a gelatinous membrane containing *otoliths* (crystals of calcium carbonate) and are surrounded by supporting cells. These receptors send *static* impulses centrally and provide information about the position of the head in space; these impulses also influence muscle tone.

The three semicircular canals are connected with the utriculus. Each ends in a widening or ampulla containing a receptor called a *crista* (Fig. 3.39). The hair cells of each crista ampullaris are embedded in a gelatinous material that forms a high cupula containing no otoliths. The hair cells of the crista are sensitive to the movement of the endolymph within the semicircular canals. They are *kinetic* receptors. The impulses produced by the receptors in the labyrinths constitute stimuli in the reflex arcs that coordinate the muscles

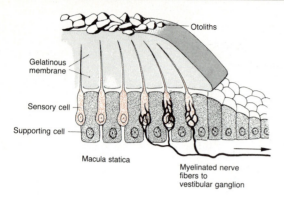

Fig. 3.38 Macula statica.

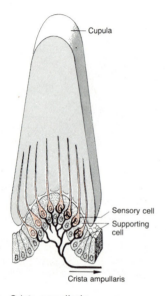

Fig. 3.39 Crista ampullaris.

of eyes, neck, and body in such a way that equilibrium is maintained regardless of position and movement of the head.

The *vestibular ganglion* (Scarpa's ganglion) is located in the internal acoustic meatus and contains bipolar cells. All its peripheral fibers are in contact with the receptors in the vestibular apparatus, and its central fibers form the vestibular nerve. Together with the cochlear nerve, the vestibular nerve passes through the internal acoustic meatus toward the pontocerebellar angle, where it enters the brainstem at the pontomedullary junction on its way to the vestibular nuclei near the floor of the fourth ventricle.

The vestibular nuclear complex (Fig. 3.**40**) is composed of:

1. The *superior vestibular nucleus* (Bechterew's nucleus).
2. The *lateral vestibular nucleus* (Deiter's nucleus).
3. The *medial vestibular nucleus* (Schwalbe's nucleus).
4. The *inferior vestibular nucleus* (Roller's nucleus).

The fibers of the vestibular nerve divide before terminating at the cell groups of the vestibular nuclei from which the second neurons extend (see Fig. 3.**40b**). The precise anatomic pattern of the afferent and efferent fibers in these nuclei has not been fully clarified.

Some fibers of the vestibular nerve transmit impulses directly via the juxtarestiform tract, which is located next to the inferior cerebellar peduncle and runs to the flocculonodular lobe of the cerebellum (archicerebellum). Efferent stimuli from the *fastigial nucleus* (archicerebellum) turn through the *uncinate fasciculus of Russell* back to the vestibular nuclei and via the vestibular nerve to the hair cells of the labyrinth, exerting a regulatory, predominantly inhibitory, influence (see Fig. 3.**37**).

The *archicerebellum* also receives secondary fibers from the superior, medial and in-

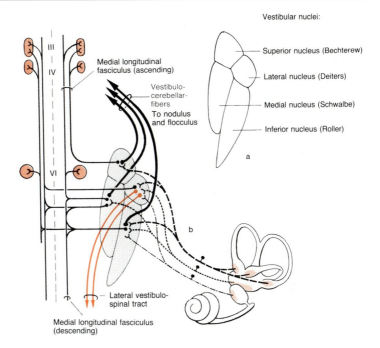

Fig. 3.40 Central connections of vestibular nuclear complex.

ferior vestibular nuclei (see Figs. 3.37 and 3.40b). It returns efferent stimuli directly to the vestibular nuclear complex and to spinal motor neurons via cerebelloreticular and reticulospinal connections. In the lateral vestibular nucleus (Deiter's nucleus), the important *lateral vestibulospinal tract* originates. It descends ipsilaterally in the anterior funiculus to gamma and alpha spinal motoneurons down as far as the sacral segments. This tract has a facilitating influence on extensor reflexes and keeps muscle tone throughout the body sufficiently high to maintain equilibrium.

Fibers of the *medial vestibular nucleus* (*Schwalbe's nucleus*) join the medial longitudinal fascicle on either side, connect with motor cells of the anterior horn of the cervical segments, and descend as the *medial vestibulospinal tract* into the rostral portion of the thoracic spinal cord. These fibers are situated near the anterior median sulcus of the cervical cord. They form the *sulcomarginal fasciculus*, which descends and terminates in the rostral portion of the thoracic cord. These fibers influence the muscle tone of the neck in conformity with various positions of the head. They are probably also part of reflex arcs that help maintain equilibrium by initiating compensatory movements of the arms.

Together with the flocculonodular portion of the cerebellum, the vestibular nuclei form a complex which is extremely important for equilibrium and tonus of the skeletal musculature. There are additional systems subserving equilibrium, spinocerebellar and cerebrocerebellar, which will be discussed in Chapter 4 (Cerebellum).

All vestibular nuclei are connected with the nuclei of the ocular motor nerves by the medial longitudinal fasciculi. Some fibers have been shown to connect with the interstitial Cajal's nucleus and Darkschewitsch's nucleus and to continue to the thalamus (see Fig. 3.37).

The receptors in the semicircular canals can be stimulated by rotation or by irrigation of the external auditory canal with warm or cold water. The result is a *nystagmus* in the plane of the corresponding semicircular canal. Cold water (30°C) or warm water (44°C) produces a movement of the endolymph in the semi-circular canals in, respectively, one direction or the other, which stimulates the receptors (cristae ampullares). Movement of the endolymph also occurs in the rotation test. Subjective consequences are rotatory vertigo and nausea; objective changes are nystagmus, a tendency to fall, gait deviation, diffuse sweating, paleness, and possibly vomiting.

Impairment of the Vestibular System

Irritation of the vestibular apparatus and its central connections first produces *vertigo*, giving the feeling that one is turning around one's own axis or that the surroundings are rapidly turning. This feeling produces insecurity in walking and standing and a tendency to fall. Because the vestibular apparatus is connected with autonomic centers in the reticular formation of the brainstem (see Fig. 3.**51a**), there may also be nausea, retching, vomiting, and, possibly, profuse sweating and pallor.

The following experiment will produce the feelings of a patient suffering from an attack of vestibular irritation (for example, an attack of *Menière's disease*): Place an object such as a coin on the floor. While standing over it, bend forward approximately 30° so that you can see the coin. While looking at the coin, make five or six rapid turns around your axis to the right, stop suddenly, stand erect, and stretch your arms out in front. What happens? You have the feeling that you are turning to the left, that you may fall to the right, and that the arms deviate to the right. Because of the danger of falling, you should not engage in this experiment without another person being present. There is also a possibility of severe nausea and even vomiting. There will be nystagmus contralateral to the direction of rotation. Because the head is held forward during the experiment, the horizontal semicircular canals are in the plane of rotation. Therefore, the fast rotation causes movement of the endolymph in these canals. As you suddenly stop rotating, the fluid continues to move in the same direction for a while, because of its inertia, and stimulates the cristae. This causes the illusion that you are still turning around.

It is evident that during the experiment impulses originating in the semicircular canals reach the motor nuclei of the eye muscles (nystagmus), the spinal cord (insecurity and tendency to fall while walking and standing), and the autonomic centers in the reticular formation (sweating, paleness).

The *static labyrinth* (maculae staticae in utriculus and sacculus) controls the distribution of the level of skeletal muscle tone necessary for counteracting gravity and maintaining upright posture. The *kinetic labyrinth* (cristae ampullares) probably influences the position of the eyes so that optical orientation in space is guaranteed during whatever movements the head may perform. As was mentioned earlier, other systems join in this task. Thus, if the labyrinths fail but optical and proprioceptive systems are still intact, one is still able to move about with little restriction. If it is dark and the walking surface is uneven, however, one will be rather helpless.

The vestibular system must have connections with the cerebral cortex, because one is consciously aware of one's own position in space and of disorders in vestibular function. The vestibulocortical pathways, however, have not been fully identified. The cortical projection is most likely contralateral. It has been assumed that the cortical field for vestibular sensations occupies an area in the temporal lobe, but according to more recent investigations, it is probably located in the immediate vicinity of the central region, more precisely, in the area representing the head.

One's own position in space can be judged correctly only if visual, proprioceptive, and vestibular signals are immediately registered centrally and integrated with one another.

Because the right and left labyrinths are exceptionally well tuned to each other, the information they render about position in space should be identical in a healthy person. Vestibular information becomes disproportionate if the function of one of the labyrinths is reduced because of disease. Vertigo, loss of balance, and nystagmus will develop.

Nystagmus

A spontaneous nystagmus with one slow and one fast component is always abnormal and points to an alteration in the labyrinths and their central connections. The slow component is the actual sign of irritation, whereas the fast component constitutes only a jerk-like, reflexive return of the eyes to their original position. It is common practice to name the direction of the nystagmus according to that of the fast reflex component.

Peripheral nystagmus occurs if the labyrinths or the vestibular nerves are diseased; *central nystagmus*, if the vestibular nuclei or their central pathways are damaged.

Peripheral impairment may have the following causes: labyrinthitis, Menière's syndrome from endolymphatic hydrops, perilymphatic fistula, trauma of a labyrinth (petrous bone fracture), labyrinth apoplexy, vertebrobasilar insufficiency, toxic injury of the labyrinth from streptomycin or other drugs, and neurinoma within the internal acoustic meatus.

Similar to the cause of trigeminal neuralgia and facial spasm, Menière attacks have been found to be triggered by a blood vessel that was attached to the proximal, nonmyelinated root of the eighth nerve. Operative relocation of the vessel brought an end to the attacks (Jannetta, 1975; Samii, 1981; Wigand et al., 1983).

Central impairment may be caused by circulatory lesions (softening, bleeding) in the vertebrobasilar territory, multiple sclerosis, syphilis, tumors, or other conditions.

Vagal System (VII Intermediate, IX, X, Cranial XI)

Glossopharyngeal Nerve (IX)

The glossopharyngeal nerve has so much in common with the intermediate, vagus, and cranial accessory nerves that it is advisable to discuss them together under the heading "vagal system" to avoid unnecessary repetition. The nerves are mixed and share, for example, the *nucleus ambiguus* and the *nucleus of the solitary tract* (see Figs. 3.3 and 3.4 and Table 3.1).

The glossopharyngeal nerve is joined by the vagus and accessory nerves as it leaves the cranium via the *foramen jugulare*. At the foramen it has two ganglia, the *intracranial ganglion superius* and the *extracranial ganglion inferius*. After passing through the foramen the nerve proceeds between the internal carotid artery and the internal jugular vein to the stylopharyngeal muscle. Between this muscle and the styloglossal muscle the nerve extends to the base of the tongue and supplies the mucosa of the pharynx, the tonsils, and the posterior third of the tongue. It has the following branches (Figs. 3.41 and 3.42):

1. *Tympanic nerve:* It originates from the extracranial inferior ganglion, passes through the middle ear and the tympanic (Jacobson's) plexus, and continues via the minor petrosal nerve and the otic ganglion to the parotid gland (see Fig. 3.34). It is the sensory nerve for the mucosa of the middle ear and the eustachian tube.

2. *Stylopharyngeal branches:* They supply the stylopharyngeal muscle.

3. *Pharyngeal branches:* Together with branches of the vagus nerve, they form the pharyngeal plexus. They innervate the striated musculature of the pharynx.

4. *Carotid sinus branches:* They accompany the internal carotid artery to the carotid sinus and to the glomus caroticum.

5. *Lingual branches:* They pick up taste impulses from the posterior third of the tongue.

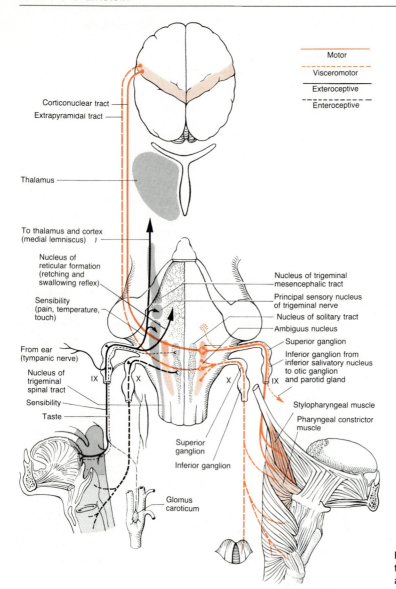

Fig. 3.41 Central connections of glossopharyngeal and vagus nerves.

Impairment of the glossopharyngeal nerve

Isolated damage to the glossopharyngeal nerve is rare. In most instances the vagus and accessory nerves are also damaged.

Causes of glossopharyngeal impairment are, among others, fracture of the base of the skull, thrombosis of the sigmoid sinus, tumors of the base of the posterior fossa, aneurysms of vertebral and basilar arteries, meningitides, neuritis, progressive bulbar paralysis, and syringobulbia.

Syndrome of impairment of the glossopharyngeal nerve. This syndrome includes the following signs and symptoms:

1. loss of taste sensation (*ageusia*) in the posterior third of the tongue
2. absence of retching reflex and palatal reflex

Cranial Nerves 127

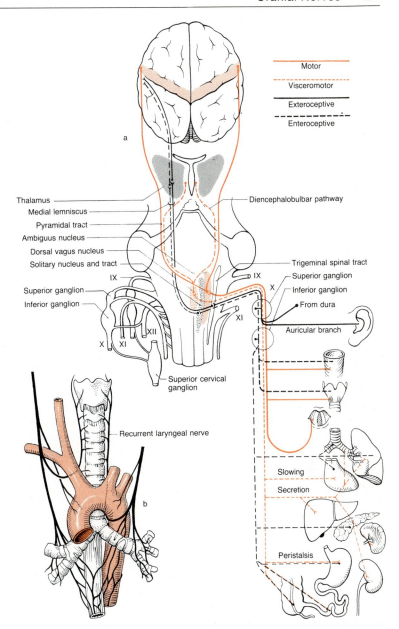

Fig. 3.42 Vagus nerve.

3. anesthesia and analgesia in the rostral portion of the pharynx, in the region of the tonsils, and in the base of the tongue
4. mild disorder of swallowing (*dysphagia*)

Glossopharyngeal neuralgia. Neuralgia of the glossopharyngeal nerve is a particular disease entity. Similar to that in neuralgia of the trigeminal nerve, the pain is paroxysmal and excruciating. Its onset is sudden and its duration is usually brief. The pain most often commences at the base of the tongue, in the area of the tonsils, or in the soft palate and radiates into the ear. The paroxysms can be triggered by swallowing, chewing, coughing, or speaking. If the pain persists, a malignant tumor of the pharynx should be suspected. As with the trigeminal neuralgia, it is also possible that the pain is triggered by a blood vessel pressing on the proximal, non-myelinated root of the glossopharyngeal nerve. Operative relocation of the vessel is said to have cured the condition (Jannetta, 1977).

Vagus Nerve (X)

The vagus nerve also has two ganglia, the *ganglion superius or jugulare* and the *ganglion inferius or nodosum*. Both are situated in the area of the foramen jugulare.

The vagus nerve represents the nerve of the fourth and subsequent branchial arches. Caudally from the ganglion inferius (nodosum), it descends along the internal carotid artery and the common carotid artery and arrives in the mediastinum via the superior thoracic aperture. The right nerve passes over the subclavian artery, and the left over the aortic arch and behind the root of the lungs. From that point on both nerves are in close touch with the esophagus, the fibers of the right nerve being attached to the posterior aspect and those of the left nerve to the anterior side of the esophagus. Together they form the esophageal plexus. Terminal branches pass with the esophagus into the abdominal cavity via the diaphragmatic esophageal hiatus.

Branches of the vagus nerve

On its way from the superior ganglion to the abdominal cavity, the vagus nerve gives off the following branches (see Figs. 3.**41**, 3.**42** and 5.**25**):

1. *Dural branch:* This branch originates from the ganglion superius, returns through the foramen jugulare, and supplies the dura of the posterior fossa.
2. *Auricular branch:* Descending from the ganglion superius, this branch supplies the skin of the posterior aspect of the ear and the posterior wall of the external auditory meatus. It is the only branch of the vagus nerve that supplies skin.
3. *Pharyngeal branch:* Together with the fibers of the glossopharyngeal nerve and the cervical sympathetic chain, these fibers enter the pharyngeal plexus and provide motor innervation to the musculature of pharynx and soft palate.
4. *Superior laryngeal branch:* This nerve runs from the inferior ganglion to the larynx. Its external branch innervates the constrictor muscles of the pharynx and the cricothyroid muscle. Its internal sensory branch carries impulses from the area from the mucosa of the larynx down to the vocal cords and the mucosa of the epiglottis. The nerve also carries taste fibers from the epiglottis and parasympathetic fibers for the glands of the mucosa.
5. *Recurrent laryngeal branch:* On the right the recurrent branch loops around the subclavian artery, and on the left around the arch of the aorta (see Fig. 3.**42**b). Thereafter the two branches ascend between trachea and esophagus until they reach the larynx. They provide motor innervation to all the muscles of the larynx except the cricothyroid muscle. Their sensory portions are responsible for the mucosa of the larynx below the level of the vocal cords.
6. *Superior cervical cardiac branches and thoracic cardiac branches:* These branches go together with sympathetic fibers via the cardiac plexus to the heart.
7. *Bronchial branches:* These form the pulmonary plexus in the wall of the bronchi.
8. *Anterior and posterior gastric, hepatic, celiac, and renal branches:* All these branches join the celiac and superior mesenteric plexuses (anterior and posterior branches, respectively) and together with sympathetic fibers supply the viscera

of the abdominal cavity (stomach, liver, pancreas, spleen, kidneys, and adrenals, as well as small intestines and the first portion of the colon). These branches of both vagus nerves are intermingled with fibers of the sympathetic nervous system in the abdominal cavity and cannot be clearly differentiated from them.

Syndrome of impairment of the vagus nerve

Causes of vagus nerve impairment can be both intracranial and peripheral. *Intracranial causes* include tumor, hematoma, thrombosis, multiple sclerosis, syphilis, amyotrophic lateral sclerosis, syringobulbia, meningitis, and aneurysm. *Peripheral causes* are neuritis (from alcohol, diphtheria, lead, arsenic), tumor, glandular disease, trauma, and aneurysm of the aorta.

Bilateral complete paralysis of the vagus nerve is rapidly fatal. Unilateral complete interruption of the nerve produces the following syndrome: The ipsilateral soft palate droops down, and speech is nasal. Because the pharyngeal constrictor muscle is paralyzed, the soft palate is pulled to the healthy side during phonation. Paralysis of vocal cords produces hoarseness. In addition, there may be some dysphagia and occasional tachycardia and arrhythmia.

Damage to the recurrent laryngeal nerve, with paralysis of the laryngeal muscles except for the cricothyroid muscle, is not rare and produces a transient hoarseness (aneurysm of aorta). Bilateral paralysis adds respiratory difficulties.

Accessory Nerve (Cranial XI)

The accessory nerve has cranial and spinal roots (Fig. 3.**43**). The cranial roots are axons of neurons in the ambiguus nucleus located next to neurons that belong to the vagus nerve. This *cranial* portion of the accessory nerve should actually be considered a part of the vagus nerve, because it shares a nucleus with the vagus and is similar in its function.

This cannot be said about the *spinal* portion of the accessory nerve. Actually, the cranial division separates itself from the spinal division and joins the vagus nerve in the jugular foramen. The spinal roots will be discussed later.

Nucleus Ambiguus

The nucleus ambiguus is composed of the motoneurons of the glossopharyngeal, vagus, and cranial accessory nerves (see Figs. 3.**41**, 3.**42**, and 3.**43**). It receives supranuclear impulses from both cerebral hemispheres via the corticonuclear tract. Therefore, unilateral interruption of central fibers produces no significant loss of function. The axons of the nucleus accompany the glossopharyngeal, vagus, and cranial accessory nerves and innervate the musculature of the soft palate, that of the pharynx and larynx, and the striated muscles of the rostral portion of the esophagus. The nucleus ambiguus receives afferent impulses from the trigeminal spinal nucleus and from the nucleus of the solitary tract. These nuclei are parts of reflex arcs that originate in the mucosa of the respiratory and digestive tracts and trigger coughing, retching, and vomiting.

Parasympathetic Motor Nuclei

The *dorsal nucleus of the vagus nerve* and the *inferior salivatory nucleus* are the parasympathetic motor nuclei (Fig. 3.**41**). The superior salivatory nucleus is the parasympathetic nucleus for the intermediate nerve (Fig. 3.**34**).

The axons of the dorsal vagus nucleus are the preganglionic fibers of the vagus nerve for the various ganglia in head, thoracic, and abdominal areas. Short postganglionic fibers send the motor impulses to the smooth muscles of lungs and intestines, down to the splenic flexure of the colon, and to the heart muscles. Stimulation of these parasympathetic fibers slows heart rate, constricts the smooth bronchial muscles, and promotes secretion of the mucosal glands of the

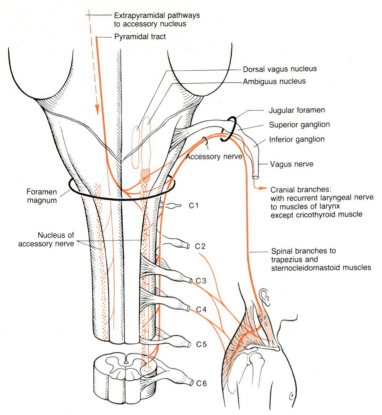

Fig. 3.43 Accessory nerve.

bronchi. In the intestinal tract peristalsis and glandular secretion in stomach and pancreas are activated.

The dorsal nucleus of the vagus nerve receives afferent impulses from the hypothalamus, the olfactory system, autonomic centers in the reticular formation, and the nucleus of the solitary tract. These connections are important parts of reflex arcs controlling cardiovascular, respiratory, and alimentary functions. Impulses from baroceptors in the wall of the carotid sinus are transmitted by the glossopharyngeal nerve and subserve arterial blood pressure regulation. Chemoreceptors in the glomus caroticum participate in the regulation of oxygen tension in the blood. Receptors in the arch of the aorta and in the para-aortic bodies have a smiliar function; they transmit their impulses via the vagus nerve.

The parasympathetic motor fibers that originate in the inferior salivatory nucleus and innervate the parotid gland via the glossopharyngeal nerve have already been discussed.

Visceral Afferent Fibers of IX and X

Special afferent visceral fibers of the glossopharyngeal nerve originate from pseudounipolar cells in its extracranial ganglion inferius; those of the vagus nerve, in its ganglion inferius (nodosum). Both carry impulses from taste receptors in the posterior third of the tongue and in the area of the epiglottis. *The glossopharyngeal is the principal nerve for taste.* The central processes of the ganglionic nerve cells proceed via the solitary tract to the nucleus of the tract, where the taste impulses from the anterior two-thirds of the tongue arrive via the intermediate nerve (see Fig. 3.33). From the nucleus of the solitary tract, taste impulses are carried centrally over the thalamic ventral posteromedial nucleus to the cortical taste area at the foot of the posterior central convolution.

Other afferent visceral fibers of the glossopharyngeal nerve come from its ganglion superius, those of the vagus nerve, from its ganglion nodosum. They carry sensory impulses from the mucosa of the posterior third of the tongue, of the pharynx (IX) and of the viscera in thorax and abdominal cavity (X) (see Figs. 3.41 and 3.42).

Somatic Afferent Fibers of IX and X

The glossopharyngeal nerve fibers of its ganglion superius relay pain and probably also temperature sensations in the mucosa of the posterior third of the tongue, of the rostral pharynx, of the eustachian tube, and of the middle ear to the nucleus of the spinal trigeminal tract. The vagus nerve and fibers of its ganglion jugulare transmit these sensations for the mucosa of the caudal portion of the pharynx and larynx, for the skin behind the ear and of part of the external auditory canal, for the tympanic membrane, and for the dura of the posterior fossa.

Fibers transmitting touch sensations from all these areas probably terminate in the principal sensory nucleus of V. They go to the posterior central convolution via the medial lemniscus and thalamus.

Accessory Nerve (Spinal XI)

The spinal division of the accessory nerve originates in a cell column of the ventrolateral anterior horns of C2–C5 or even C6 (see Fig. 3.43). The axons first ascend in the lateral funiculus for one or two segments before they leave the cord laterally and dorsally from the dentate ligament. Several roots located between the segmental anterior and posterior roots join to form a common stem. Rostrally the stem passes through the foramen magnum into the cranium and unites with the cranial portion of the nerve; the nerve then leaves the cranium through the foramen jugulare. The cranial accessory nerve becomes part of the vagus nerve, and the spinal accessory nerve is now called the *ramus externus*. This external branch descends in the neck and provides motor innervation to the sternocleidomastoid and trapezius muscles. In addition, there are spinal somatic efferent fibers from segments C2–C4. The relative contributions of the accessory nerve and the spinal nerves of C2–C4 to the innervation of the trapezius muscle is still open to dispute. Some authors believe that the accessory nerve innervates predominantly the caudal part of the muscle; others assume that it serves mostly the rostral portion. Injury to the accessory nerve is followed by an atrophy involving predominantly the rostral part of the muscle. The ramus externus also carries some afferent fibers and neurons that transmit proprioceptive impulses centrally.

Syndrome of impairment of accessory nerve

Impairment may be caused by central (intramedullary, intracerebral) or by peripheral lesions.

Central impairment. The neurons of the spinal accessory nerve receive impulses over the corticospinal and corticonuclear tracts of both sides but predominantly of the opposite side. Consequently, a cerebral hematoma or infarct produces a contralateral spastic paresis of the sternocleidomastoid and trapezius muscles but the paresis is usually not extensive and may be overlooked. In addition, the neurons receive extrapyramidal impulses (spasmodic torticollis, chorea) and reflex impulses via the tectospinal and vestibulospinal tracts and the medial longitudinal fasciculus.

If the anterior horns of C1 to C4 are unilaterally destroyed (poliomyelitis, trauma, asymmetrical syringomyelia), there will be a complete ipsilateral, flaccid paralysis of the sternocleidomastoid and trapezius muscles.

Peripheral impairment. A unilateral interruption of the external ramus of the accessory nerve outside the foramen jugulare affects the sternocleidomastoid and trapezius muscles to different degrees. The sternocleidomastoid shows flaccid paralysis, whereas the trapezius is paretic only in its rostral portion because it is also innervated by the spinal motor roots of C3 and C4. If the damage is located distally from the sternocleidomastoid muscle, only the trapezius muscle will be paretic. Such damage is occasionally iatrogenic and the result of a surgical removal of a lymph node at the posterior margin of the sternocleidomastoid for histologic examination. Sensory deficits do not occur, because the spinal accessory nerve has only motor function.

Diagnostic signs. A unilateral paralysis of the sternocleidomastoid muscle causes great difficulty in turning the head to the opposite side. A bilateral paralysis makes it almost impossible to hold up the head. In the supine position the patient is unable to raise his head. A paresis of the trapezius muscle produces a hanging shoulder and a caudolateral displacement of the scapula on the paretic side. It is difficult to raise the arm laterally to more than 90°, because under normal conditions the trapezius muscle supports the anterior serratus muscle in this movement. The diagnosis of paralysis of the accessory nerve can be made simply by ascertaining visually the atrophic state of the sternocleidomastoid and the drop of the shoulder.

The spinal part of the accessory nerve receives impulses via the corticonuclear and corticospinal tracts, predominantly via those of the opposite side. A cerebral hematoma or infarct may produce a contralateral spastic pareses of the sternocleidomastoid and trapezeus muscles. It is not very impressive because of the ipsilateral impulses and is sometimes overlooked. Among others, there are also extrapyramidal impulses (spasmodic torticollis, chorea) and reflex connections via the tecto- and vestibulospinal tracts and the medial longitudinal fascicle.

Causes of accessory nerve damage. Aside from those mentioned above, the causes may be head and neck injury with or without skull fracture, polyneuritis, amyotrophic lateral sclerosis, posterior fossa tumor (particularly in the area of the foramen magnum), and developmental anomalies at the craniospinal junction.

Hypoglossal Nerve (XII)

The nuclei of the hypoglossal nerves are located in the lower medulla oblongata on either side of the midline and next to the floor of the fourth ventricle, where they produce the hypoglossal trigone (Fig. 3.**44**; see Figs. 3.**1b**, 3.**2**, and 3.**3**). Each nucleus is made up of several groups of motoneurons, and each group innervates its own tongue muscle. Developmentally, the neurons are identical to the motoneurons of the spinal anterior horns. The hypoglossal is a somatic efferent nerve. Its axons proceed ventrally toward the anterior lateral sulcus between pyramid and inferior olive. There they come to the surface in multiple thin bundles (see Fig. 3.**1**), which soon unite to form the nerve. The nerve leaves the cranium through its own canal, the *canalis hypoglossi*, above the lateral margin of the foramen magnum (see Figs. 3.**6** and 3.**44**). Deep within the neck it passes in between the internal jugular vein and the internal carotid artery and is accompanied by fibers of the three upper cervical segments (*ansa hypoglossi*). These fibers do not unite with the hypoglossal nerve; rather, they soon separate and innervate the muscles of the hyoid bone (thyrohyoid, sternohyoid, omohyoid).

The hypoglossal nerve innervates the muscles of the tongue: the styloglossus, hyoglossus, and genioglossus. Voluntary innervation travels via the corticonuclear tract, which, coming from the precentral cortex, accompanies the corticospinal tract on its way through the internal capsule.

The hypoglossal nucleus receives impulses predominantly from the contralateral corticonuclear tract. In addition, afferent fibers

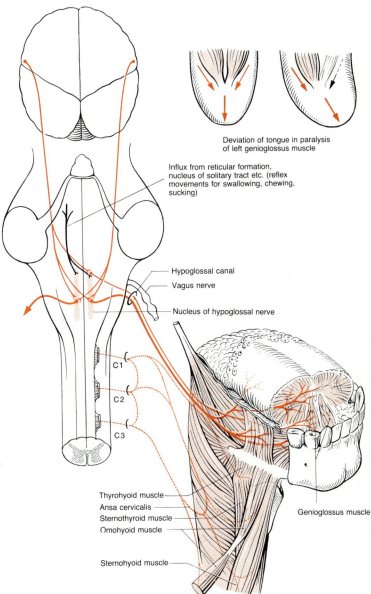

Fig. 3.44 Hypoglossal nerve.

from the reticular formation, from the nucleus of the solitary tract (taste), from the midbrain via the tectospinal tract, and from the trigeminal nuclei are components of reflex arcs subserving swallowing, chewing, sucking, and licking.

A unilateral supranuclear interruption of innervation has no major consequences, because the nuclei also receive some ipsilateral impulses and the muscles of the tongue are tightly interwoven across the midline. In a unilateral spastic paresis, the extended tongue usually deviates slightly to the paretic side. The two genioglossal muscles move the tongue forward. If one of them is weak, the stronger, healthy muscle pushes the tongue to the paretic side (see Fig. 3.**44**). In the presence of a hemiplegia there is some initial dysarthria but no disorder of swallowing (dysphagia). Causes of a combined hemiplegia and unilateral supranuclear hypoglossal palsy are, among others, hematoma, infarct, tumor, and multiple sclerosis. If the supranuclear paralysis is bilateral, there is severe impairment of speaking and swallowing (pseudobulbar paralysis).

Alterations in the nuclear areas of the hypoglossal nerves may involve both nuclei, because of their proximity. The result may be a bilateral, flaccid paresis with atrophy and fasciculation of the tongue muscles. In cases that have progressed further, the paralyzed tongue lies flaccid on the floor of the mouth and displays strong fasciculations. Speaking and swallowing are severely impeded. Among the possible causes are bulbar paralysis, amyotrophic lateral sclerosis, syringobulbia, poliomyelitis, and vascular disease.

Alterations in the peripheral hypoglossal nerve have the same sequelae as does nuclear involvement except that the paralysis is usually unilateral. Possible causes are basal fracture of the skull, aneurysm, tumor, and diverse toxic substances (alcohol, lead, arsenic, carbon monoxide, and others).

Combined Impairment of IX through XII

Progressive bulbar paralysis

This syndrome develops in the course of amyotrophic lateral sclerosis and syringobulbia, which is often a rostral extension of cervical syringomyelia. The underlying pathologic change consists of a degenerative loss of neurons in motor nuclei of several cranial nerves, mainly IX to XII. The nuclei of the facial nerves may also be involved. The degenerative process often ascends from the cervical cord but may commence in the brainstem. A disorder of speech (*dysarthria, anarthria*) is usually the first sign. Soon swallowing becomes impaired (ambiguus nucleus), the tongue develops atrophy with fasciculation, and signs such as nystagmus, ptosis, and facial paresis follow.

In bulbar paralysis from poliomyelitis, involvement of the brainstem nuclei is irregular in location and intensity. Signs develop rapidly. If the vagus nuclei become bilaterally involved, death invariably occurs.

Pseudobulbar paralysis

This syndrome stems from bilateral interruption of the corticonuclear tracts, most often caused by cerebral arteriosclerosis. The result is bilateral spastic paresis of the motor cranial nerves IX to XII. Dominant signs are *dysarthria* and *dysphagia*. There is a tendency to *forced laughter* and *forced crying*, possibly caused by bilateral interruption of descending cortical fibers carrying inhibitory impulses.

Internal Structure of the Brainstem

For a satisfactory understanding of the signs and symptoms caused by local lesions or disease processes of the brainstem, one should

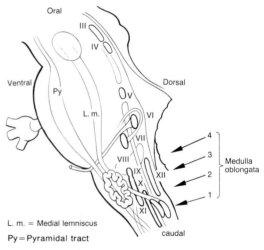

Fig. 3.**45** Levels of cross-sections of medulla oblongata shown in Figure 3.**46**.

Internal Structure of the Brainstem

consider the topography of the pathways of the brainstem and their nuclei; the location and function of additional gray structures, such as the reticular formation, the olivary bodies, the red nucleus, and the substantia nigra; and their interconnections and relationships to cerebral, cerebellar, and spinal structures.

Figs. 3.45 through 3.48 illustrate the topographical relationships of nuclei and of ascending as well as descending pathways on

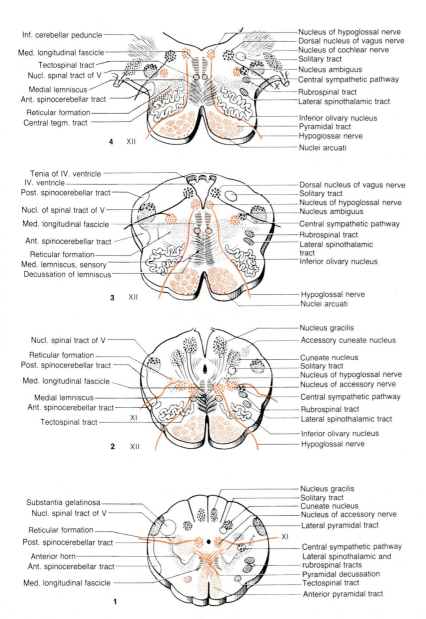

Fig. 3.46 Cross-sections of medulla oblongata at levels indicated by arrows in Figure 3.45.

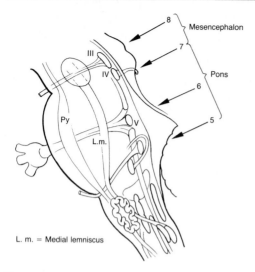

Fig. 3.47 Levels of cross-sections of pons and mesencephalon shown in Figure 3.48.

cross-sections of the brainstem. Figs. 3.**49** and 3.**50** present the spatial relationships of the various structures on lateral and dorsal views of the brainstem shown longitudinally.

Medulla Oblongata

Figs. 3.**45** (1) and 3.**46** (1) show a cross-section through the decussation of the pyramidal tract. The arrangement of gray and white matter is considerably different from that described for the spinal cord. The anterior horns can still be recognized but are rather small; they contain the motoneurons for C1 and for roots of the accessory nerve (XI). The descending corticospinal tracts forming the pyramid cross in front of the central canal and become the *lateral pyramidal tracts* of the spinal cord. The areas of the posterior funiculi contain, medially, the nuclei graciles and, laterally, the cuneate nuclei. Their impulses coming up the gracilis and cuneate tracts are relayed to the second neurons that transmit them to the contralateral thalamus via the medial lemniscus. The impulses coming from the lower extremities are transferred to the nucleus gracilis, and those of the upper extremities to the cuneate nucleus, in somato-topic order. This order is maintained in the medial lemniscus, in the thalamus, and in the cortex. Figs. 3.**49c** and 3.**50c** illustrate the meandering course of the medial lemniscus. In Fig. 3.**50c** the most lateral fibers represent the leg, and the more medial fibers the arm.

The lateral spinothalamic tract (pain, temperature) as well as the anterior spinothalamic tract (touch, pressure) maintain approximately the same position they have in the spinal cord. The same is true of the spinotectal tract as it goes to the quadrigeminal area. Fibers of the spinal reticular formation terminate in the *lateral reticular nucleus*, a relatively large group of neurons which lies rostral and dorsal to the inferior olive. The spinal reticular fibers transmit sensory impulses from skin and viscera. In the cord they are somewhat diffusely arranged or are attached to the spinothalamic tract. The posterior spinocerebellar tract, which originates in *Clarke's column* (*nucleus thoracicus*) and ascends ipsilaterally in the cord, keeps its position in the lower medulla (see Fig. 3.46). Then it shifts more and more dorsally and enters the cerebellum together with the olivocerebellar tract via the inferior cerebellar peduncle (see Figs. 3.**49b** and 3.**50b**). The partially crossed anterior spinocerebellar tract runs rostrally through medulla and pons and enters the cerebellum through the superior cerebellar peduncle (brachium conjunctivum) and the superior medullary velum (see Figs. 3.**49b** and 3.**50b**).

The nuclear complex of the inferior olive extends through the rostral three-fourths of the medulla dorsal to the pyramids. It consists of the principal nucleus of the inferior olive and a medial as well as a dorsal accessory olivary nucleus. The principal nucleus constitutes a much-folded bag-like sheet of gray matter with its opening or hilus facing the midline. The axons of the many small, characteristic neurons of the principal nucleus leave through the hilus, cross the midline as the olivocerebellar tract, and become a main component of the inferior cerebellar peduncle. They terminate throughout the

Internal Structure of the Brainstem

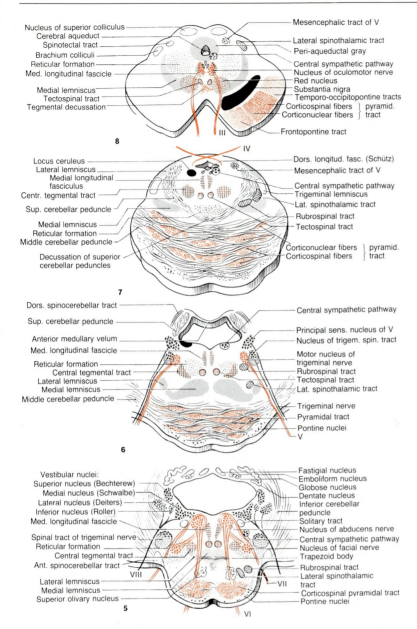

Fig. 3.48 Cross-sections of pons and mesencephalon at levels indicated by arrows in Figure 3.47.

cortex of the neocerebellum. The main afferent fiber tract of the olivary complex is the *central tegmental tract*. It carries impulses from the red nucleus of the midbrain, the periaqueductal gray matter, the reticular formation, and the striatum. Cerebral cortical impulses take the corticoolivary tract, which descends together with the corticospinal tract. The olivocerebellar tract belongs to the system controlling the precision of voluntary

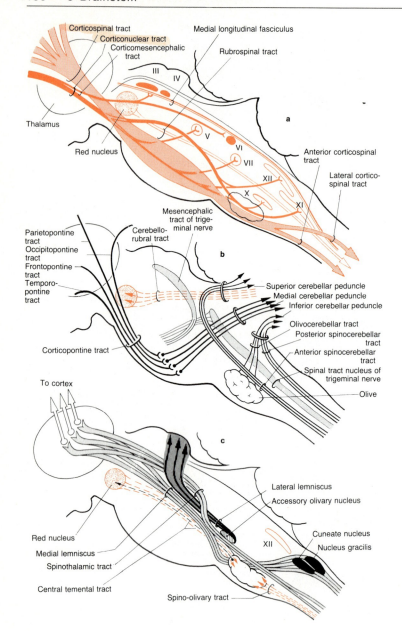

Fig. 3.49 Lateral view of **a** efferent pathways, **b** cerebellar pathways, and **c** afferent pathways through medulla oblongata, pons, and midbrain.

movements, as will be discussed in Chapter 4 on the cerebellum and in Chapter 6 on the basal ganglia and extrapyramidal system.

Interruption of afferent impulses traveling through the central tegmental tract or direct damage to the inferior olive produces rhythmical jerking of the soft palate, the pharynx, and, perhaps, the diaphragm (*myorhythmias, myoclonias, singultus*). The most frequent cause is an infarct above the area of the olive interrupting the central tegmental tract.

Internal Structure of the Brainstem

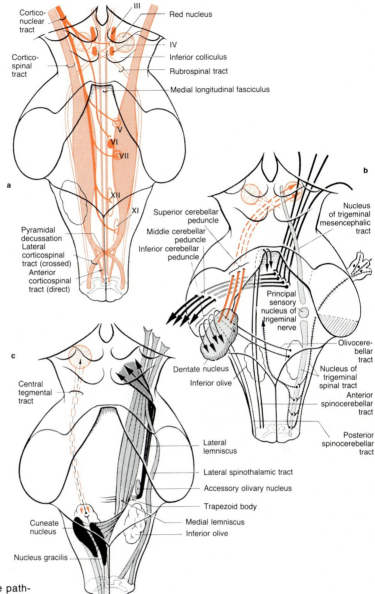

Fig. 3.**50** Dorsal view of the pathways shown in Fig. 3.**49**.

The accessory olives are phylogenetically older than the principal olivary nuclei. They connect with the archicerebellum and maintain equilibrium.

The course of the corticospinal and corticonuclear tracts can be seen on the cross-sections in Fig. 3.**48** and particularly in Figs. 3.**49a** and 3.**50a**.

The rubrospinal tract passes through the medulla oblongata and accompanies the lateral corticospinal tract on its way to the spinal cord. This pathway is also visible in

Figs. 3.**49a** and 3.**50a**. The tract originates in the red nucleus and soon crosses to the other side in the ventral tegmental (Forel's) decussation.

Neurons in the mesencephalic tectum give rise to the tectospinal tract, which turns around the periaqueductal gray matter, crosses the midline in the dorsal tegmental (Meynert's) decussation, and continues caudally near the midline. It gradually shifts ventrally and laterally. In the medulla oblongata it is located in the ventrolateral portion. On its way through the brainstem it gives off collaterals to the nuclei of the ocular motor nerves, to the nucleus of the facial nerve, and to the cerebellum before it terminates in the cervical cord.

The superior colliculi receive optical stimuli from the retina and auditory stimuli from the inferior colliculi. If these stimuli are strong, they pass to tectonuclear and tectospinal pathways and cause reflex closure of the eyes, averting of the head, and perhaps raising of the arms in a protective posture.

As was mentioned earlier, the cortex of the occipital lobes is connected with the superior colliculi. These pathways and the tectospinal tracts control the automatic pursuit movements of eyes and head that occur when tracking a visual object.

It can be noted on the various cross-sections of the brainstem that groups of neurons are diffusely interspersed among the various nuclei and ascending and descending pathways. These cell groups vary in size and form clusters in places. The neurons are interconnected with a net-like system of fibers; for this reason, these cell groups are referred to as the *reticular formation*. In the spinal cord its cells are located between the posterior and lateral horns (see Fig. 1.**21**). In medulla, pons, and midbrain they occupy the central portions of either half of the tegmentum. The great importance of these cells was first emphasized by Moruzzi and Magoun (1949). We shall discuss it later.

The *dorsal nuclei of the vagus nerves* are noteworthy structures of the medulla oblongata. They form the vagus trigone, an elevation in the floor of the fourth ventricle (see Fig. 3.**1b**). Their neurons have autonomic motor functions, functions they share with their relatives, the neurons of the lateral horns of the spinal segments T1 through L2.

The nucleus of the solitary tract is situated more laterally and receives sensory impulses. Taste impulses carried by fibers of cranial nerves VII, IX, and X travel to the rostral portion of the nucleus. Its caudal portion receives impulses from viscera in chest and abdomen. This portion has contacts with the dorsal nucleus of the vagus nerve and with visceral centers in the reticular formation as well as with neurons of this formation that send efferent impulses to autonomic neurons in the lateral horns of the spinal cord. Thus, the vagal dorsal nucleus and the nucleus of the solitary tract are components of reflex arcs controlling cardiovascular, respiratory, alimentary, and other vegetative functions (Fig. 3.**51a**).

Some nuclei have been discussed earlier in this chapter, among them the hypoglossal, ambiguus, and vestibular nuclei and the spinal nucleus of the trigeminal nerve. It is noteworthy that three pathways share their location on either side of the midline of the medulla: the medial longitudinal fascicles (dorsal), the tectospinal tracts (intermediate), and the medial lemnisci (see Fig. 3.**46**).

Pons

The pons consists of two parts, base and tegmentum. The *base* contains numerous groups of neurons, the *nuclei pontis*, and many crossing fiber bundles that form the middle cerebellar (pontocerebellar) peduncles on each side. These peduncles convert the pons into a bridge connecting the cerebellar hemispheres over the ventral portion of the fourth ventricle. Hence, Varolius (1543–1575) gave it the name *pons*. The fibers of each peduncle are axons of the neurons of the pontine nuclei in the contralateral half of the base. Here, these second neurons receive the ipsilateral corticopontine fibers descending from frontal, parietal, and temporal areas of the cortex. After crossing, the second neurons project to the cortex of the cerebellum. The pontine nuclei receive additional impulses from collaterals of the pyramidal tracts.

Exact duplicates of all discharges in the cerebral cortex causing voluntary movements are simultaneously transmitted to the cerebellar cortex by the nuclei pontis. The activities of the cerebellar cortex initiated in this way are immediately relayed to the dentate nucleus and from there via the superior cerebellar peduncles (brachia conjunctiva) to the thalamus and back to the cerebral cortex. This feedback circuit regulates the fine tuning and precision of voluntary movements. As the pontocerebellar fibers cross the base of the pons, they divide the corticospinal tracts into numerous small fascicles (see Fig. 3.**48**). Near the medulla oblongata the fascicles unite again and form the rather compact pyramids.

The structure of the *tegmentum* of the pons is similar to that of the medulla. The medial lemniscus at this point is a transverse band of ascending fibers spread out along the ventral border of the tegmentum (see Figs. 3.**48** and 3.**50c**). Because of its 90° rotation, the fibers coming from the cuneate nucleus are now located medially and those from the nucleus gracilis laterally. Thus, the somatotopic arrangement from leg to trunk to arm to neck extends at this point in a lateral-to-medial direction. The lateral spinothalamic tract and the auditory lateral lemniscus are located farther laterally. The lateral lemniscus is the rostral extension of the trapezoid body in the lower part of the pons (Figs. 3.**48a** and 3.**50c**). This body represents the crossing of the axons originating in the cochlear nuclei. The lateral lemniscus carries crossed and some uncrossed auditory fibers to the inferior colliculi (see Fig. 3.**36b**). The vestibular nuclear complex has the most lateral location, near the floor of the fourth ventricle. The lateral vestibular nucleus gives origin to the vestibulospinal tract. As do the other three vestibular nuclei, it communicates with somatomotor and visceromotor nuclei of the brainstem via the medial longitudinal fasciculis (see Fig. 3.**40**).

The spinal division of the trigeminal nerve terminates in the middle third of the pons. Rostrally, the principal sensory nucleus follows. Ventrolateral to it is the nucleus of the trigeminal motor root for the innervation of the masticatory muscles. The neurons of the spinal trigeminal nucleus (pain and temperature) and those of the principal sensory nucleus (*epicritic sensitivity*) form the ventral trigeminothalamic tract, which crosses on its way to the thalamus. Some fibers of the principal nucleus proceed uncrossed via the dorsal trigeminothalamic tract. The nucleus of the mesencephalic division of the trigeminal nerve extends rostrally into the midbrain. Its sensory neurons form a single line around the periaqueductal gray matter. This nucleus differs from the other trigeminal nuclei in that its neurons, although located in the midbrain, are first neurons and correspond to the first neurons of the other two trigeminal nuclei, located in the gasserian ganglion. The afferent fibers of these mesencephalic neurons are attached to receptors in masticatory muscles and mandibular joints and transmit proprioceptive impulses.

Mesencephalon (Midbrain)

The midbrain is the thinnest (about 1.5 cm), most rostral part of the brainstem. On cross-section (see Fig. 3.**48**) it can be subdivided into four parts:

1. the tectum, the most dorsal part, represented by the quadrigeminal plate; its ventral border is an imaginary transverse line across the aqueduct
2. the tegmentum, located between the substantia nigra and tectum
3. the substantia nigra
4. the cerebral peduncles or crura cerebri

The lamina quadrigemina consists of two superior and two inferior colliculi. These colliculi are very differentiated, seven-layered grisea, which have numerous afferent and efferent connections. They are described in a cursory way only.

The inferior colliculi constitute relay stations for numerous fibers of the auditory pathway, the lateral lemniscus (see Figs. 3.**49** and 3.**50**). These auditory fibers continue over the brachia of the inferior colliculi to the medial geniculate body and from there to the auditory cortex of the temporal lobe in the sylvian fissure (transverse convolutions; Heschl's gyrus).

The nuclei of the superior colliculi receive fibers of the optic tract and from the occipital cortex, the spinal cord (spinotectal tract), and the inferior colliculi. The superior colliculi send out fibers to the spinal cord (tectospinal tract), cranial nerve nuclei (tectonuclear tract), the red nucleus, and the reticular formation.

The connections between the inferior and superior colliculi are part of a reflex arc responsible for turning the eyes and head in the direction of a noise. Retinal fibers that enter the superior colliculi via the lateral geniculate body are part of a reflex arc that closes the eyes and possibly averts the head upon presentation of a sudden visual stimulus. The tectonuclear and tectospinal tracts are important in this reflex.

The pretectal nuclei, consisting of two small groups of neurons, are located within the tectum rostrolateral to the superior colliculi. They are relay stations for fibers that come from the retina, circle around the periaqueductal gray matter, and terminate at the parasympathetic Edinger-Westphal nuclei. These nuclei are part of a reflex arc that widens or narrows the pupils in response to the intensity of light.

The *red nuclei* occupy the center of each half of the tegmentum. Their color is caused in part by their dense capillary network and in part by their iron content. The caudal half of each nucleus is magnicellular; the rostral half is parvicellular. Afferent impulses come from the cerebellar emboliform and dentate nuclei via the *superior cerebellar peduncles (brachia conjunctiva)*. The fibers that originate from the phylogenetically older emboliform nucleus are part of reflex arcs that help control posture and motion. The fibers coming from the dentate nuclei, which are particularly well developed in man, are part of cerebellar reflex arcs that connect with the cerebral cortex via the thalamus and control the smooth and precise performance of voluntary movements. Many of these fibers terminate in the parvicellular portion of the red nucleus. All cerebellorubral fibers cross in the decussation of the brachia conjunctiva in the lower midbrain. Other afferent impulses that reach the red nucleus come from the cerebral cortex (corticorubral tract) and the tectum of the midbrain. All impulses received by the red nucleus become efferent via the rubrospinal and rubroreticular pathways, which influence the spinal motoneurons. Both tracts cross early in the ventral tegmental (Forel's) decussation. In addition, rubroolivary efferent fibers in the central tegmental tract report back to the cerebellum.

The mesencephalic *trigeminal tract*, the *medial* and *trigeminal lemnisci*, and the *spinothalamic tract* occupy the lateral portion of the tegmentum. The nuclei of the *trochlear nerves* are located in front of the periaqueductal gray matter of the lower midbrain on either side of the midline. The axons of the nerve cells swing around the periaqueductal gray matter and cross in the tectum behind the inferior colliculi. As the only cranial nerves, the trochlear nerves cross and emerge thereafter at the dorsal aspect of the tectum. They then encircle the lower midbrain from behind and run beneath the rim of the tentorium to the cavernous sinuses.

The nuclei of the *oculomotor nerves* and their accessory parasympathetic Edinger-Westphal and Perlia's nuclei are situated in front of the periaqueductal gray matter at the level of the superior colliculi. They are located on either side of the midline and medially from the medial longitudinal fascicles.

Before leaving the midbrain, in the interpeduncular fossa, the fibers of the nerves swing around and partially through the red nuclei.

The *medial longitudinal fasciculus* constitutes a collection of various fiber systems that carry impulses from the vestibular nuclei. The bundle descends to the spinal cord and upward through pons and midbrain near the midline, beneath the floor of the fourth ventricle and ventrally to the central periaqueductal gray matter. Some of the fibers terminate in the nuclei of abducens, trochlear, and oculomotor nerves and connect them. These fibers also connect with nuclei of the reticular formation (interstitial Cajal's nucleus and Darkschewitsch's nucleus).

The *central sympathetic tract* probably has its origin in nuclei of the hypothalamus and in the reticular formation. In the midbrain and pons, it passes close to the aqueduct and the floor of the fourth ventricle. In the medulla oblongata it occupies the lateral portion. From there it continues to the lateral horns of the spinal cord. Interruption causes Horner's syndrome.

The *substantia nigra* is a large motor territory located between the tegmentum and the cerebral peduncle (crus cerebri). Its dark color is caused by the melanin pigment in its neurons, which accumulates gradually during childhood and adolescence. The substantia nigra is part of the extrapyramidal motor system, which will be discussed later in detail (page 226).

The *cerebral peduncles* are made up almost solely of descending pathways: corticospinal or pyramidal, corticonuclear, and corticopontine tracts (see Figs. 2.**8** and 3.**48**). After passing through the internal capsule, these fiber bundles converge immediately to form the peduncles. The corticospinal and corticonuclear fibers are bordered on both sides by corticopontine fibers (see Fig. 3.**48**).

The *reticular formation* pervades the tegmentum of the entire brainstem and fills the spaces between cranial nerve nuclei and olivary bodies and between ascending and descending fiber tracts with groups of neurons and axons (Fig. 3.**51a**; see Figs. 3.**46** and 3.**48**). Its neurons receive afferent impulses from the spinal cord, cranial nerve nuclei, cerebellum, and cerebrum. They send efferent impulses to the same structures. One group of reticular nuclei influences spinal motor action as well as autonomic functions via descending fibers. Other nuclei of the reticular formation, particularly those located in the midbrain, project to more rostrally located centers, mainly via intralaminar nuclei of the thalamus and, more directly, via the subthalamus. These nuclei receive collaterals from various ascending fiber groups (spinothalamic tract, spinal trigeminal tract, nucleus of the solitary tract, vestibular and cochlear nuclei, and optic and olfactory systems). They transmit various impulses polysynaptically to widespread areas of the cerebral cortex, where they have an activating effect. Stimulation of these reticular nuclei in a sleeping animal causes awakening. Based on investigations by Moruzzi and Magoun (1949) and numerous other authors, it is now believed that in man this division of the reticular system is important for maintaining the *state of consciousness*, the state of *attentive alertness*, and the rhythm of *wakefulness and sleep*. This division is called the *ascending reticular activating system*. If it is damaged, disorders of consciousness to the degree of total loss of consciousness or coma will result. There are, however, still some unanswered questions; it may be assumed without doubt that more than one area of the brain is involved in producing unconsciousness.

The descending reticular pathways (ventral and lateral reticulospinal tracts) originate in nuclei that have an activating (facilitory) as well as an inhibitory effect on the spinal motor neurons. These nuclei are influenced by the cerebral cortex, particularly the frontal cortex, by the cerebellum, and by the basal ganglia. They are part of the extrapyramidal system. The *activating* impulses originate in the lateral portions of the reticular forma-

3 Brainstem

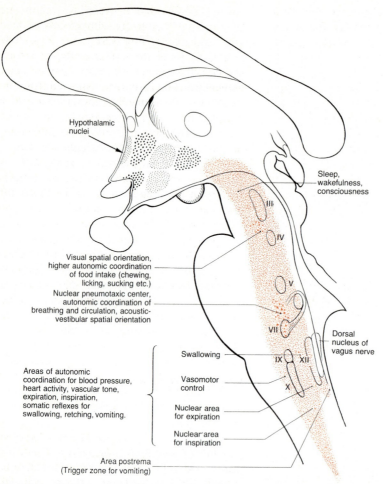

Fig. 3.51a Reticular formation. Its most important regulatory centers in medulla oblongata, pons, and midbrain.

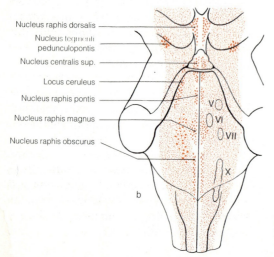

Fig. 3.51b Reticular formation. View from dorsal showing the rapheal nuclei.

tion, mainly in those of pons and midbrain. They are transmitted via the reticulospinal and vestibulospinal tracts in the anterior lateral funiculus of the spinal cord. The *inhibitory* impulses come from reticular nuclei in the ventromedial portion of the medulla oblongata. They are transmitted polysynaptically to the spinal motor neurons over the lateral reticulospinal tract, located near the corticospinal pathways. Both the facilitory and the inhibitory systems use intercalated neurons to send their impulses to gamma cells. The reticular formation plays a large role in keeping muscle tone adequate for walking, standing, and maintaining equilibrium, because of its influence on the spinal reflex arcs.

Many neurons of the reticular formation have *autonomic* functions. These neurons are scattered throughout pons and medulla, which explains their close connections with somatic cranial nerve nuclei (see Fig. 3.**51a**). These autonomic neurons receive impulses from the hypothalamus and transmit them to cranial as well as spinal nerves.

Salivation is controlled by the superior and inferior salivatory nuclei. As was mentioned earlier, a flow of saliva may be triggered by reflex upon tasting or smelling. Salivation may cease, however, and the mouth become dry purely as a result of emotions. Salivation also stops as soon as a person falls asleep.

Neurons of other reticular nuclei *control blood pressure*. The carotid sinus sends out afferent impulses over the glossopharyngeal and vagus nerves to these nuclei in the medulla oblongata (autonomic centers for blood pressure, cardiac activity, and width of blood vessels), which are located in the vicinity of the nuclei of IX and X. Efferent impulses from the vagus nerve inhibit the heart and the pulse rate. Other impulses travel over the spinal cord and inhibit groups of neurons in the sympathetic system, controlling the width of the blood vessels. Consequently, vasodilation occurs. Reticular nuclei dorsal to the inferior olives control respiration; there is a center for expiration and another for inspiration. Other reticular nuclei control or coordinate the movement of the intestines. Swallowing is a complicated reflex process. The various muscles participating in this act must be innervated in the proper strength and sequence if food is to be transported from the mouth to the stomach. A *swallowing center* near motor nuclei of cranial nerves in the medulla oblongata is in charge of coordinating the activity of various nerves innervating the muscles participating in swallowing. A center for *retching* exists in the same area. In or near the *area postrema* is the center for *vomiting*. The *locus coeruleus* in the tegmentum of the rostral pons appears to coordinate respiration and circulation (*pneumotactic nuclei*). The midbrain contains an area of higher order for the oral movements concerned with the uptake of food, such as chewing, licking, and sucking (see Fig. 3.**51a**).

Blood Supply of the Brainstem

Arteries

The two *vertebral arteries* are the chief suppliers of blood for brainstem, cerebellum, and upper cervical cord. They are the first branches of the subclavian arteries, originating at the level of the upper margin of the first ribs. On their way to the transverse processes of the seventh cervical vertebra, they are located behind the internal jugular veins, the vertebral veins, the sympathetic tracts, and the inferior cervical sympathetic ganglia. The fibers of these ganglia accompany the arteries that ascend further through the transverse foramina of the rostral six cervical vertebrae. Thereupon, they wind around the massa lateralis of the atlas and pierce the posterior atlanto-occipital membrane (see Fig. 8.**33**). The arteries enter the posterior cranial fossa on either side of the medulla oblongata and converge in front of the pyramids to form the basilar artery in front of the pontomedullary junction (Fig. 3.**52**).

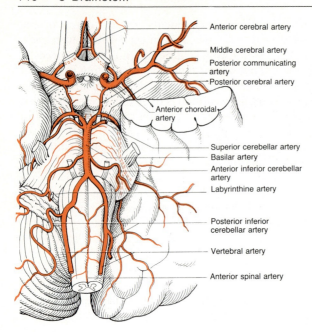

Fig. 3.**52** Arterial supply of brainstem (basal view).

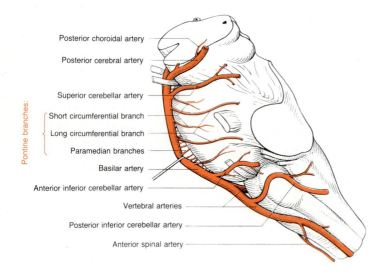

Fig. 3.**53** Arterial supply of brainstem (lateral view).

The *vertebral arteries* give off the following branches within the cranium before forming the basilar artery:

1. Descending branches that form the anterior spinal artery.
2. Descending posterior spinal arteries.
3. The paramedial and lateral fossa arteries of the medulla oblongata, supplying the paramedian and middle thirds of each half of the medulla, respectively. (These arteries may derive from the basilar or inferior anterior cerebellar artery.)

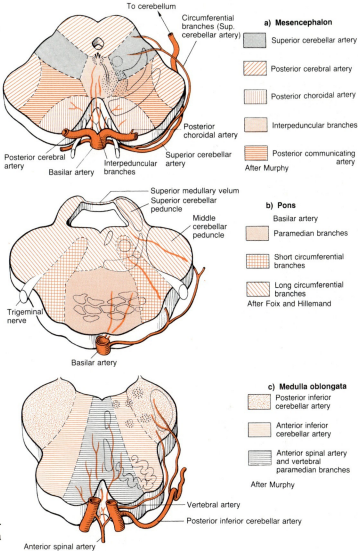

Fig. 3.54 Arterial supply territories with brainstem. **a** mesencephalon, **b** pons, **c** medulla oblongata

4. The inferior posterior cerebellar arteries. The first branches of these arteries supply the dorsolateral thirds of the medulla oblongata (see Fig. 3.54c).

The *basilar artery* is the principal supplier of the pons, giving off to each half of the pons paramedian as well as short and long circumferential branches (Figs. 3.53 and 3.54b). The paramedian branches of the rostral basilar artery enter the floor of the interpeduncular fossa and supply not only the uppermost base of the pons on either side of the midline but also the paramedian parts of the upper half of the pontine tegmentum by descending through the *rostral foramen cecum* at the end of the interpeduncular fossa. Similarly, paramedian branches extending from the caudal basilar artery at the junction of the vertebral arteries turn around the caudal base of the pons and enter the caudal foramen cecum, i.e. the rostral dead end of the medial longitudinal fissure between the pyramids. These branches supply the paramedian portion of the tegmentum of the caudal half of the pons. The lateral two-thirds of base and tegmentum are supplied by pairs of short and long circumferential branches.

The *anterior inferior cerebellar artery* descends from the caudal half of the basilar artery. Before supplying cerebellar structures, it gives off branches to the middle third of each side of the rostral medulla oblongata and to the base of the pons near the medulla (Fig. 3.**54c**; see Fig. 3.**53**). In most cases it gives rise also to the labyrinthine or internal auditory artery, which proceeds through the internal auditory canal to supply the inner ear. Occasionally the artery is a branch of the inferior posterior cerebellar artery or of the basilar artery itself. An obstruction of this artery produces *deafness*.

The *superior cerebellar artery* descends from the basilar artery just before it divides into the two posterior cerebral arteries. On its course to the cerebellum, it follows the pontomesencephalic junction into the rostral pontocerebellar fissure. After looping once or twice, it emerges from the fissure along the rostral margin of the cerebellum. Within the fissure it gives off branches to the superior cerebellar peduncle (brachium conjunctivum), where it passes through the tegmentum of the rostral pons. Other small branches supply the inferior colliculi of the quadrigeminal plate and the dorsolateral tegmentum of the lower midbrain. This is illustrated in Fig. 3.**54a**, which also shows the other territories supplied by the posterior communicating artery and by stem and branches (interpeduncular, posterior choroid) of the posterior cerebral artery. Because the arteries mentioned are subject to some variation, the supply territories shown are likely to differ somewhat from case to case. Anastomoses may very well be the cause of overlapping or variation of the territories.

Correspondingly, clinical syndromes can be expected to vary along with differences in the extent of ischemic lesions stemming from stenosis, embolism or thrombosis.

Veins

The veins of the brainstem form a rich network of anastomoses. Those of the medulla oblongata, including veins of the wall of the fourth ventricle, communicate with veins of the rostral spinal cord and with the caudal cerebellar veins, which drain into the transverse sinus or superior petrosal sinus together with veins of the lower pons. Veins of the medulla oblongata also connect with the venae flocculares, which collect blood from the ventral portion of the cerebellum and drain into the superior or inferior petrosal sinuses. Veins of the ventral portion of the pons connect with veins in the interpeduncular fossa of the midbrain, which drain via the basal veins of Rosenthal into the great vein of Galen. Veins of the lateral portion of the pons form collecting veins that run rostrally within the lateral sulci of the midbrain and also communicate with the basal veins as they pass around the midbrain, as do the rostromedial cerebellar veins and the veins of the midbrain (Figs. 8.**49**, 8.**50**, and 8.**51**).

Syndromes Caused by Circulatory Disorders

Syndromes related to *vertebrobasilar insufficiency* and *impaction of tentorium and foramen magnum* are discussed in the section on the cerebral circulatory system (page 291). Here, focal brainstem syndromes that have been described in the literature are of interest.

All these syndromes are the result of local infarcts, occurring always in certain preferred areas and destroying particular nuclei and pathways. These syndromes, some of which carry names, are illustrated in Fig. 3.**55** through 3.**63**. Infarcts habitually vary in size. Therefore, the syndromes often vary depending on which additional structures are damaged. In order to help the reader understand variations of each syndrome, the names of the structures involved inside and outside each lesion and the corresponding symptomatology are provided in each figure. The lesions used as examples are arbitrarily outlined by circles.

Fig. 3.55. *Syndromes of three lesions producing contralateral hemiplegia.* The three lesions indicated by black circles have in common that they interrupt one pyramidal tract, resulting in a contralateral spastic hemiplegia. Each lesion damages additional structures near the pyramidal tract (III, VII, XII). The signs produced by the failure of these structures permit diagnosis of the level of each lesion within the brainstem, that is, whether the lesion is in midbrain, pons, or medulla oblongata.

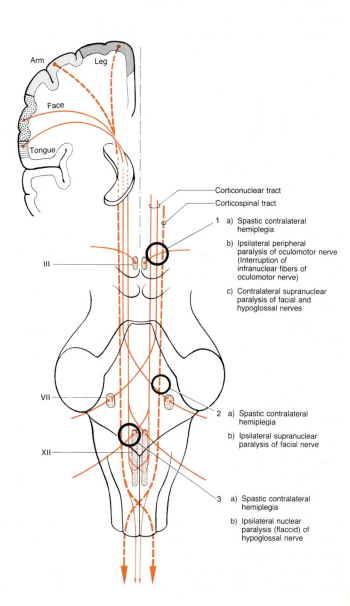

Fig. 3.55 Three brainstem lesions causing spastic contralateral hemiplegia. Additional signs permit specific topical diagnosis.

3 Brainstem

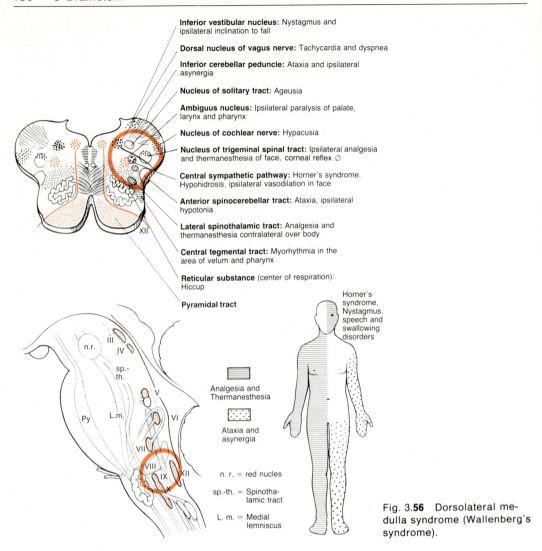

Fig. 3.56 Dorsolateral medulla syndrome (Wallenberg's syndrome).

Fig. 3.56. *Dorsolateral medulla oblongata (Wallenberg's) syndrome.* The most frequent cause is obstruction of the inferior posterior cerebellar artery or of the vertebral artery. Symptomatology: sudden onset with vertigo, nystagmus (inferior vestibular nucleus and inferior cerebellar peduncle), nausea and vomiting (reticular formation, area postrema), dysarthria and dysphonia (nucleus ambiguus), and singultus (respiratory center in the reticular formation).

Fig. 3.57. *Medial medulla oblongata (Dejerine's) syndrome.* Cause: usually obstruction of the paramedian branches of the vertebral or basilar artery. The lesion is occasionally bilateral. Symptomatology: ipsilateral flaccid paralysis of hypoglossal nerve; contralateral hemiplegia (not spastic) with positive Babinski's sign; contralateral posterior tract hypesthesia for touch, vibration, and position sensation; nystagmus if lesion extends to medial longitudinal bundle.

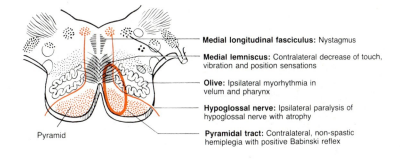

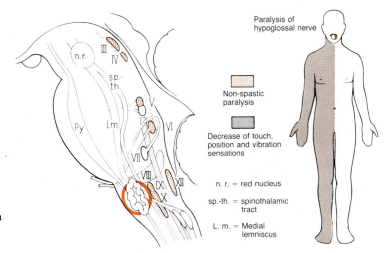

Fig. 3.57 Medial oblongata syndrome. (Dejerine's syndrome.)

Fig. 3.58. *Ventrocaudal pons (Millard-Gubler or Foville's) syndrome.* Cause: obstruction of circumferential branches of basilar artery. Symptomatology: ipsilateral paralysis of abducens nerve (peripheral) and facial nerve (nuclear), contralateral hemiplegia, analgesia, thermanesthesia, and hypoesthesia for touch, vibration, and position sensation.

Fig. 3.59. *Syndromes of caudal pontine tegmentum.* Cause: obstruction of short and long circumferential branches of the basilar artery. Symptomatology: ipsilateral nuclear paralysis of abducens and facial nerves; nystagmus (medial longitudinal bundle); inability to look to the side of the lesion; ipsilateral hemiataxia and asynergia (middle cerebellar peduncle); contralateral analgesia and thermanesthesia (lateral spinothalamic tract); hypesthesia for touch, vibration, and position sensation (medial lemniscus); ipsilateral myorhythmias of soft palate and pharynx (central tegmental tract).

Fig. 3.60. *Syndrome of rostral pontine tegmentum.* Cause: obstruction of long circumferential branches of basilar artery, seldom of superior cerebellar artery. Symptomatology: ipsilateral sensory loss in face (interruption of all fibers of the trigeminal nerve), ipsilateral paralysis of muscles of mastication (trigeminal motor nucleus), hemiataxia, intention tremor, adiadochokinesia (superior cerebellar peduncle), sensory loss for all qualities over contralateral portion of body except face.

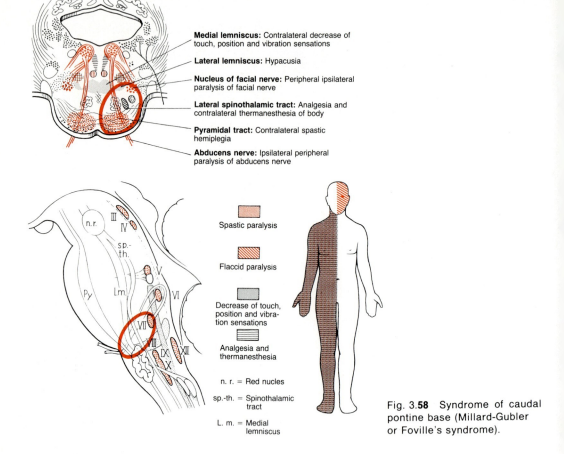

Fig. 3.58 Syndrome of caudal pontine base (Millard-Gubler or Foville's syndrome).

Fig. 3.61. *Syndrome of midpontine base.* Cause: obstruction of paramedian and short circumferential branches of the basilar artery. Symptomatology: ipsilateral flaccid paralysis of masticatory muscles, ipsilateral hypesthesia as well as analgesia and thermanesthesia of face, ipsilateral hemiataxia and asynergia, contralateral spastic hemiparalysis.

Fig. 3.62. *Red nucleus (Benedikt) syndrome.* Cause: obstruction of interpeduncular branches of basilar or posterior cerebral artery or both. Symptomatology: ipsilateral paralysis of oculomotor nerve associated with mydriasis (interruption of root fibers of III within midbrain); contralateral hypesthesia for touch, vibration, position, and discrimination (damage to medial lemniscus); contralateral hyperkinesia (tremor, chorea, athetosis) caused by damage to red nucleus; contralateral rigor (substantia nigra).

Fig. 3.63. *Cerebral peduncle (Weber) syndrome.* Cause: obstruction of interpeduncular branches of posterior cerbral artery or posterior choroid artery, or both. Symptomatology: ipsilateral paralysis of oculomotor nerve, contralateral spastic hemiparalysis, contralateral rigor (parkinsonism, substantia nigra), contralateral dystaxia (corticopontine tract); possibility of cranial nerve involvement caused by interruption of supranuclear pathways to VII, IX, X, and XII.

Blood Supply of the Brainstem 153

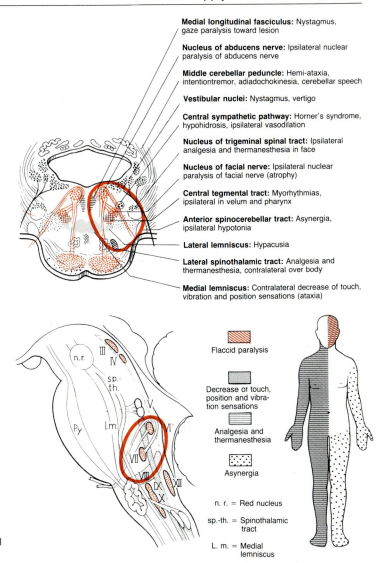

Fig. 3.59 Syndrome of caudal pontine tegmentum.

Fig. 3.64. *Miniature infarcts of base of pons syndrome.* Cause: multiple, small, and usually old cystic infarcts in one or both halves of the base in the presence of arteriosclerosis of the basilar artery which may be associated with diabetes mellitus. Symptomatology: pseudobulbar paralysis with articulation and swallowing disorders caused by interruption of supranuclear fibers of cranial motor nerves.

There are usually additional ischemic lesions in the cerebral hemispheres, quite often in the basal ganglia.

Fig. 3.65. *Pontine apoplexy syndrome.* Cause: rapidly expanding hematoma of arterial origin with tendency to rupture into the fourth ventricle resulting from hypertensive vascular disease or rupture of an arterio-

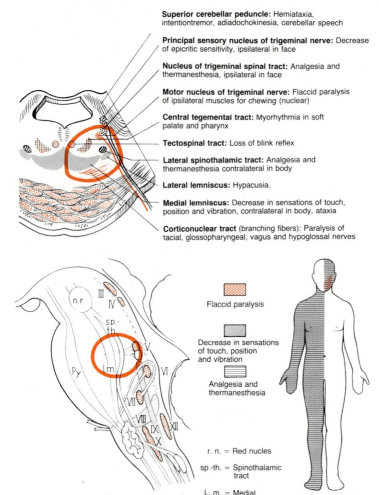

Fig. 3.60 Syndrome of rostral pontine tegmentum.

venous angioma. Symptomatology: apoplectiform onset of hemiplegia or tetraplegia, disorder of respiration, increase in systemic blood pressure, central hyperthermia. Rupture into the ventricle produces decerebrate rigidity and coma. The lesion is usually fatal within 24 hours.

Diseases of the brainstem are, of course, not limited to the vascular system. There are many other pathologic conditions known to involve the brainstem acutely or gradually, such as multiple sclerosis, encephalitides, syphilis, tuberculosis, and tumor ranging from gliomas to metastases of carcinomas and sarcomas.

Syndromes Caused by Tumors

Tumors may originate outside and grow into the brainstem. For example, a pineal germinoma may grow into the midbrain and produce signs of midbrain involvement and of hypertensive internal hydrocephalus stemming from compression of the aqueduct. Other tumors may come from the cerebellum or the wall of the fourth ventricle.

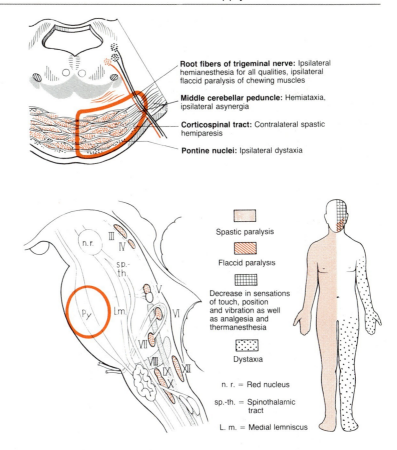

Fig. 3.61 Syndrome of midpontine base.

The most frequent intrinsic pontine tumors are the *gliomas* occurring in children and adolescents rather than in adults. The pons gradually enlarges, forcing the basilar artery to arch over its ventral surface. The first signs are usually occipital headaches and pain in the neck, associated with vomiting and vertigo. Papilledema may be absent for quite some time. Involvement of the abducens nerves may cause diplopia and a disorder of conjugate movements. Because of the longitudinal growth of the tumor, other cranial nerves may become damaged. Eventually sensory and motor disorders develop in face and extremities and are often associated with disorders of equilibrium. The life of the patient is endangered by respiratory crises and central hyperthermia. The symptomatology usually progresses slowly, which speaks against a lesion of circulatory origin. A sudden exacerbation may be caused by bleeding into the tumor or a sudden increase in intraventricular pressure when the fourth ventricle and its exits become blocked.

In rare instances a tumor, most likely a *meningioma*, may grow into the foramen magnum and compress the medulla oblongata and the rostral portion of the cervical cord. It may damage caudal cranial nerves (XI and XII) and increase the intracranial pressure, resulting in occipital headaches. Spastic signs, motor paresis, and sensory disorders may develop later. Pressure on the cervical cord and its anterior spinal artery may result in flaccid paralysis of the extremities.

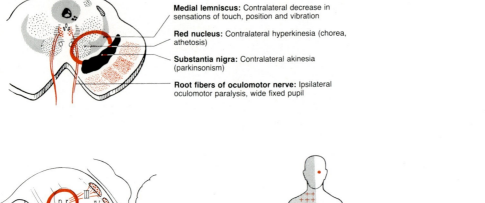

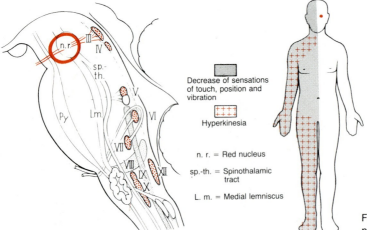

Fig. 3.62 Syndrome of lower red nucleus (Benedikt's syndrome).

Fig. 3.66. *Parinaud's or sylvian aqueduct syndrome.* Cause: a tumor, usually a *pinealoma*, presses on the superior colliculi of the midbrain, or an alteration, such as a *periaqueductal astrocytoma*, involves the pretectal region near the aqueduct (Cajal's interstitial nucleus).

This syndrome consists of a paralysis of conjugate upward movement of the eyes in the absence of paralysis of convergence. The *doll's head maneuver* is positive for vertical eye movements; in forward bending of the head, the eyes move conjugately upward reflexively. As the tumor grows into the tegmentum of the midbrain, there will be additional nuclear paresis of III with reflex pupilloplegia and paresis of IV. Compression of the aqueduct causes hypertensive hydrocephalus of lateral and third ventricles. Damage to the inferior colliculi produces hearing loss. There is a tendency to fall backward and to the opposite side.

Ataxia is caused by involvement of the superior cerebellar peduncle (brachium conjunctivum) and the cerebellum. Occasionally, tentorial herniation provokes attacks of decerebrate rigidity. As the tumor grows into the hypothalamus and third ventricle, hypothalamic symptoms may develop (diabetes insipidus and others).

Syndromes of Tentorium and Foramen Magnum Impaction

A few introductory remarks on the topography of the tentorium and its incisure are appropriate.

Blood Supply of the Brainstem

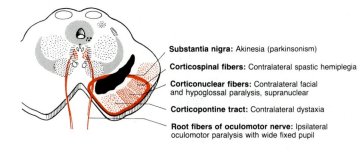

Substantia nigra: Akinesia (parkinsonism)

Corticospinal fibers: Contralateral spastic hemiplegia

Corticonuclear fibers: Contralateral facial and hypoglossal paralysis, supranuclear

Corticopontine tract: Contralateral dystaxia

Root fibers of oculomotor nerve: Ipsilateral oculomotor paralysis with wide fixed pupil

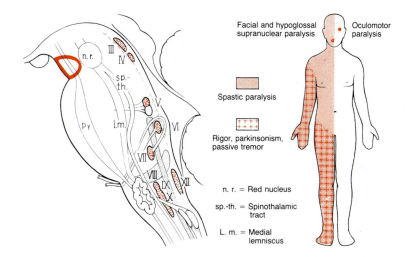

Fig. 3.**63** Syndrome of peduncle of midbrain (Weber's syndrome).

n. r. = Red nucleus
sp.-th. = Spinothalamic tract
L. m. = Medial lemniscus

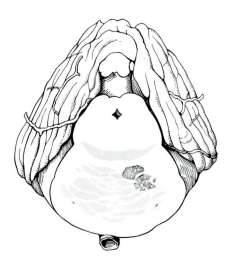

Fig. 3.**64** Focal cystic softenings in base of pons after occlusion of a short circumferential branch of the basilar artery (drawn from specimen).

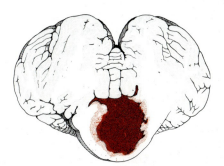

Fig. 3.**65** Pons hematoma with breakthrough into fourth ventricle (drawn from specimen).

158   3 Brainstem

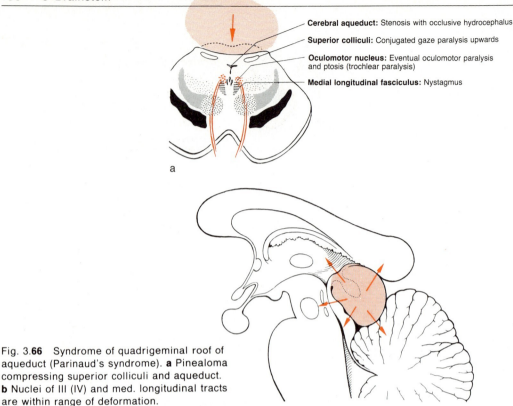

Fig. 3.66 Syndrome of quadrigeminal roof of aqueduct (Parinaud's syndrome). **a** Pinealoma compressing superior colliculi and aqueduct. **b** Nuclei of III (IV) and med. longitudinal tracts are within range of deformation.

The dural duplication called the tentorium cerebelli serves as tent-like partition between cerebellum and cerebrum. Along its periphery it is attached to the ridges of the petrous bones and the dural wall of the transverse sinuses. The top of the tent is located just beneath the splenium of the corpus callosum. Caudally and along the dorsal midline, the falx joins the tentorium, and both form the straight dural sinus that drains the blood collected by the *great vein of Galen* into the *torcular Herophili* or confluence of superior longitudinal and right and left transverse sinuses (see Figs. 8.**50** and 8.**53**).

In front of its top the tentorium has its opening or incisure, which extends rostrally as far as the body of the sphenoid bone (Fig. 3.**67**). The incisure is the passageway for the midbrain, the most rostral segment of the brainstem, for blood vessels, and for the cerebrospinal fluid as it circulates through the aqueduct of the midbrain into the fourth ventricle and from the cisterns around medulla and pons into the basal cistern, from where most of cerebrospinal fluid flows through supratentorial cisterns and smaller subarachnoid spaces to its points of resorption, the pacchionian granulations of the arachnoid (see Chapter 7).

The *basal cistern* occupies the incisure in front of the midbrain. It continues posteriorly on either side between midbrain and tentorial margin as the *cisterna ambiens*. Behind the midbrain the two cisternae ambientes join the large *cistern of the great cerebral vein* or *transverse cistern* (Fig. 7.**3**).

The basal cistern contains the posterior portion of the arterial (Willis') circle and its branches supplying hypothalamus and much

Blood Supply of the Brainstem

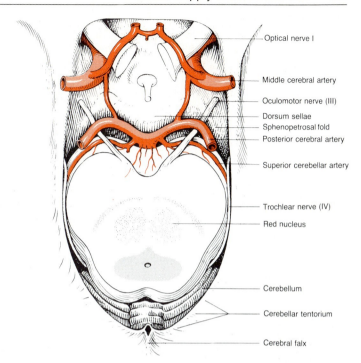

Fig. 3.**67** Topography of midbrain and associated structures within the tentorial opening (view from above).

of thalamus and midbrain, the anterior choroid arteries, the basal (Rosenthal's) veins, the pituitary stalk connecting the tuber cinereum and pituitary gland, both oculomotor nerves, and, more laterally beneath the tentorial margin, the trochlear nerves. Its dorsal wall is formed by optic chiasm and tracts, tuber cinereum, and mamillary bodies. The cisternae ambientes harbor stems and branches of the posterior cerebral arteries, the superior cerebellar arteries, the basal veins on their course to the great vein of Galen and the trochlear nerves on their way from the medullary velum to the cavernous sinuses. The transverse cistern (see Fig. 7.**3**) contains branches of the posterior cerebral arteries; the basal, internal cerebral, and occipital veins as they drain into the great cerebral vein; and the pineal gland. The culmen of the cerebellar vermis often extends into the supratentorial space and protrudes into the transverse cistern from below.

Under normal conditions the incisure of the tentorium provides ample space for unimpeded function of the structures within or near it. It becomes easily crowded and impacted, however, in the presence of a space-occupying alteration located either above or below the tentorium. Impaction from a supratentorial lesion is by far more frequent and dangerous than one from an infratentorial alteration. The supratentorial lesion, be it a tumor, an intracerebral, subdural, or extradural hematoma, or an abscess, is usually unilateral.

There may first be a displacement of brain structures across the midline, in other words, a herniation of these structures through the opening of the falx toward the other side. This may be sufficient for the shifting uncus of the ipsilateral parahippocampal gyrus to press the oculomotor nerve against the posterior sphenopetrosal fold, which the nerve crosses before it enters the cavernous sinus (Fig. 3.**67**). The parasympathetic fibers of the nerve are known to be particularly vulnerable to this pressure: the ipsilateral pupil becomes dilated after initial miosis and shows poor

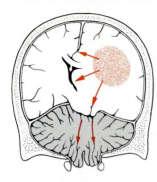

Fig. 3.**68** Space-occupying process in right cerebral hemisphere with impaction of tentorial opening and foramen magnum. (Compression of midbrain; herniation of tonsils into foramen magnum.) (After Kautzky and Zülch, Neurologisch-Neurochirurgische Röntgendiagnostik, Springer, Berlin 1955.)

and, later, no accommodation or contraction to light. Lateral displacement of the ipsilateral parahippocampal gyrus will force the midbrain across the midline toward the contralateral margin of the tentorium. This still minor disfiguration of the midbrain may lower the state of awareness of the patient and produce a purposeless restlessness.

Eventually the ipsilateral pallidum, internal capsule, and thalamus move in a caudal direction and the parahippocampal gyrus herniates over the tentorial margin toward the subtentorial space (Fig. 3.**68**). The mamillary bodies become wedged into the narrowed interpeduncular fossa. The midbrain is now under severe pressure, causing coma. The midbrain may be so severely shifted against the contralateral margin of the tentorium that the descending motor fibers in the compressed peduncle are injured (Fig. 3.**69**; Fig. 3.**70** shows normal anatomical relationships for comparison). The hemiplegia produced by the injury is not contralateral but ipsilateral to the site of the space-occupying lesion, because the injured pyramidal fibers cross further down in the lower medulla to the ipsilateral side (*crus syndrome of Kernohan*, 1929). During the caudal shift of the midbrain, the oculomotor nerve becomes endangered in a second area. This time it may be pressed upon by the stem of the posterior cerebral artery where it emerges from the interpeduncular fossa and briefly dives beneath the artery on its way through the basal cistern (see Fig. 3.**67**).

Impaction interferes with the functioning of structures of the midbrain and adjacent areas by the mechanical, distorting stress to which they are subjected and, more important, by hemorrhages and necrosis resulting from circulatory deficiencies caused by compression of blood vessels.

Compression of stem or branches of the posterior cerebral artery leads to usually hemorrhagic infarction of lower temporal and occipital cortex, often including the calcarine cortex. Pressure exerted along the tentorial margin on arteries of Ammon's horn is responsible for selective neuronal loss of neurons terminating in Ammon's horn sclerosis. Similar pressure exerted on pallidum branches of the anterior choroidal artery is the cause of infarction of the medial segment of this gray structure. Compression of the arteries entering the nervous tissue through the posterior perforated substance of the interpeduncular fossa produces thalamic lesions and, most important, edema and secondary hemorrhages and areas of necrosis in midbrain and rostral tegmentum of pons (Figs. 3.**71**). The hemorrhages usually commence in the midline of the lower midbrain. They are often erroneously referred to as *Duret's hemorrhages*. These are small, perivenous hemorrhages in the wall of the fourth ventricle which Duret had produced in dogs by blows to the unprotected dura of the parietal area.

In the presence of bilateral suptratentorial space-occupying lesions or swelling of the cerebral hemisphere, the midbrain is under pressure from both parahippocampal gyri and becomes elongated on cross-section. The interpeduncular fossa is narrow. Compression of the exit of the third ventricle and aqueduct may be responsible for increased

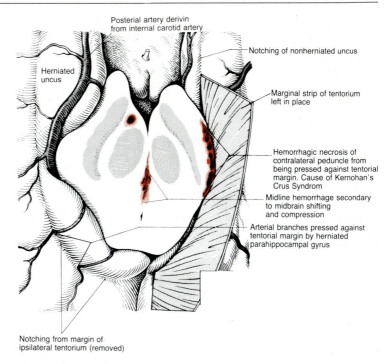

Fig. 3.**69** Severe herniation of right uncus and parahippocampal gyrus caused by subdural hematoma over right cerebral hemisphere. Wedging of mamillary bodies into narrowed interpeduncular fossa promoted secondary midline hemorrhage. Shifting of midbrain against contralateral tentorial margin caused hemorrhagic necrosis of left peduncle responsible for Kernohan's crus syndrome. (Drawn from specimens.)

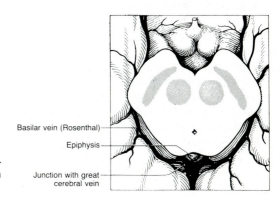

Fig. 3.**70** Normal anatomical relationships of midbrain and surrounding structures for comparison with Figure 3.**69**.

pressure of cerebrospinal fluid in lateral and third ventricles. By pressing on the chiasm the latter may produce bitemporal hemianopsia. By ballooning the tuber cinereum it may cause *diabetes insipidus* among other hypothalamic signs. If there is no caudal shift of the midbrain, secondary hemorrhages and necroses are usually absent in this structure.

If the patient does not die from central respiratory failure, he has a chance to recover from signs of tentorial impaction as the press-

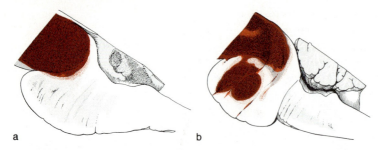

Fig. 3.**71** Hemorrhages in upper brainstem secondary to impaction of tentorial opening seen on longitudinal sections (drawn from specimen). **a** Secondary midline hemorrhages in midbrain caused by vascular compression in interpeduncular fossa. Extension into tegmentum of pons. **b** Secondary hemorrhage in midbrain and tegmentum of pons associated with hemorrhage in base on pons caused by kinking of paramedial branches of basilar artery (drawn from specimen).

ure on the midbrain recedes. Severe destruction of the midbrain by secondary changes may be survived, but the patient will remain in coma for the rest of his life.

Decerebrate Rigidity

Compression of the midbrain may produce extension spasms accompanying decerebration or decerebrate rigidity (Fig. 3.72). The head is bent backward (opisthotonus), the arms are extended and rotated inward, the hands and fingers are flexed, the legs are stretched out and rotated inward, and the feet and toes are bent in the equinovarus position. Decerebration occurs if the compression of the midbrain interrupts the passage of central inhibitory impulses that normally act on lower motor reflex arcs. In experimental animals – for example, in cats – transection of the midbrain between superior and inferior colliculi produces decerebrate rigidity and a strong hypertonia of extensor muscles of head and extremities as long as the rostral and lateral portions of the reticular formation and the nuclei of the vestibular nerves remain intact.

The most frequent unilateral space-occupying lesions that occur above the tentorium are intracerebral hematomas of natural causes (rupture of diseased arteries or of vascular malformations), swelling of a larger infarct during the first one to six days, tumors, and traumatic extradural, subdural, and intracerebral hematomas. Swelling of both cerebral hemispheres is the most common cause of bilateral compression of the midbrain. Acute shock of whatever nature is the most frequent cause of generalized brain swelling.

With space-occupying lesions in the posterior fossa, such as cerebellar hematomas (see Fig. 4.**10**), the culmen of the vermis and its

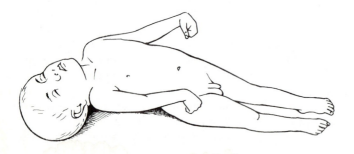

Fig. 3.**72** Decerebrate rigidity with extension spasms.

surrounding tissue may shift high up into the supratentorial space (see Fig. **4.11**). It pushes the midbrain ventrally towards the basal cistern. The oculomotor nerves are not endangered by this posterior impaction; therefore, pupillary changes described earlier as a result of pressure on the nerves are missing. Instead, there may be other disorders of oculomotion, particularly if there is also pressure on the tegmentum of the pons. There is no early unconsciousness and decerebrate rigidity. Pyramidal signs may be present and be related to an impaction of the foramen magnum by herniation of the cerebellar tonsils. As the tonsils shifts into the posterior portion of the foramen magnum, they often press the medulla oblongata against the ventral margin of the foramen magnum, exposing the pyramids to local compression. The pyramid ipsilateral to the cerebellar lesion may be subjected to more pressure than the other, and this may account for asymmetry in motor signs. In addition, there may also be hypesthesia or anesthesia on one or both sides of the body. In acute cerebellar lesions, such as hematomas, the great danger is paralysis of respiration. In contrast to the respiratory failure from midbrain compression, respiratory standstill of medullary origin is often sudden and unexpected. The patient may be responding or even be alert up to the onset of the failure. It is obvious that in the presence of a tentorium and foramen magnum impaction, a lumbar puncture is extremely risky and may, in fact, trigger a fast, fatal deterioration.

Apallic Syndrome

Apallic means lack of function of the cerebral pallium or cortex. Midbrain damage from tentorial impaction is probably responsible for the first phase of the so-called apallic syndrome. Continued deep coma after severe head injury suggests compression of the midbrain, which produces the additional signs of flexor or extensor spasms, rigidity, oculomotion, disorders, and unilateral or bilateral signs of pyramidal tract disorders.

After this phase has passed, it may take several weeks until signs of generalized cerebral damage appear. Deep coma improves to *coma vigil*, characterized by fleeting periods of wakefulness. The patient's eyes are open, but he does not react to environmental stimuli. Pyramidal and extrapyramidal signs are present: *akinesia* or *hyperkinesia* with pseudospontaneous movements, myoclonia and repetitive movements, forced grasping, postural retention, and oral reflex automatisms. Death may occur from an *autonomic crisis* with increasing blood pressure, tachycardia, respiratory disorder, hyperthermia, and profuse sweating and salivation.

If this phase is survived, improvement may follow, and the patient may gradually regain contact with the surroundings. Residual to overall brain damage, however, a severe psychoorganic syndrome usually remains, in combination with various focal neurologic signs. There will be defective recent and past memory, a weakness in concentration, a lack of initiative, changes in personality, and a regressed intelligence. Occasionally, improvement may be astonishing, however, particularly in younger patients.

It appears that one of the causes of this apallic syndrome is morphologic and functional damage to the mesencephalic reticular formation. In addition, there may be generalized damage to the white matter of the cerebral hemispheres as sequela of former swelling. After transient cardiac arrest the cerebral cortex on either side of the arterial borderzones can be expected to be injured and most severely in the parietooccipital areas because they are most remote from the heart.

4 Cerebellum

External Architecture

Cerebellum and brainstem occupy the posterior cranial fossa, which has as its roof the tentorium that separates the cerebellum from the cerebrum (see Fig. 8.53). Each substructure of the brainstem is connected with the cerebellum by pairs of peduncles. These are the *superior cerebellar peduncles* or *brachia conjunctiva* at the level of the midbrain, the *middle cerebellar peduncles* or *brachia pontis* at the level of the pons, and the *inferior cerebellar peduncles* or *corpora restiformia* at the level of the medulla oblongata.

In contrast to the surface of the cerebrum, that of the cerebellum has a rippled appearance, because all cerebellar convolutions are of the same small diameter and run parallel to each other as folia separated by rather narrow sulci (Fig. 4.1). Numerous rows of these folia are aggregated into various subdivisions, which are separated from each other by deeper fissures. The hemispheres are connected by one cortical subdivision which, because of its wormlike configuration, is known as *vermis*, an upright structure almost circular on sagittal section. Its continuity is interrupted only ventrally, by the fourth ventricle. There, the rostral end of the vermis is called the *lingula*, and the caudal end bordering the ventricle is called the *nodulus* (Fig. 4.2). The cortex of the nodules extends bilaterally into characteristic subdivisions, called *flocculi*, which are located caudolaterally from the middle and inferior cerebellar peduncles and separated from them by lateral recesses of the fourth ventricle. These recesses communicate with the subarachnoid space in the pontocerebellar angle by the *foramina of Luschka*. At the site of the foramina the choroid plexus can be seen protruding like a miniature bouquet (Bochdalek's flower basket).

Early anatomists divided hemispheres and vermis into many parts and gave them a variety of descriptive names. This partitioning of the cerebellar cortex has no functional or clinical relevance. It now appears to be sufficient to differentiate phylogenetically three major subdivisions of the cerebellum:

1. The *archicerebellum* (flocculonodular lobe). This subdivision represents the oldest portion of the cerebellum, which consists only of the *flocculi and nodules of the vermis* (see Fig. 4.2). The archicerebellum is intimately related to the vestibular system.

2. The *paleocerebellum* consists of the anterior lobe rostral to the primary fissure, including the lingula, central lobule, and culmen of the vermis, the contiguous paravermian zone bilaterally, the pyramis and uvula of the lower vermis, and the paraflocculus and the cerebellar tonsils. The paleocerebellum receives afferent impulses predominantly from spinocerebellar pathways.

3. The *neocerebellum*, also referred to as the posterior lobe, consists of all portions of vermis and hemispheres situated between the primary and posterolateral fissures. It is the largest and phylogenetically youngest portion of the cerebellum. Its development is closely related to that of the

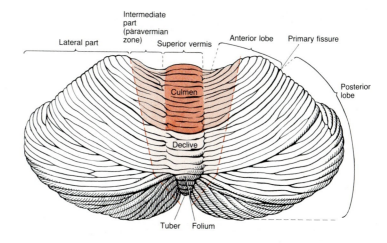

Fig. 4.1 Cerebellum (dorsal view).

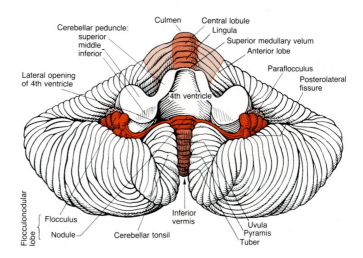

Fig. 4.2 Cerebellum (ventral view).

cerebral cortex and to the erect posture of the primates. Skilled motor movements, initiated by the cerebral motor cortex, are modified by the neocerebellum. Analogously to the development of the cerebral neocortex, the neocerebellum overshadows the older portions of the cerebellum in volume.

The three subdivisions of the cerebellum may be designated on the basis of the main source of their afferent impulses as the *vestibulocerebellum, spinocerebellum,* and *pontocerebellum.*

Internal Architecture

A few remarks on the internal structure of the cerebellum are needed prior to discussing the anatomic and functional relationships between the cerebellum and other portions of the central nervous system.

The cortex of the cerebellum consists of only three layers: the molecular layer, the Purkinje cell layer, and the granular layer (Fig. 4.3).

The *molecular layer* contains scattered small neurons (*stellate and basket cells*); dendritic arborizations of several types of cells,

4 Cerebellum

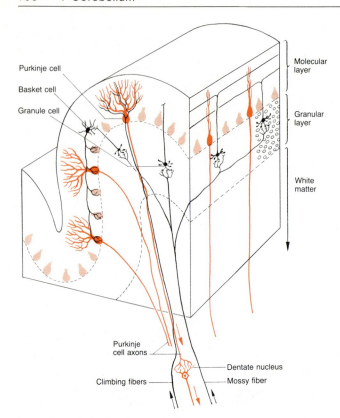

Fig. 4.3 Organization of cerebellar cortex with afferent and efferent connections.

particularly Purkinje cells; and numerous thin axons, most from the very small granule cells of the granular layer. The *Purkinje cell layer* contains only these rather large cell bodies, or perikarya, side by side in a single sheet. In contrast, the granule cells of the *granular layer* are not larger than lymphocytes and are tightly packed. Scattered in between are individual larger neurons, the *Golgi-type II cells*. The unmyelinated axons of the granule cells ascending to the molecular layer run only parallel to the longitudinal axis of each convolution or folium. In contrast, the dendrites of the Purkinje cells and of the basket cells extend only in planes perpendicularly to the longitudinal axis of each folium, in other words, parallel to the vermis (see Fig. 4.3).

The *Purkinje cells* are the only cerebellar neurons capable of transmitting efferent impulses from the cerebellar cortex. The axons originate at the base of each cell and pass through granular layer and white matter on their way to deep cerebellar nuclei. Their dendrites receive comprehensive information from various parts of the central nervous system. Some information arrives directly, and some indirectly, via relay stations; some is stimulating, whereas some is inhibiting. This information travels over fibers of different neurons. These fibers carry names such as *climbing fibers, mossy fibers, basket fibers, tangential fibers, and parallel fibers*. Mossy fibers almost exclusively transmit impulses from spinal cord and vestibular and pontine nuclei by using granule cells of the granular layer as mediators. Climbing fibers transmit impulses from the inferior olivary nuclei directly to the dendrites of the Purkinje cells.

Each cerebellar hemisphere has four paired nuclei: the *fastigial, globose, emboliform, and dentate nuclei*. Fig. 3.**48** shows these nuclei on a cross section through pons and cerebellar white matter. Fig. 4.4 illustrates their location on sagittal sections through the cerebellum.

The first three nuclei are located in the roof of the fourth ventricle. The *fastigial nucleus* is located next to the gable end of the fastigium (Latin for "roof"). It is phylogenetically the oldest of the nuclei and receives afferents from the archicerebellum—more specifically, the lobus flocculonodularis—and additional fibers from the vermis. Its efferent fibers run direct via the inferior cerebellar peduncle to the vestibular nuclei (fastigiobulbar or cerebellobulbar tracts). Numerous fibers cross to the other side of the cerebellum, loop around the contralateral superior cerebellar peduncles and reach the reticular formation and vestibular nuclei via the *uncinate bundle of Russell*.

The *globose* and *emboliform nuclei* lie slightly lateral to the fastigial nucleus. These nuclei receive afferents from the paravermian region of the paleocerebellum. Their efferents project to the contralateral red nucleus via the superior cerebellar peduncles (see Fig. 4.4).

The *dentate nucleus* is the largest of the four and is located in the central portion of the white matter of the cerebellar hemisphere. It receives impulses from the Purkinje cells of the entire neocerebellar and of part of the paleocerebellar cortex. The efferent fibers course through the superior cerebellar peduncle, cross to the opposite side at the pontomesencephalic border, and terminate in the contralateral red nucleus and in the ventrolateral nucleus (V.o.p.) of the thalamus (see Fig. 5.5). The thalamic fibers project to the primary motor cortex (Brodmann's areas 4 and 6).

All impulses entering the cerebellum terminate in the cerebellar cortex or via certain collaterals in the cerebellar nuclei. These afferents originate in cerebral cortex, in brainstem (vestibular nuclei, reticular formation, inferior olive, accessory cuneate nucleus), and in spinal cord. The *inferior cerebellar peduncle* (restiform body) constitutes the passageway of the following afferent fibers:

1. Fibers of the vestibular nerve and nucleus, terminating at the flocculonodular lobe (relayed to fastigial nucleus).
2. The olivocerebellar tract, originating in the contralateral inferior olive and terminating as climbing fibers directly at the dendrites of the Purkinje cells of the entire cerebellum.
3. The posterior spinocerebellar tract, which originates in Clarke's column (nucleus thoracicus) next to the base of the posterior horn (see Fig. 1.19). Impulses transmitted by this tract originate mainly in muscle spindles and are carried to the paravermian zone of the anterior and posterior lobes of the cerebellum. This tract consists of the fastest-conducting fibers in the entire nervous system.
4. Fibers originating in the accessory cuneate nucleus joining and adjoining those of the posterior spinocerebellar tract. These fibers transmit impulses received by the accessory cuneate nucleus from nuclei in the middle and rostral portions of the cervical cord above the level of Clarke's column; they ascend in the lateral part of the cuneate fascicle.
5. Fibers from the reticular formation of the brainstem (not shown in Fig. 4.4).

As an efferent pathway the fastigiobulbar or cerebellobulbar tract passes through the *inferior cerebellar peduncle* on its way to the vestibular nuclei. Its fibers represent the efferent limb of a vestibulocerebellar modulating feedback circuit through which the cerebellum influences spinal cord motor activity via the vestibulospinal tract and the medial longitudinal fasciculus.

The *middle cerebellar peduncle* (brachium pontis) essentially consists of masses of crossed pontocerebellar fibers. They belong to the neurons of pontine nuclei that are the second neurons of the fibers of the corticopontine tracts or bundles.

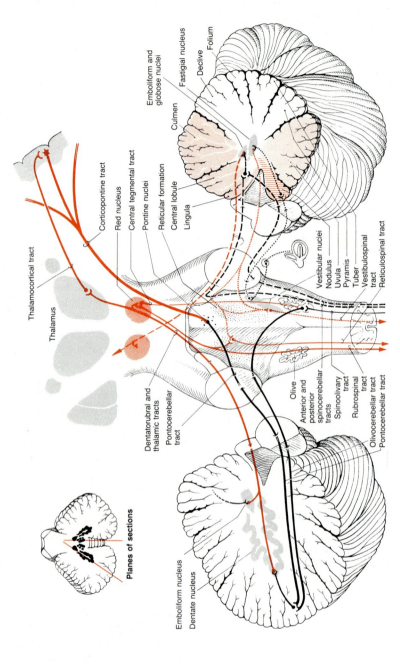

Fig. **4.4** Afferent and efferent pathways of cerebellum (left, through dentate nucleus; right, through vermis). Inset shows planes of cuts.

The *superior cerebellar peduncle* (brachium conjunctivum) contains efferent fibers originating in neurons of the dentate, emboliform, globose, and fastigial nuclei. These fibers project to the contralateral red nucleus, the ventrolateral (V.o.p.) and centromedian nucleus of the thalamus, and the reticular formation of the brainstem. Postsynaptic thalamocortical fibers project to the cortex, from where corticopontine fibers descend. In this way an important feedback loop is closed. It extends from cerebral cortex to pontine nuclei to cerebellar cortex to dentate nucleus and from here back to thalamus and cortex. (Fig. 4.5; see Fig. 4.4).

An additional feedback loop is formed by the *triangle of Guillain-Mollaret*. It extends from the red nucleus to the inferior olive via the central tegmental tract, and from there to the cerebellar cortex, to the dentate nucleus, and back to the red nucleus (Fig. 4.6). In this way the cerebellum indirectly modulates motor activity of the spinal cord by its connections with the red nucleus and the reticular formation, from which the descending

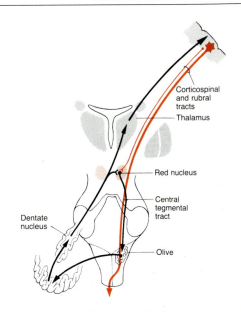

Fig. 4.6 Cerebellar feedback circuit via inferior olive for using Guillain-Mollaret triangle (red nucleus, central tegmental tract, olive, cerebellum, red nucleus).

rubrospinal and reticulospinal tracts originate. The effect of the cerebellar actions is ipsilateral because of a double decussation of the fibers within this system. Fibers deriving from the dentate nucleus cross to the contralateral red nucleus. The fibers of the descending rubrospinal tract cross again in Forel's decussation shortly after leaving the red nucleus.

The superior cerebellar peduncle contains only one *afferent* pathway, the anterior spinocerebellar tract, which terminates in the paleocerebellum, as does the posterior spinocerebellar tract. Both spinocerebellar tracts convey proprioceptive impulses from peripheral receptors, such as the muscle spindles, Golgi tendon organs, and pressure receptors. More specifically, impulses from muscle spindles are conducted predominantly by the posterior spinocerebellar tract, whereas those originating in the Golgi tendon organs are conveyed mainly by the anterior spinocerebellar tract.

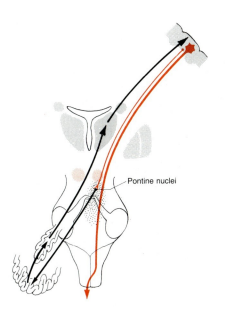

Fig. 4.5 Cerebellar feedback circuit via pontine nuclei.

The cerebellum thus receives sensory information from all parts of the central nervous system by way of three cerebellar peduncles and is connected with all motor pathways because its nuclei serve as efferent partners in regulating feedback circuits. Although the cerebellum is in contact with the cerebral cortex through the thalamocortical fibers, its activities are not accompanied by awareness. This is one of the reasons why it is difficult to determine the normal function of the cerebellum. What is known about this structure is derived from an integration of embryologic, comparative anatomic, and experimental data with clinical findings concerning circumscribed lesions in well-defined segments of the cerebellum.

Function

The cerebellum acts as a coordination center for the maintenance of equilibrium and muscle tone by being part of complex regulatory and feedback mechanisms. It also enables the somatic muscular system to accomplish discrete, skilled movements. It has been suggested that it functions like a computer in screening and coordinating its sensory inputs and modulating its motor outputs.

The *archicerebellum* receives information on the spatial position of the head from the vestibular system and on the movements of the head through kinetic impulses from receptors in the semicircular canals. These early messages enable the cerebellum to modulate synergistically the spinal motor impulses at all times, securing equilibrium, regardless of position or movement of the body.

Damage to the flocculonodular lobe results in disturbance of equilibrium and in unsteadiness in standing (*astasia*) and walking (*abasia*). The gait becomes broad-based and reeling, reminiscent of the unsteadiness of an inebriate (*truncal* or axial ataxia). The ataxia does not increase when the eyes are closed, in contrast to an ataxia caused by posterior tract disease. Cerebellar ataxia is not related to an abnormal decrease of consciously registered proprioceptive sensations but rather is the result of an inability of muscle groups to act in coordination, called *asynergia* (*flocculonodular syndrome*).

Damage to the *nodulus* abolishes reactions to caloric and rotational tests of vestibular function. Patients in whom the nodules and part of the uvula have been removed are no longer susceptible to motion sickness. Identical loss of function follows an interruption of pathways going to or leaving the flocculonodular lobe. Equilibrium is maintained by the following reflex arc: impulses originating in the labyrinth travel directly as well as indirectly over the vestibular nuclei to the archicerebellum and continue to the fastigial nucleus; from there efferent impulses return to the lateral vestibular nucleus (Deiter's) and to the reticular formation. Via the vestibulospinal and reticulospinal tracts, and via the medial longitudinal bundle the impulses reach the anterior horn cells and modify their activity. Injury to this system may lead to nystagmus but does not produce additional cerebellar signs and symptoms.

The *paleocerebellum* receives afferent impulses from the spinal cord via the anterior and posterior spinocerebellar tracts and from the accessory cuneate nucleus via the cuneocerebellar tract. Efferent impulses from the paleocerebellum modulate activity of the antigravity musculature and provide the intensity of muscle tone required for maintaining equilibrium while standing or moving. The spinal impulses project to the cortex of the paleocerebellum in a somatotopic pattern, representing in each cerebellar hemisphere the ipsilateral half of the body. The cortex of the paravermian areas projects to the emboliform and globose nuclei; the cortex of the vermis projects to the fastigial nuclei.

Efferent fibers of neurons in the deep cerebellar nuclei cross in the superior cerebellar peduncle to reach the contralateral red nucleus. The descending rubrospinal and rubroreticular tracts cross again and modulate the activity of motor neurons in brainstem and spinal cord, which are located ipsilateral to the cerebellar nuclei but contralateral to the red nucleus. Impulses ascending from the cerebellar nuclei also project to the centromedian nucleus of the thalamus and from there to caudate nucleus and putamen (striatum), thereby influencing the extrapyramidal system. The combined effect of the paleocerebellum and archicerebellum results in control of skeletal muscle tone and in smooth, synergistic coordination of agonist and antagonist muscle groups subserving normal gait and stance. Lesions of the paleocerebellum produce truncal ataxia. It is rare, however, for lesions to be limited to the paleocerebellum. For this reason, and because there is some functional overlap between paleocerebellum and neocerebellum, it is impossible in many cases to relate clinical deficits to a circumscribed area of the cerebellum.

The *neocerebellum* receives afferent impulses indirectly from extensive areas of cerebral cortex, particularly from Brodmann's motor areas 4 and 6, via the *corticopontocerebellar pathway*. It also receives a large contingent of afferent fibers from the inferior olives (*olivocerebellar tracts*), which in turn receive impulses from the red nucleus via the central tegmental tracts, as mentioned earlier (see Fig. 4.6). The cerebellum receives information on each planned voluntary movement in advance. It modifies and corrects by inhibition all pyramidal and extrapyramidal motor impulses via the *dentatothalamocortical pathway*, which terminates where the motor impulses originate (see Figs. 4.4 and 4.5).

All voluntary and involuntary movements become smooth and precise because of the related action of the neocerebellum and because the motor activities in the spinal periphery are immediately and continuously reported to the cerebellum via the extremely fast conducting spinocerebellar pathways. This information enables the cerebellum to adjust and compensate instantly inaccuracies or errors in the performance of voluntary movements. The rapidity with which the cerebellum processes its input information is probably what enables us to perform previously learned and difficult combinations of movements effortlessly whenever necessary. It is also possible that the cerebellum, acting like a computer, stores various movement patterns acquired during the course of an individual's life and keeps them available for instant retrieval. A sudden loss of cerebellar function never leads to a loss of voluntary movement; it only severely compromises the harmonious orchestration of the voluntary muscle innervation.

Signs of Neocerebellar Dysfunction

The following findings can be expected with neocerebellar disease:

1. **Ataxia:** This ataxia involves the limbs, particularly the distal extremities, and is associated with deviations of gait and stance toward the side of the lesion.
2. **Dysmetria:** The inability to gauge distance correctly, resulting in premature arrest of movement or overshooting (past pointing or hypermetria).
3. **Asynergia:** Loss of coordination in the innervation of muscle groups needed for the performance of precise movements. Individual muscle groups function independently and are incapable of complex orchestrated movement patterns (decomposition of movement).
4. **Dysdiadochokinesia:** (adiadochokinesia): Rapid alternating movements of agonist/antagonist muscles cannot be performed. Alternating movements, such as rapid pronation and supination of the hands, are slow, hesitating, and arrhythmic.
5. **Intention tremor:** An action tremor that is evident when an object is pointed at. It becomes more severe as the finger or toe approaches the object. This tremor is usually associated with damage to the dentate nucleus or superior cerebellar peduncle.
6. **Rebound phenomenon:** Caused by an inability to adjust promptly to changes in muscle tension. For example, a patient's

arm pressed against the hand of the examiner cannot immediately relax when the examiner withdraws his hand but follows the hand with an uncontrolled hitting motion.

7. **Hypotonia:** Flabbiness and rapid exhaustion (*asthenia*) of the ipsilateral musculature as a result of alterations in tonic innervation. The deep tendon reflexes tend to be sluggish and to have a reverberating quality.
8. **Scanning speech:** Asynergia of the muscles of speech results in slow, hesitant, and poorly articulated speech with inappropriate emphasis on individual syllables that cause some words to be uttered explosively.
9. **Inability to discriminate weight:** An object whose weight is being judged is always believed to be lighter when held in the hand ipsilateral to the cerebellar lesion. This phenomenon is probably related to ipsilateral hypotonia and asthenia.

It has been shown in animal experiments that specific functional deficits can be correlated with damage to certain precise cerebellar areas. In disease states of the cerebellum, however, such correlations are unusual. The cerebellum must always act in its entirety to maintain equilibrium and muscle tone during each movement or for sustaining a posture and to assure smoothness, coordination, and precision in each voluntary and involuntary movement.

Topical diagnosis of cerebellar lesions is complicated for the following reasons: (1) It is rare that lesions are limited to one specific functional area of the cerebellum. (2) Slowly progressing lesions, such as benign tumors, may produce few or no clinical symptoms for some time, because of the ability of the remaining cerebellar parenchyma to compensate for the damaged area. (3) Other portions of the brain are apparently also capable of compensating for deficits in cerebellar functions, although damage to the deep cerebellar nuclei leaves little likelihood of compensation or restitution of function.

Blood Supply of the Cerebellum

Arteries

In discussing the arteries of the brainstem (page 142), we mentioned that vertebral and basilar arteries give off three paired, larger arteries to the cerebellum: the superior, the inferior anterior, and the inferior posterior cerebellar arteries (Figs. 4.7, 4.8, and 4.9; see Figs. 3.52 and 8.34).

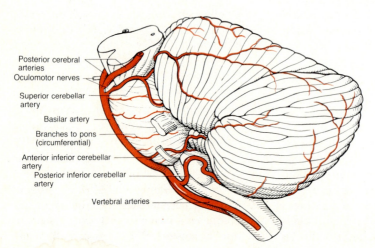

Fig. 4.7 Blood supply of cerebellum (lateral view).

Blood Supply of the Cerebellum

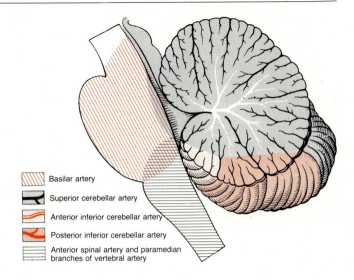

Fig. 4.8 Areas of blood supply of brainstem and cerebellum.

- Basilar artery
- Superior cerebellar artery
- Anterior inferior cerebellar artery
- Posterior inferior cerebellar artery
- Anterior spinal artery and paramedian branches of vertebral artery

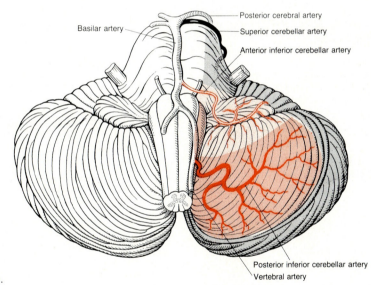

Fig. 4.9 Blood supply of cerebellum (view from below).

Superior Cerebellar Arteries

These arteries leave the rostral basilar artery shortly before it terminates by branching into the posterior cerebral arteries. They follow the pontomesencephalic junction on either side on their way into the rostral pontocerebellar fissure. Here they give off small branches to the tectum of the lower midbrain and larger branches to the superior cerebellar peduncles. These branches run opposite to the course of the peduncular fibers on their way to the cerebellar nuclei, particularly the dentate nuclei. They also supply the ventral vermis and paravermian areas on either side before they emerge from the fissure in the form of several branches that supply the rostral and rostroventral portions of both hemispheres as well as the rostral vermis. These branches, as do the branches of the other two cerebellar arteries, run over the crest of the cerebellar convolutions without looping into sulci as cerebral arteries do. Instead they give off small branches into almost every sulcus. Branches supplying the rostral vermis and the paravermian areas may at first be within the posterior portion of the tentorial incisure, depending on the individual size of this opening and the degree of normal protrusion of the vermis into the opening. Thereafter they cross the tentorial margin on their way to dorsal and lateral parts of the rostral hemispheres.

This topographic feature renders the branches vulnerable to compression during impaction of the posterior incisure by the culmen of the vermis. The result is incomplete and even complete infarction of the cortex of the rostral cerebellum and sometimes that of the rostral vermis (see Fig. 4.11).

Inferior Anterior Cerebellar Arteries

These arteries descend from the caudal half of the basilar artery in a not necessarily symmetrical fashion. Their supply territories are the smallest of the three cerebellar arteries and consist of cortex and white matter of the flocculus and adjacent ventral cerebellar convolutions. The internal auditory arteries supplying the inner ear are important branches of these arteries. Occasionally, the auditory arteries descend directly from the basilar artery.

Inferior Posterior Cerebellar Arteries

These arteries are branches of the vertebral arteries. On their way to the fissure between medulla oblongata and cerebellar tonsils, they extend a few branches to the dorsolateral medulla oblongata; these branches are involved in Wallenberg's syndrome (see Fig. 3.56). From a loop within the fissure, branches ascend to supply the caudal portions of the cerebellar nuclei and also some cortex of the inferior vermis. Thereupon the arteries divide into several branches which supply cortex and white matter of the caudal half of the cerebellum, including the tonsils.

The three cerebellar arteries are interconnected by anastomoses.

Veins

Each cerebellar hemisphere has four larger groups of veins. The first group is the rostromedial cerebellar veins, which collect blood from the rostral vermis and its vicinity and from the dentate nucleus. They terminate in the basal vein or directly in the great vein of Galen. The second group, the rostrolateral cerebellar veins, drains the rostrolateral cortex and white matter infratentorially into the transverse sinus. The third group, the caudal cerebellar veins, collects the blood of the lower portions of the hemisphere and drains into the sigmoid sinus or the superior petrosal sinus. The fourth group drains the ventral cerebellum and joins to form the venae flocculares, which connect with the superior or inferior petrosal sinus.

Circulatory Lesions

Because of the many collaterals interconnecting the cerebellar arteries, large infarct-producing cerebellar signs are rare. Small infarcts are usually not clinically apparent.

Obstruction of Superior Cerebellar Artery

Superior cerebellar artery obstruction may damage the superior cerebellar peduncle, one-half of the superior vermis, or at the least the ipsilateral paravermian area. The result may be ipsilateral ataxia with abasia and intention tremor. There also may be some signs of involvement of the mesencephalic tectum, because the artery supplies part of this structure.

Compression of Superior Cerebellar Arteries along Tentorial Margin

Fig. 4.11 shows impaction of the posterior tentorial opening caused by herniation of the

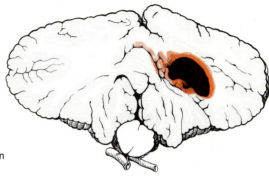

Fig. 4.10 Hematoma in cerebellum (drawn from specimen).

rostral vermis into the supratentorial space because of a space-occupying lesion in the center of the cerebellum. Such tentorial impaction also occurs in the absence of such lesions as a result of an overall swelling of the cerebellum. If there is transient systematic hypotension, the compression of the arteries along the tentorial margin may produce selective neuronal loss of Purkinje and granule cells in rostral vermis and paravermian areas, leading to ataxia, particularly of trunk and lower extremities. The ataxia is similar to that described in alcoholics, in which neuronal loss and subsequent cortical atrophy in the same area are attributed to an unknown nutritional deficiency. In both conditions there is also neuronal loss and cortical atrophy in the cerebellar tonsils or in the cortex facing the rim of the foramen magnum, indicating in both instances that the foramen magnum was also impacted (as shown in Fig. 4.10). Pressure by the tonsils may also lead to some neuronal loss in the tegmentum of the medulla oblongata and to damage to the pyramids, causing signs that may erroneously be attributed to a separate disease such as multiple sclerosis.

Cerebellar Hematoma

The branches of the superior cerebellar artery supplying the dentate nucleus are vulnerable to hypertensive vascular disease. Their calibers are similar to those of the striate body branches of the middle cerebral artery, and

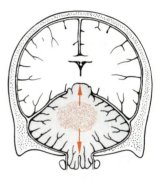

Fig. 4.11 Space-occupying effects in the posterior fossa by cerebellar lesion: impaction of tentorial opening and of foramen magnum. (After Kautzky and Zülch, Neurologisch-Neurochirurgische Röntgendiagnostik, Springer, Berlin 1955.)

they are the most frequent source of apoplectic intracerebral hematomas (Fig. 4.11), most of which occur in persons more than 50 years of age. Accompanied by edema, the bleeding reduces impaction of the tentorial opening as well as of the foramen magnum (Fig. 4.10). Rapidly increasing supratentorial pressure is caused by hypertensive hydrocephalus stemming from compression of the aqueduct, fourth ventricle, or foramen of Magendi. If not immediately diagnosed and operatively drained, such major hemorrhage is almost invariably fatal. After initial severe headaches, nausea, vomiting, and vertigo, the patient lapses into coma and experiences tonic extensor seizures, breakdown of circulatory regulation, and, finally, fatal respiratory arrest.

Smaller hematomas can be survived. They may involve only one cerebellar hemisphere and produce ipsilateral clinical signs consisting of ataxia of arm and leg, and tendencies to fall to the side of the lesion and to walk, with eyes closed, toward the side of the lesion.

Complaints concern occipital headaches, vertigo, nausea, and vomiting. If the cerebellar nuclei are severely damaged, the cerebellar sign may slowly improve but do not completely disappear. It should be pointed out that the cerebellar signs can be demonstrated only if the patient is conscious and able to perform voluntary movements.

A cerebellar hematoma is occasionally the result of rupture of an arteriovenous angioma. In rare instances an aneurysm of the inferior posterior cerebellar artery within the cerebellomedullary fissure may bleed into the cerebellum. Profuse apoplectic bleeding may also occur within a cerebellar metastasis of a carcinoma or sarcoma. The metastasis may be so small that it produced no signs or symptoms.

Cerebellar Tumors

Intrinsic tumors follow the circulatory alterations just described in frequency of occurrence. They are rarely limited to a specific area of a cerebellar hemisphere and usually involve adjacent and even more remote areas by invading or displacing and compressing them. Slow-growing tumors are insidious. They may produce no signs for quite some time because of the ability of the still intact cerebellum to compensate for deficits stemming from the damage inflicted to one or another of its segments. Therefore, when cerebellar signs and symptoms first appear, the tumor is often much larger than expected. The patient may complain only of some unsteadiness while standing or walking and a tendency to sway or deviate to one particular side. A slight unsteadiness may be found upon performing the Romberg's test, and also when asking the patient to walk by putting one foot in front of the other along a line (tightrope dancers's walk). Nystagmus may or may not be present. Papilledema usually has not yet appeared. In general, patients do not consult a physician until occipital headaches become severe and are associated with vomiting. At that time the tumor may already be too large to be removed at operation without considerable risk.

It is always good practice to assume the presence of a slow-growing cerebellar tumor and to initiate diagnostic procedures (such as computer tomography and angiography) if unsteadiness in gait and stance have existed for some time, even if other cerebellar signs and evidence of increased intracranial pressure are absent.

Two intrinsic tumors occur most often in childhood or adolescence. They are the cerebellar astrocytoma and the medulloblastoma.

Cerebellar Astrocytoma

This tumor may develop as a rather solid tumor mass in one hemisphere, in the vermis, or in the wall of the fourth ventricle with main extensions into ventricle and main pressure exerted on the tegmentum of the pons. It usually does not infiltrate surrounding tissues as do astrocytomas of the cerebrum. In fact, the tumor may remain relatively small and may be surrounded by a huge, smoothwalled cyst that contains clear or stained, and somewhat gelatinous fluid. In such a case it is not the tumor but the surrounding cyst that is the space-occupying lesion. Expansion of the cyst may be the cause of signs.

Medulloblastoma

This malignant tumor occurs only in the cerebellum. When it develops in childhood, the vermis and the flocculonodular lobe are its preferred site. Consequently, the child walks with a broad-based gait, staggering and swaying from one side to the other. Only when the tumor grows into the hemispheres or compresses them do other cerebellar signs and symptoms, such as ataxia, dysmetria, asynergy, adiadochokinesia, intention tremor, hypotonia, and finally nystagmus, gradually develop. Growth of the tumor into the cerebellar peduncles and from there into the brainstem produces additional cranial nerve deficits. Obliteration of the aqueduct, fourth ventricle, or foramen of Magendi complicates the clinical situation by causing increased intracranial pressure from a noncommunicating hypertensive hydrocephalus. The medulloblastoma tends to spread throughout the subarachnoid space and may extend over the cerebrum as well as along the spinal cord. In young adults it usually commences in one of the hemispheres, not at the midline.

Angioblastoma (Lindau's Disease)

This usually nodular tumor consists of capillaries, is benign in its growth, and is usually seen in young and middle-aged adults. It is of diagnostic interest that this tumor is often associated with angiomatosis of the retina (Hippel's disease). The condition called Lindau–von Hippel disease is often accompanied by capillary nevi in skin, multiple cysts in kidneys and pancreas, and occasionally a renal cell carcinoma, which may metastasize. A combination of cerebellar hemangioblastoma and pheochromocytoma also has been reported. Occasionally, the tumor grows to a large, space-occupying size. In about 60 percent of the cases, however, the tumor is small and is attached as a seemingly hemorrhagic nodule to the wall of a large, well-defined cyst which accounts for whatever signs are present. Symptoms are usually mild and may consist primarily of pain in the neck and occipital region, a result of an increase in intracranial pressure. It is of diagnostic interest that capillary hemangioblastomas are known to be associated with erythrocythemia. After resection of the neoplasm, the number of erythrocytes returns to normal but increases with recurrence of the tumor.

Metastatic tumors

Only rarely is the clinical pattern of a cerebellar tumor caused by a metastasis. In most instances additional metastases are present within the cerebrum and produce signs so impressive that cerebellar signs are easily overlooked. Figs. 4.12 and 4.13 illustrate the cerebellar metastases found at postmortem examination in two instances. Despite the large size of these metastases cerebellar involvement was not diagnosed, because the clinical findings were dominated by paralysis and aphasia caused by cerebral metastases. If, however, an elderly person relatively quickly and convincingly develops the symptoms of a cerebellar space-occupying lesion, a metastasis is to be considered the most likely cause. Roentgenography of the lung may support the tentative diagnosis.

Acoustic Neurinoma

Tumors originating outside the cerebellum may also be the cause of cerebellar signs. One of these tumors is a neurinoma or schwannoma of the acoustic nerve (VIII); the other is an ependymoma originating in the wall of the fourth ventricle.

An acoustic neurinoma, shown in Figs. 4.14 and 8.32, usually derives from the Schwann cells of the vestibular portion of cranial nerve VIII and occupies the pontocerebellar angle. It may slowly grow to consider-

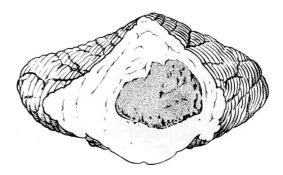

Fig. 4.12 Metastasis of a thyroid carcinoma (drawn from specimen).

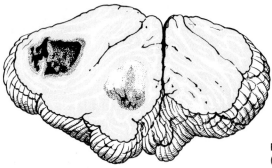

Fig. 4.13 Metastases of a bronchial carcinoma (drawn from specimen).

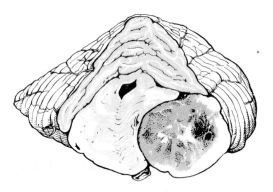

Fig. 4.14 Acoustic neurinoma in pontocerebellar angle (drawn from specimen).

able size, compressing pons, medulla oblongata, cerebellum, and adjacent cranial nerves. It grows into the internal auditory canal like a plug, gradually widening the entrance so much that its distension can be seen on roentgenographic examination.

The first sign of this tumor is usually deafness. The patient may not be aware of the hearing loss until he happens to use only the involved ear, for example, by holding a telephone receiver to the ear that he normally does not use when telephoning. The loss of hearing escapes attention because it develops gradually, with the slow growth of the tumor. This slow development is probably also the reason that vestibular signs, such as vertigo, are rare at the beginning. Hearing noises in the diseased ear is a frequent complaint. As the tumor expands, it may damage cranial nerves V to XI. There may be ipsilateral peripheral facial weakness, paresthesia or anesthesia in the corresponding half of the face, and later, loss of taste and swallowing disorders. Cerebellar signs may develop late. The gait may become unsteady and staggering, and grasping becomes insecure. Compression of the aqueduct or fourth ventricle may produce increased intracranial pressure from the development of a noncommunicating hydrocephalus. As this occurs, the patient will complain of headaches, nausea, and vomiting. If the pressure is not relieved by operation, loss of consciousness will be followed by death from central respiratory failure.

As long as the patient complains only of difficulties in hearing and noises in one ear, it is difficult to make the correct diagnosis of an acoustic neurinoma, because these complaints accompany many other diseases. If unilateral inner ear deafness is accompanied by poor or no response of the labyrinth to caloric stimulation, however, it is necessary to employ all diagnostic means that will help to clarify whether a pontocerebellar angle tumor is present. Similar signs may be produced by a large intra-arachnoidal cyst or a cystic bulging of the ventral portion of a lateral recess of the fourth ventricle; either may occupy the pontocerebellar angle. Such signs may also be caused by a diffuse vertebrobasilar aneurysm.

Ependymoma

This tumor originates in the ependyma covering the ventricle wall. Seventy percent of intracranial ependymomas derive from the wall of the fourth ventricle, particularly from its caudal portion and from the wall of one of its lateral recesses. The tumor usually grows slowly. In addition to obstructing the fourth ventricle or aqueduct, the tumor may compress and displace cerebellar structures such as the inferior vermis. Occasionally, the tumor shows malignant growth and may invade the cerebellum. Ependymomas are seen in every age group; the largest number of infratentorial ependymomas, however, occur during the first decade of life. Therefore, ependymoma should always be considered in the differential diagnosis of a space-occupying posterior fossa lesion in infancy and adolescence.

Other Cerebellar Diseases

Less frequent than tumors are degenerative diseases (including cerebellar heredoataxia, olivopontocerebellar atrophy, and late atrophy, particularly of the paleocerebellum, as seen in alcoholics) and inflammatory processes, including cerebellar abscess and encephalitis. In multiple sclerosis, lesions in the cerebellar white matter and in peduncles are often responsible for intention tremor, ataxia, and scanning speech.

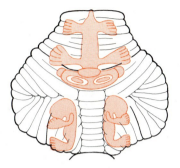

Fig. 4.15 Somatotopic organization of cerebellar cortex according to evoked potentials produced by sensory stimuli. (From Kahle, W.: Taschenatlas der Anatomie, Vol. 3, Thieme, Stuttgart, 1979.)

Addendum

As was mentioned earlier, the cerebellum receives information from virtually all parts of the nervous system and, in turn, exercises its influence via its efferent connections. There is a somatotopic order in its connections with the cerebrum. This became known in experiments with evoked potentials on various species of animals, including primates. Consequently, it is assumed that the somatotopic principle is operative also in the human cerebellar cortex (Fig. 4.15).

5 Diencephalon

The diencephalon follows the rostral midbrain. At their junction the axis of spinal cord and brainstem, also called *Meynert's axis*, tilts forward at an angle of approximately 110° and becomes the cerebral frontooccipital axis (*Forel's axis*). Accordingly, the term *rostral* or *oral* becomes synonymous with *frontal* or *anterior*; *caudal* becomes synonymous with *occipital* or *posterior* for all cerebral structures. The term *ventral* refers to the base of the cerebrum; the term *dorsal*, to its convexity.

As illustrated in Figs. 5.1 and 5.2, the diencephalon extends on either side of the third ventricle from the *rostral lamina terminalis* to the *pineal gland (epiphysis)*. Ventrally, it borders on the *basal cistern* and midbrain; dorsally, on the *tela choroidea* of the choroid plexus in third and lateral ventricles. Laterally, it is adjacent to the internal capsules. The dorsal portion of the wall of the third ventricle is formed by the thalamus, and the wall below its sulcus hypothalamicus by the hypothalamus. In front of the rostral thalamus the interventricular *foramen of Monro* is formed by the knee of the *fornix*. The *mamillary bodies* as well as the *tuber cinereum* and the *infundibulum* connecting it with the posterior pituitary gland are framed by the optic chiasm, the optic tracts and the cerebral peduncles of the midbrain. In 70 to 80 percent of cases, the thalami are connected by the *massa intermedia*, called gray or soft commissure, containing the nucleus commissuralis. The diencephalon is composed of the following structures:

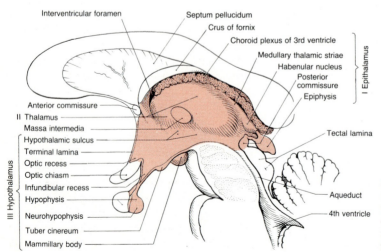

Fig. 5.1 Sagittal section through brainstem, showing transition from mesencephalon to diencephalon and structures in the area of the wall of the 3rd ventricle.

Thalamus 181

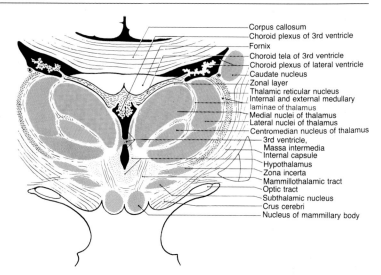

Fig. 5.2 Section through diencephalon.

1. **Epithalamus:** This structure comprises the habenular nuclei, the habenular commissure, the pineal gland, and the posterior commissure.

2. **Thalamus:** These two large, symmetrical gray structures make up four-fifths of the diencephalon.

3. **Hypothalamus:** The hypothalamus consists of various nuclei separated from the thalamus by the sulcus hypothalamicus of the wall of the third ventricle. This periventricular gray structure is characterized by poor myelination. It is the center of the autonomic nervous system (see Figs. 5.13 and 5.14). The fiber column of the fornix passes in a ventrocaudal direction through the hypothalamus on its way to the mamillary body, a component of the limbic system.

4. **Subthalamus:** The main structure of the subthalamus is the subthalamic nucleus (corpus subthalamicum Luysi), a small, elliptic structure that lies dorsolateral to the mamillary body and in front of the substantia nigra. The pallidum (globus pallidus), although separated by the internal capsule, is also considered part of the subthalamus. It will be discussed in Chapter 6, dealing with basal ganglia and extrapyramidal motor system.

The pituitary gland, connected with the hypothalamus by the pituitary stalk, is considered in the section on the autonomic nervous system.

Thalamus

The term *thalamus* stands for the large, egg-shaped, symmetrical gray matter complexes on either side of the third ventricle, each having a cross-sectional size of approximately 3×1.5 cm. Instead of representing a uniform mass of neurons and fibers, each thalamus is subdivided into different neuronal aggregations or nuclei. Each subdivision has its own afferent connections and is in contact with different portions of the cerebrum. As can be seen grossly, layers of white, myelinated fibers (*internal medullary laminae*) subdivide each thalamus into major gray areas: a *lateral nucleus* which is the largest; a *medial nucleus* which extends to the wall of the third ventricle; and an *anterior nucleus* which is the smallest and is located near the foramen of Monro. Some smaller groups of cells lie within the medullary laminae separating the lateral and medial nuclei. The largest of these groups is called the *centromedian nucleus* (see Figs. 5.2 and 5.4). The caudal portion of the thalamus is called the *pulvinar*. Attached to its ventral surface

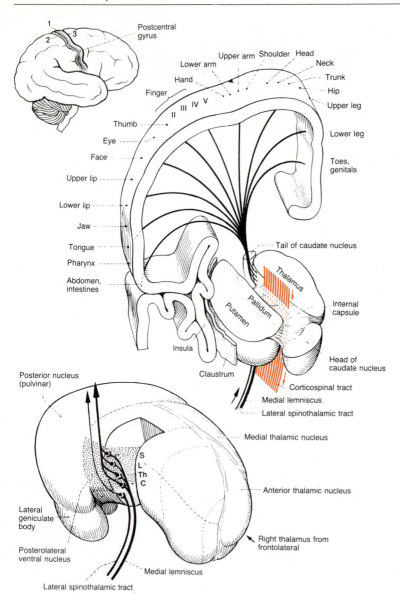

Fig. 5.3 Somatotopic arrangement of somatosensory neurons is postcentral gyrus and in thalamus.

are the *medial geniculate body* (*hearing*) and, slightly separated from it, the *lateral geniculate body* (*vision*). The lateral border of the thalamus, separating it from the internal capsule, is formed by the external medullary lamina, to which a thin layer of neurons, the *reticular thalamic nucleus*, is attached (see Fig. 5.2).

The three large nuclei have been cytologically and functionally subdivided further. At present, 120 subgroups have been counted. The most important of them are illustrated in Fig. 5.4. Because there is still no full agreement on classification and nomenclature, the anatomic names according to the Nomina Anatomica are entered in red and the clinically oriented nomenclature of Hassler, which will be used here, is entered in black.

In the previous chapters we followed the various ascending tracts that reach the thalamus from spinal cord, brainstem, and cerebellum. For all incoming impulses, with the exception of olfactory stimuli, the thalamus is the central relay station, in which the impulses are transferred to the final thalamocortical neurons.

Fig. 5.5 demonstrates the various end stations, where the diverse afferent pathways terminate, and the areas of origin of the corresponding central neurons connecting the thalamus with well-defined cortical areas.

The thalamic neurons receive impulses from spinal cord and brainstem (for example, via the medial lemniscus) in somatotopic order and transmit the impulses to the cerebral cortex in exactly the same point-to-point order (Figs. 5.3, 5.5).

Thalamic nuclei that receive impulses from well-defined areas of the periphery of the body and transmit these impulses to correspondingly circumscribed areas of the cerebral cortex (primary projection areas) are called *specific* thalamic nuclei. This term also includes the secondary and tertiary portions of the sensory systems of the thalamus, which project to the association fields of the cerebral cortex. In contrast, *nonspecific* thalamic nuclei receive afferent impulses from several different sensory organs, usually after a crossover in the reticular formation. The impulses of the nonspecific nuclei make a detour through basal ganglia and travel over a nonspecific projection system to almost all cortical areas, including the so-called association fields.

All somatosensory pathways (medial lemniscus, spinal thalamic tract, trigeminothalamic tract, and others) have a relay station in the lateral ventroposterior thalamic complex, more specifically, in the nucleus ventrocaudalis internus (*V.c.i.* or *VPM* nucleus), nucleus ventrocaudalis parvocellularis (*V.c.pc.* nucleus), nucleus ventrocaudalis externus (*V.c.e.* or *VPL* nucleus) and nucleus ventralis intermedius (*V.i.m.* nucleus) (Fig. 5.5). The axons from neurons in these nuclei terminate in the well-circumscribed architectonic areas 3a, 3b, 1, and 2 of the somatosensory cortex.

Taste impulses originating in the solitary nucleus arrive in the medial portion of the nucleus ventrocaudalis internus (*V.c.pc.i.* or *VPM* nucleus) and are relayed to the ventral or foot portion of the posterior central region just above the insula (see Fig. 3.33).

Other specific thalamic nuclei are the lateral and medial geniculate bodies. The lateral geniculate body receives visual impulses via the optic tract and transmits these impulses via the optic radiation to the visual cortex (area 17) in *retinotopic order* (Fig. 5.6; see Fig. 3.9). The medial geniculate body receives auditory impulses via the lateral lemniscus and transmits them in *tonotopic order* via the acoustic radiation to the auditory cortex (area 41; Heschl's transverse convolutions) in the temporal lobe (Fig. 5.6 and see Fig. 3.36).

The oral ventral nucleus (*V.o.p.* nucleus) receives impulses from the dentate nucleus and red nucleus by way of the dentatothalamic tract (see Figs. 4.4, 4.5, and 4.6) and transmits them to the cortical motor field (Fig. 5.5). The nucleus ventralis oralis anterior (*V.o.a.* nucleus) and the nucleus ventralis anterior (*VA* nucleus) receive afferent impulses from the pallidum and project to the premotor cortex (areas 6aα and 6aβ).

The nucleus anterior, nucleus dorsalis, nucleus medialis, and pulvinar belong to the secondary and tertiary groups (see Figs. 5.6 and 5.7) that project to the association fields. These nuclei usually receive their afferent impulses not directly but over relay stations in the primary projection nuclei of the thalamus.

Anterior nucleus (Fig. 5.7): The neurons of this nucleus have reciprocal connections with the mamillary body and fornix via the *mamillothalamic fascicle* (*tract of Vicq d'Azyr*). The

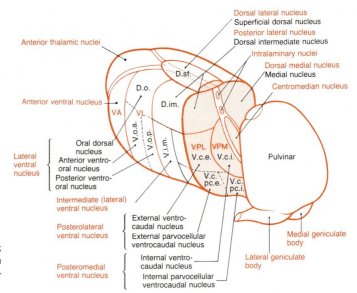

Fig. 5.4 Thalamus nuclei. Black letters: Functional organization (after Hassler), Red letters: Nomina Anatomica.

anterior nucleus projects point to point to area 24 of the *cingulate gyrus*, a part of the limbic system. The *limbic system* is composed of, among other structures, the cortex of the hippocampus of the parahippocampal gyrus, the dentate gyrus, and the cingulate gyrus. This system facilitates an exchange of impulses among mesencephalic, diencephalic, and neocortical structures. It is assumed to be related to the emotional and instinctive behaviors of self-preservation and propagation of the species (MacLean, 1958). The function of the hippocampus is believed to be important for the deposition of recent memories.

Lateral dorsal nucleus: This nucleus is composed of the oral and intermedial dorsal nuclei (see Fig. 5.6). The oral dorsal nucleus (D.o.) project in a reciprocal fashion point to point to the association fields in the prefrontal cortex, the intermedial dorsal nucleus (D.i.m.) to that in the parietal cortex caudal to the postcentral gyrus (see Fig. 5.6).

Dorsal nucleus: This superficial nucleus (see Fig. 5.6, *D.sf.*) receives its afferent impulses from the pallidum and projects to the caudal portion of the cingulate gyrus, area 23 (see Figs. 5.7, 8.9b).

Medial Nucleus: This nucleus has two-way point-to-point projections to the association areas of the prefrontal lobe, rostral to the premotor region (see Fig. 5.6). The nucleus receives its afferent impulses from other thalamic areas (ventral and intralaminary nuclei), hypothalamus, midbrain nuclei, and pallidum. Destruction of this nuclear territory by tumor or any other disease process produces a frontal lobe syndrome with personality changes like those described following leukotomy by coagulation of frontal white matter. The visceral impulses coming from the hypothalamus probably influence *mood*, leading to feelings of *happiness* or *depression*, for example.

Posterior nucleus (pulvinar): This thalamic area projects reciprocally point to point to the association fields in parietal as well as occipital lobes (see Fig. 5.6). This area of association is surrounded by somatosensory, visual, and acoustic projection fields and

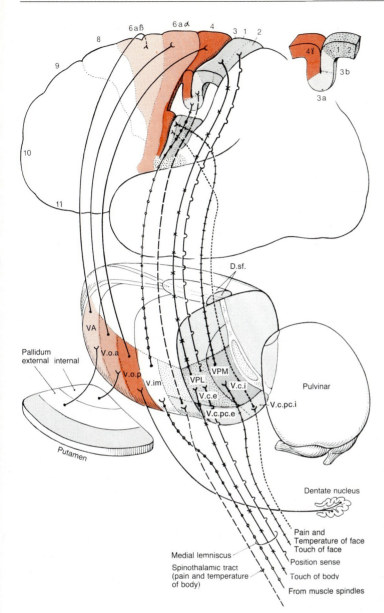

Fig. 5.5 Neuronal connections of ventrolateral nuclei of thalamus with cerebral cortex (after Hassler).

probably plays an important role in interconnecting these different kinds of incoming sensory information. The pulvinar receives its afferent impulses from other thalamic nuclei, particularly from the intralaminar nuclei.

Intralaminar nuclei: These nuclei form the main portion of the nonspecific projection system of the thalamus. They are located within the internal medullary lamina and receive impulses in part from ascending fibers of the reticular formation of the brainstem and in part from fibers originating in thalamic nuclei. They do not project to the cerebral cortex but to the caudate nucleus, putamen, and pallidum of the extrapyramidal

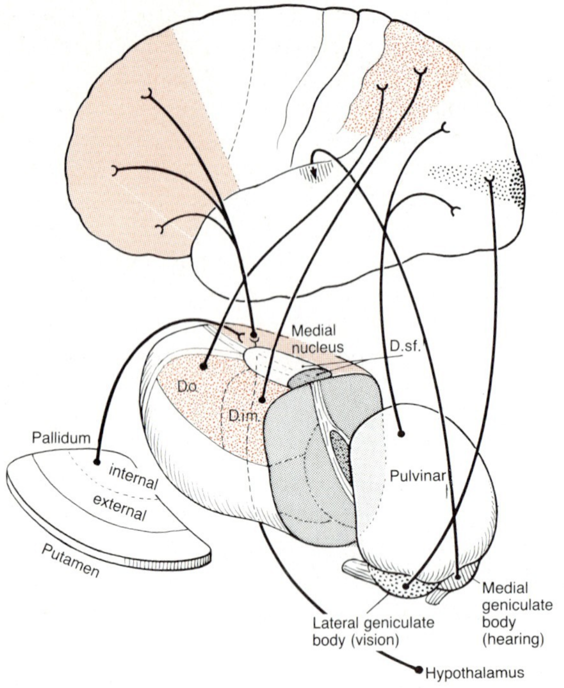

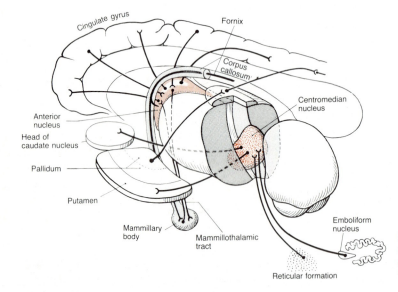

Fig. 5.6 Connections of dorsal, medial, and posterior nuclei (pulvinar), and of medial and lateral geniculate bodies of thalamus with cerebral cortex.

Fig. 5.7 Afferent and efferent neurons of anterior and centromedian nuclei of thalamus.

system and probably also in a diffuse pattern to all thalamic nuclear complexes, which transmit impulses to large secondary areas of the cerebral cortex. The *centromedian nucleus* is an important part of this intralaminar complex, which represents the thalamic portion of the ascending reticular activating system. A nonthalamic portion of this arousal system probably runs over subthalamus and hypothalamus.

Function

The function of the thalamus is a rather complex issue, as is suggested by the presence of its numerous, individually differentiated nerve cell groups and its many different afferent as well as efferent connections. First, the thalamus is the large subcortical depot for the many exteroceptive and proprioceptive impulses arriving from external as well as internal stimuli. It is also a large relay station that transmits to the cerebral cortex all the impulses received from receptors of skin and internal organs, from visual and auditory pathways, and from hypothalamus, cerebellum, and brainstem (reticular formation). Some of the thalamic pathways connect with the striatum, but the great majority connect with the cerebral cortex. All impulses reaching the cerebral cortex must pass through the thalamus in order to enter awareness. Therefore, the thalamus has been called the *"gate to consciousness"*.

In addition to serving as a relay station, the thalamus is the important center in which the different afferent impulses from various parts of the body become coordinated and integrated and colored by affect. The various elementary feelings, such as pain, displeasure, well-being and others, are attached to sensations in the thalamus and then transferred to the cortex. Certain elementary sensations, such as pain, heat, and cold, are probably felt in the thalamus, because there is awareness of pain after ablation of the sensory cortex.

Because of its connections with the extrapyramidal system, the thalamus constitutes a coordination center, playing an important role in the origin of expressive, affective movements that occur as reactions to painful and other emotionally influential stimuli.

Because the connections between thalamus and cortex run both ways, the thalamus also receives information from the motor cortex. By its collateral circuit with the extrapyramidal system, it has a modifying influence on motor actions not unlike that of the cerebellum.

Finally, the thalamus is, as mentioned earlier, a very important part of the *ascending reticular activating system*. Stimulation of individual thalamic nuclei of this system activates only individual, specific areas of the cerebral cortex. Stimulation of nonspecific thalamic nuclei and of the mesencephalic reticular formation, however, activates the entire cerebral cortex. Thus, it is posited that this thalamic system has two functions: 1. It activates the entire cerebral cortex in a nonspecific way. 2. It may be able to activate only very specific cortical areas. This would explain why it is possible to concentrate on specific thoughts while suppressing others.

Signs and symptoms of thalamic damage have been identified by studying thalamic infarcts from vascular obstructions.

Dejerine and Roussy were the first to describe a *thalamus syndrome* in detail, in 1906. It consists of:

1. contralateral disorders of peripheral sensations and even more extensive disorders of deep sensations;
2. astereognosis and hemiataxia;
3. spontaneous pain in the contralateral half of the body;
4. mild, transient hemiplegia without spastic contractions;
5. choreoathetotic movements.

This syndrome has been most often observed in infarcts involving the thalamogeniculate artery, which supplies the ventral posterolateral nuclear area.

Blood Supply

The arterial supply of the thalamus has been systematically studied by Foix and Hillemand (1925) and others. The posterior cerebral arteries, the posterior communicating arteries, and the anterior and posterior choroidal arteries supply the thalamus. Details of the arterial supply are shown in Fig. 5.**8**. The venous drainage of the ventral portion of the thalamus takes place via the

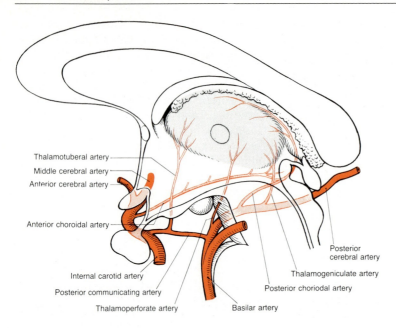

Fig. 5.8 Arterial supply of thalamus.

basal vein of Rosenthal, and that of the dorsal thalamus via the internal cerebral vein. Both veins drain into the great vein of Galen (see Fig. 8.**51**).

Syndrome of Thalamic Disorders

Signs and symptoms of thalamic disease vary greatly depending on the type of the disorder. The complete thalamus syndrome is rare. Signs that may be found as a result of unilateral or bilateral involvement of the thalamus are:

1. Contralateral hypesthesia, usually involving trunk and extremities more severely than the face. Decrease in deep sensations is particularly severe. The threshold for perceiving touch, pain, and temperature is usually elevated. If it is extremely high, even light stimuli produce unpleasant sensations in the form of irradiating, burning, piercing, tearing pain (*hyperpathia*). Regular visual or acoustic stimuli, such as melodious music, may be irritating and displeasing. Spontaneous, ineffable pain or parethesias in the contralateral half of the body are common. They are often exacerbated by emotions or exhaustion. Analgesics often provide no relief. Instead, an antiepileptic drug such as Dilantin (diphenylhydantoin) may be helpful. Otherwise, stereotactic destruction of the ventrocaudal parvicellular nucleus of the thalamus (*V.c.pc.* nucleus in Fig. 5.**4**) has been carried out in an attempt to eliminate the pain.

2. Intention tremor or hemiataxia associated with choreoathetotic movements, probably caused by damage to cerebellothalamic, rubrothalamic, or pallidothalamic fibers. Peculiar contractures may also develop, most often involving the hands (*thalamus hand*).

3. Affective disorders in the form of emotional lability and a tendency to *forced crying or laughter*, possibly related to damage to the anterior nucleus and its connections with the hypothalamus or limbic system.

4. Contralateral hemiparesis, often transient if the internal capsule is involved only by perifocal edema.

Syndromes of Thalamic Circulatory Disorders

Of the various circulatory thalamic syndromes described in the literature, two will be mentioned briefly, and a third interesting syndrome will be described with case history.

Posterolateral thalamic syndrome (Dejerine and Roussy, 1906) is the result of an obstruction of the thalamogeniculate artery. It represents the classic thalamus syndrome: usually transient contralateral hemiparesis, persistent contralateral hemianesthesia for touch and particularly for deep sensations, decrease in pain and temperature sensations, spontaneous pain in the involved areas, mild hemiataxia and astereognosis, and contralateral choreoathetotic restlessness.

One-sided anterolateral thalamic syndrome is usually caused by unilateral obstruction of branches of the thalamoperforating artery. The syndrome includes tremor at rest or intention tremor, choreoathetotic movements, and possibly thalamus hand. No sensory disorders and no thalamic pain occur.

Bilateral ventromedial thalamic syndrome is caused by a bilateral infarction of the ventromedial thalami. This unusual syndrome is illustrated by the following case (Fig. 5.9).

Case report: A 37-year-old woman suddenly collapsed while shopping and was immediately taken to a hospital. At first she was unresponsive. During the subsequent days, unconsciousness improved to somnolence. She could be awakened for brief periods, during which she was oriented and recognized her relatives. Speech was slurred. Initial hypertension improved, but hyperglycemia did not respond to therapy. When awake, the patient was able to take liquids. Her response to neurologic testing was poor. There were bilateral positive Babinski's signs but no papilledema. Cerebrospinal fluid was normal. Death occurred twelve days later as a result of circulatory collapse.

Postmortem examination (Professor W. Krücke, Max-Planck Institute for Brain Research, Frankfurt/Main) showed dark-colored symmetrical, butterfly-shaped infarcts involving the ventromedial thalami centered around the nonspecific nuclei of the internal medullary laminae and extending into the left mamillary body, the wall of the exit of the third ventricle, and the rostral red nuclei. Histologically, the lesion showed the characteristics of the second phase of infarction,

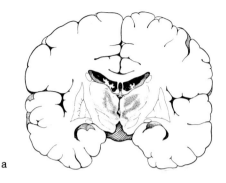

a

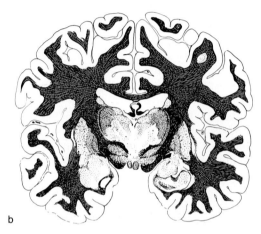

b

Fig. 5.9 Necrotic foci in both thalami. **a** Large, symmetrical, butterfly-shaped softening of thalami (in resorption) centered around the nonspecific nuclei of internal medullary laminae with extension into left mamillary body, wall of exit of 3rd ventricle, and rostral red nucleus. Cause: Obstruction of a larger artery in the posterior basal cistern (possibly embolism of an unknown primary tumor or circumscribed calcified granulomatous endarteritis). (Drawn from specimen.) **b** Myelin preparation from section shown in **a**.

with resorption of the necrotic tissue by phagocytes. One of the larger arteries in the posterior basal cistern was found to be obstructed by a thromboembolus in a state of organization with formation of shell-like calcifications. Possibly secondary vascular alterations within the infarction consisted of separation of the intima in small arteries and the formation of multiple fresh, sometimes hyaline thrombi in small arteries and veins. An additional small infarct of the same age involved cortex and white matter of the left third temporal convolution.

Characteristic thalamus signs could not be elicited in this patient because of the severe somnolence; this uninterrupted sleepiness was clearly the result of the bilateral destruction of the thalamic components of the ascending reticular activating system. Schaltenbrand (1969) published a similar case report; in that patient small infarcts in the medial thalami had produced somnolence lasting for weeks.

Tumors of the Thalamus

Tumors very rarely produce a complete thalamus syndrome. If some signs are present, they are mild, even in the presence of considerable thalamic damage. Occasional patients may be virtually asymptomatic. Compression of the third ventricle or its entrance to the aqueduct may produce early noncommunicating hydrocephalus of the lateral ventricles, masking specific thalamic symptoms. Fig. 5.10, drawn from specimen from the first patient in the case reports that follow, demonstrates a circumscribed oligodendrocytoma in the medial left thalamus causing such internal hydrocephalus. The tumor extends posteriorly to the superior colliculi, displaces the pineal gland, and compresses the posterior third ventricle and the entrance to the aqueduct. The enlargement of the lateral ventricle is asymmetrical. The characteristically rounded lateral angles of the ventricles press against the deep cerebral white matter.

Case report: A 27-year-old woman had had peculiar, vertigo-like attacks for the previous two years. She would suddenly slump without losing consciousness. These attacks became more frequent and tended to occur when she rose from a sitting position. They did not impair her efficiency at work. Headaches were rare. Occasionally she would vomit in the morning. Tinnitus occurred for a period of time. Physical examination and cerebrospinal fluid were normal. Neurologic examination revealed the head to be held in a rigid position. Pupils did not react to light. The right optic nerve was atrophic, and the left slightly prominent. Tendon reflexes of the arms were more brisk on the right side than on the left. There was bilateral intention tremor and slight ataxia, more on the right side than on the left. Position sense was decreased in the right fingers. The patient exhibited a positive Babinski's sign on the left side. Position sense in toes was decreased, and there was a tendency to fall backward. Mentally she was indolent, slow, and usually somewhat somnolent. Roentgenography revealed calcifications in the area of the pineal gland. Ventriculography showed considerable hydrocephalus of lateral ventricles. The patient refused operation. Three months later she died during an epileptic attack.

The seizure-like states of acute collapse or slumping that were the dominant neurologic sign were probably mesencephalic in origin. They probably represented an acute loss of

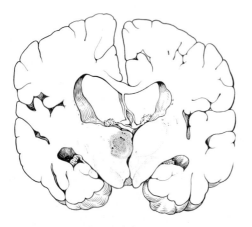

Fig. 5.10 Oligodendroglioma in left thalamus (drawn from specimen).

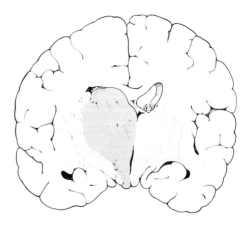

Fig. 5.11 Astrocytoma of left thalamus (drawn from specimen).

labrinthine or postural reflexes and were similar to affective catalepsy, often associated with narcolepsy. True thalamic signs were scant: there was only some disorder in the position sense in the fingers of the right hand and in the toes. Intention tremor and a mild ataxia were evidenced, more pronounced on the right side than on the left.

In a second patient the entire left thalamus was taken over by an astrocytoma, shown in Fig. 5.11. The tumor displaced the internal capsule laterally, compressed the third ventricle, bulged into the lateral ventricle, and extended caudally to the fourth ventricle, destroying the pineal gland and the quadrigeminal plate.

Case report: The 50-year-old woman, complained of fatigue for the previous nine months, had lost initiative, and was often in a depressed mood. She complained frequently of headaches and dizziness. Vision had decreased supposedly more in the right eye than in the left. Hearing was reduced on the right. She complained about constant "pressure on her mood" and about her head being "like crazy." Answers were slow, monotonous, and hesitant. There were no physical abnormalities. Neurologic examination revealed coarse horizontal nystagmus to the right; weakness of upward gaze; left abducens paresis; right pupil wider than left; nonreactive right pupil; sluggish reaction of left pupil to light; papilledema of 2 to 3 diopters in right eye and of 3 to 4 diopters in left eye; reduced right corneal reflex; hypesthesia in entire right half of face, associated with weakness of right facial and hypoglossal nerves; intention tremor and adiadochokinesia on the right; hypesthesia for all qualities in entire right half of the body; and insecurity and tendency to fall to the right backward. The patient complained of a very annoying feeling of numbness over the right half of her body and showed a lack of attention span and obvious loss of recent memory. Somnolence and stupor occurred, associated with clasping reflex and a tendency to perseveration. The patient refused operative intervention. Death from respiratory failure occurred after $4\frac{1}{2}$ months.

In addition to signs referable to the midbrain, there were unquestionable thalamic signs, such as hypesthesia for all qualities in the entire right half of the body, ataxia on the right, intention tremor, and harassing paresthesias in the right half of the body.

Just as tumors of the thalamus have a tendency to grow into the midbrain, those originating in the midbrain or at the site of the pineal gland often grow into both thalami or hypothalami. These bilateral tumors usually produce more prominent thalamic signs and may be associated with severe, ineffable pain in one half of the body and with hyperpathia to the slightest touch.

Inflammatory Disease of the Thalamus

Thalamic signs and symptoms may be the result of a focal inflammatory process, particularly if it is granulomatous and is caused, for example, by tuberculosis or syphilis. It is important to know, however, that such condition may produce no thalamic syndrome at all. The following case of a thalamus granuloma caused by **toxoplasmosis** serves as example.

Case report: A 45-year-old dentist was healthy until two years prior to his death. The disease began with severe sweating about the head and shoulder girdle. Deep breathing produced pain beneath the ribs. Liver and spleen were noticably enlarged, and the testicles were painfully swollen. Swelling of lymph nodes in neck, axillae, and groin led to the tentative diagnosis of lymphosarcoma. A giant follicular lymphoma (Brill-Symmers disease) was diagnosed histologically and subsequently treated with an antileukemia drug for some time. The swelling of the lymph nodes regressed, and the patient's condition improved considerably. Repeated examinations failed to reveal any neurologic signs. About 6 to 7 weeks prior to death, the patient developed a mild weakness of the right side of his body, particularly of the right leg. At first it did not interfere with his practice as a dentist. The paresis became stronger, however, and necessitated admission to a hospital. Here, the hemiparesis developed into a hemiplegia. Bilateral papilledema was found but was the only abnormal neurologic finding; sensibility, for example, was completely intact. The patient showed a notable euphoria, which accounted for an absence of complaints and worries on his part about his disease. Electroencephalography indicated a left temporal lesion; angiography showed some dorsal displacement of sylvian branches of the middle cerebral artery. An increase in the intracranial pressure and a slurring of speech associated with paraphasia occurred shortly thereafter, whereas word choice and comprehension remained intact. The patient

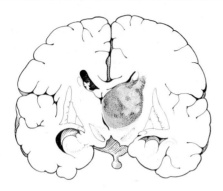

Fig. 5.12 Toxoplasmosis granuloma in the left thalamus (drawn from specimen).

became stuporous and died in coma four weeks after admission.

Postmortem examination (Department of Pathology of the University of Frankfurt/Main) showed no evidence of Brill-Symmers disease. The lymph nodes showed extensive destruction as a result of the antileukemia treatment. Examination of the brain (Professor W. Krücke, Max-Planck Institute for Brain Research, Frankfurt/Main) revealed the surprising finding of a multifocal toxoplasmic encephalitis and a large, older granuloma destroying much of the left thalamus (Fig. 5.12). Upon reexamination the lymph nodes showed alterations indicative of toxoplasmosis.

It is amazing that the large granuloma produced no neurologic deficits that could be related to thalamus dysfunction. This is in contrast to the high frequency of thalamic signs in patients with infarcts. It agrees, however, with the observation mentioned earlier that tumors, when involving only one thalamus, often fail to cause thalamic symptoms. This finding probably relates to the fact that tumor cells do not destroy all the neurons in their path so that many neuronal groups and fiber tracts remain largely intact. Thus, a thalamus syndrome can be expected only if there is total destruction of larger parts of the very cellular griseum. Space-occupying thalamic lesions often produce an early noncommunicating hydrocephalus of the lateral ventricles, as was mentioned earlier. Its signs and symptoms may make establishing a definite thalamic symptomatology difficult.

A fully developed thalamus syndrome suggests a circulatory lesion. Signs pointing to involvement of perithalamic structures, however (tegmentum of the midbrain, subthalamus, hypothalamus, internal capsule, basal ganglia), and the appearance of an occlusive hydrocephalus of the lateral ventricles in the presence of mild thalamic signs that include a visual field defect or hypacusia (damage to lateral and medial geniculate bodies, respectively) suggest a thalamic tumor or a tumor-like lesion, such as the aforementioned granuloma.

Epithalamus

The habenular nuclei, consisting of groups of neurons in the reinlike structures of the habenulae, are part of the epithalamus. They probably act as relay stations connecting olfactory impulses with the automatic centers of the brainstem (see the discussion of the olfactory system, page 80). These impulses originate in the olfactory region (septal area) and travel along the medullary striae of the thalamus and the habenular commissure to the contralateral habenular nucleus. From there they are likely transferred to the interpeduncular nucleus by the retroflex fascicle (Meynert's bundle) and further to the autonomic brainstem centers by the dorsal longitudinal bundle (see Fig. 3.7).

The *posterior commissure*, another part of the epithalamus, represents a crossing of fibers from superior colliculi and tectum of the midbrain that subserve the light reflex.

The *epiphysis* or *pineal body* is the third constituent of the epithalamus. It contains *pinealocytes* within a vascular network of connective tissue. These large, polygonal cells have a secretory function and are attached to interlobular blood vessels by agyrophilic dendrites. In the second decade of life, calcium and magnesium salts are deposited within the stroma of the epiphysis. The visibility of these deposits on routine roentgenograms permits simple determination of pineal gland displacement.

Tumors arising from the epiphysis or its immediate vicinity are generally called *pinealomas*. Those originating from the pineal parenchymal cells represent one type among these tumors, the *pineocytomas*. They are slow-growing, noninvasive tumors which occur at any age. The more important variety is called *pineal germinoma*. It tends to break out of the epiphyseal area and infiltrate the adjacent structures, which include the quadrigeminal plate and the gray matter around the third ventricle. Most of these tumors occur in the second and third decades of life. Because they press on or infiltrate the quadrigeminal plate, pinealomas are the most frequent cause of *Parinaud's syndrome* (see Fig. 3.**66**). By compressing the aqueduct, they may also produce an early noncommunicating hydrocephalus of the lateral and third ventricles. A pinealoma, usually a germinoma, occurring in childhood may cause *pubertas praecox*, for reasons not fully understood. Some believe that the pineal gland has an inhibiting influence on sexual maturity and that destruction of its parenchyma abolishes this influence. It is also possible that an irritation of the tuber cinereum of the hypothalamus by an enlarging third ventricle provides the stimulus for early sexual development (Spatz, 1953; 1962–1964).

Subthalamus

The subthalamus is the area adjacent to the thalamus through which various pathways, such as the medial lemniscus and the spinothalamic and trigeminothalamic tracts, pass on their way to the thalamus. They all enter the ventroposterior nuclear area of the thalamus (see Fig. 5.**5**). The substantia nigra and the red nucleus of the midbrain border the subthalamus.

In front of the red nucleus lies Forel's field H1, through which the dentatothalamic tract passes on its way to the posterior ventrooral nucleus of the thalamus. The fibers of the globus pallidus travel through the lenticular fascicle (Forel's bundle H2) to the anterior ventrooral nucleus and the anterior nucleus of the thalamus. Still further rostrally is the ansa lenticularis (see Fig. 6.**9**). The mesencephalic reticular formation continues rostrally to the zona incerta of the subthalamus. The most important connections between the putamen, pallidum, subthalamus, and thalamus are shown in Fig. 5.**12 A**.

The *subthalamic nucleus* or *corpus Luysi* is part of the extrapyramidal system and stays in close contact with the globus pallidus (see Fig. 5.**2**). If one of these small, elliptic nuclei

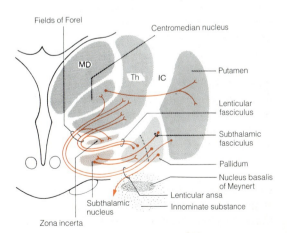

Fig. 5.**12 A** Fiber pathways in the subthalamus.
MD = Nucleus medialis dorsalis thal.
Th = Thalamus
IC = Inner capsule

is damaged, contralateral *hemiballismus* will occur. This term signifies coarse, lightning-fast, hurling, involuntary movements of the proximal portion of arms and legs. The movements are so violent that the entire body participates. Characteristically, they are present only as long as the patient is awake and stop as he falls asleep. The cause may be a circulatory lesion or a metastasis or, as in one of our patients, a small tuberculoma. The condition may be transient when occurring after a stereotactic operation.

Hypothalamus

Structure

The hypothalamus represents the cerebral center for all autonomic functions of the body. It consists of the periventricular gray matter of the third ventricle below the sulcus hypothalamicus, which extends almost horizontally below the thalamic massa intermedia (Fig. 5.**13**). The mamillary bodies are part of the hypothalamus, as are the tuber cinereum, the infundibulum, and the posterior lobe of the pituitary gland (*neurohypophysis*), which is basically a thickening of the pituitary stalk. The anterior lobe of the pituitary is glandular and is therefore referred to as the *adenohypophysis*. It developed from Rathke's pouch and is superficially attached to the neurohypophysis. Craniopharyngioma or suprasellar epidermoid cyst is said to develop from remnants of Rathke's pouch, as are the *intrasellar cysts* that are lined with cuboidal or ciliated epithelium and compress the pituitary gland.

Each hypothalamus is divided into a medial and a lateral area by the pars tecta or hidden portion of the fornix, which descends from the anterior wall of the foramen of Monro in a ventrocaudal direction to the mamillary body (Fig. 5.**14**). The lateral area contains fiber bundles, among them the medial forebrain bundle, which originates in the

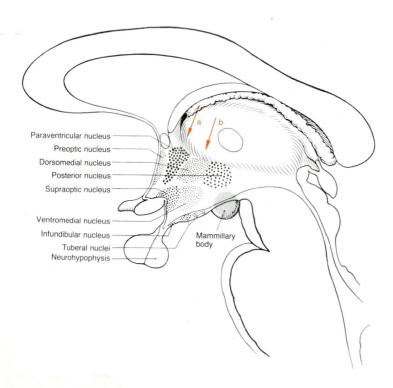

Fig. 5.**13** Autonomic hypothalamic nuclei (medial view). Red arrows a and b indicate the levels of the two coronal planes shown in Figure 5.**14**.

basal olfactory area and runs as a chain of neurons to the midbrain. The lateral nuclei of the tuber cinereum are also part of the lateral area and occupy its base. Fairly well delineated nuclei occur in the medial hypothalamic area; these are customarily subdivided into rostral, medial or tuberal, and posterior or mamillary groups (see Figs. 5.13 and 5.14).

The *preoptic, supraoptic,* and *paraventricular nuclei* are the most important structures of the rostral group. The supraoptic and paraventricular nuclei are connected with the neurohypophysis by the *supraopticohypophyseal tract*. They produce the hormones vasopressin and oxytocin, which are carried by the tract through the pituitary stalk to the neurohypophysis. More details are presented in the (subsequent) section on the relationship between hypothalamus and hypophysis.

The *medial group* of nuclei essentially consists of the *infundibular, tuberal, dorsomedial, ventromedial,* and *lateral* or *tuberomamillary nuclei*.

The *posterior group* of nuclei includes the *supramamillary, mamillary, intercalatus,* and *posterior nuclei*, among others. *Hess* called this area a *dynamogenic zone*, where impulses of the autonomic system are immediately transformed into forceful actions.

Afferent and efferent connections of the hypothalamus are numerous and rather complex. They must involve all parts of the nervous system for the hypothalamus to act as a coordination center for all autonomic processes within the body. Indeed, there are numerous connections to the cerebral cortex, particularly to that of the cingulate gyrus, frontal lobe and hippocampus, and also to the thalamus, basal ganglia, brainstem, and spinal cord.

Some of the most important **afferent connections** will be discussed in detail (Fig. 5.15).

The *medial forebrain bundle* originates in the basal olfactory area and septal nuclei. As a neuronal chain, it passes through the lateral area of the hypothalamus to the reticular formation of the midbrain, giving off fibers to the preoptic, dorsomedial, and ventromedial nuclei. This bundle constitutes a reciprocal link between olfactory and preoptic nuclei and midbrain and subserves olfactovisceral as well as olfactosomatic functions.

The *stria terminalis* originates in the amygdaloid nucleus. This fiber bundle passes caudally through the temporal white matter near the choroid plexus of the inferior ventricular horn. After swinging around the thalamus, it takes an anterior course and terminates in the preoptic area and the anterior hypothalamic nuclei. These fiber bundles supposedly carry olfactory sensations as well as affectively tinged instinctive drives.

The *fornix*, a well-outlined, myelinated bundle, comprises the axons of the large neurons of the hippocampus, first forming

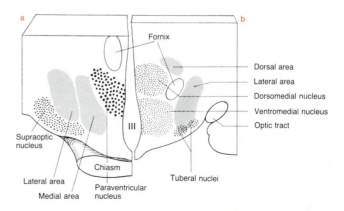

Fig. 5.14 Hypothalamic nuclei in two different coronal planes indicated by arrows in Figure 5.13.

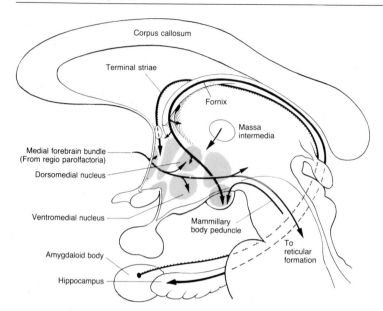

Fig. 5.15 The most important afferent hypothalamic connections.

the fimbria. The fimbria separates at the caudal portion of the hippocampus as the independent structure of the fornix. The fornix swings around the posterior thalamus and runs anteriorly near the midline towards the interventricular foramen of Monro. Over the posterior thalamus some fibers cross to the fornix of the other side, forming the *fornical* or *hippocampal commissure* (*psalterium*). Some of these fibers connect with the habenular nucleus. As closely attached columns, the fornices form the vault of the third ventricle, hence their name (fornix means "vault"). The fornices are attached to the ventral surface of the corpus callosum by the septum pellucidum, forming a partition dividing the lateral ventricles. Rostrally, the columns of the fornices form the anterior walls of the interventricular foramina of Monro by arching ventrally. As they approach the anterior commissure, each column divides into a *precommissural* and a *postcommissural fornix*. Precommissural fibers terminate in the septal (subcallosal) area, the lateral preoptic area, and the anterior part of the hypothalamus. The postcommissural fornix runs posteriorly through the hypothalamus to the mamillary body. It connects via the mamillothalamic tract with the anterior thalamic nucleus and the dorsal intralaminar nuclei. Some fibers continue caudally to the tegmentum of the midbrain. The fornix is a very important pathway within the limbic system, as will be shown later.

Visceral afferents: Visceral impulses originate in the peripheral autonomic systems and in the solitary nucleus (taste). They are transmitted to the reticular formation of the brainstem and to tegmental and interpeduncular nuclei. They reach the hypothalamus via the medial forebrain bundle (which conducts in both directions): via the dorsal longitudinal bundle, and via the peduncle of the mamillary body (see Figs. 5.15 and 5.16). Somatosensory information from erogenous zones (genitals, nipples) also takes this course to the hypothalamus, and it is here that the appropriate autonomic reactions are induced. Finally, the hypothalamus receives additional information from the medial thalamic nucleus, from the frontoorbital neocortex, and from the pallidum.

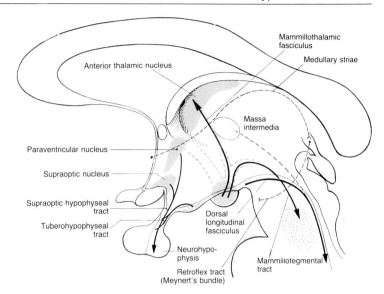

Fig. 5.16 The most important efferent hypothalamic connections.

Visceral efferents: The most important efferent pathways connecting the hypothalamus with the brainstem are the dorsal longitudinal fascicle (Schütz's bundle), which conducts in both directions, and the medial forebrain bundle. Along these pathways the hypothalamic impulses pass several relay stations, particularly in the reticular formation, until they reach the parasympathetic nuclei in the brainstem. These nuclei are the Edinger–Westphal nucleus (miosis), the salivatory nucleus (salivation), the lacrimal nucleus (tears), and the dorsal nucleus of the vagus nerve. Other impulses reach the autonomic centers in the brainstem that coordinate circulation, respiration, intake of food, and other functions. Hypothalamic impulses also influence the motor nuclei of the cranial nerves that are important for eating and drinking: the motor nucleus of the trigeminal nerve (chewing), the nucleus of the facial nerve (expressive movements of the face), the nucleus ambiguus of the vagus nerve (swallowing), and the nucleus of the hypoglossal nerve (licking) (see Fig. 3.51a). Even the spinal motor neurons receive hypothalamic impulses, via the reticulospinal tracts. These impulses play a role in the maintenance of temperature regulation (shivering of the muscles).

The *mamillotegmental fascicle* (Fig. 5.16) connects the mamillary body with the tegmentum and the reticular formation of the midbrain. The *mamillothalamic tract* (fasciculus of Vicq d'Azyr) connects the hypothalamus reciprocally with the anterior nucleus of the thalamus, which in turn connects in both directions with the cingulate gyrus. The anterior thalamic nucleus and the cingulate gyrus are important components of the *limbic system* (see Fig. 5.20). This system is believed to be important for emotional behavior pertaining to self-preservation and the propagation of the species (MacLean, 1958).

Hypothalamus and Hypophysis

Only the posterior lobe of the hypophysis, the *neurohypophysis*, has direct connection with hypothalamic nuclei, specifically with the supraoptic and paraventricular nuclei, via the supraopticohypophyseal tract (see Fig. 5.16). This tract not only transmits neuronal impulses but also carries neurosecretions, the hormones *vasopressin* and *oxytocin*, into the posterior lobe of the pituitary, where they enter the circulatory system (Fig. 5.17).

Vasopressin (antidiuretic hormone ADH) is probably produced mainly in the supraop-

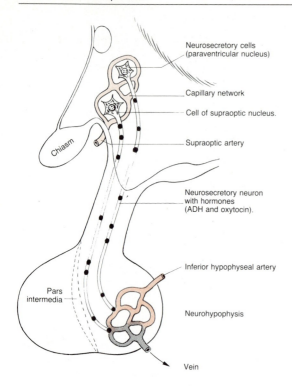

Fig. 5.17 Posterior lobe of hypophysis (neurohypophysis). Neurosecretory fibers reach the posterior lobe of the hypophysis directly.

tic nucleus. One of its functions is stimulating resorption of water by the epithelial cells of the distal portion of the uriniferous tubules of the kidney independently of solids. In this way it controls the concentration of urine. The neurons of the supraoptic nuclei serve as osmoreceptors. They are very sensitive to changes in the salinity of the surrounding tissues and regulate the water metabolism of the body. Damage to these nuclei causes *diabetes insipidus*: the patient produces large amounts of urine of low specific gravity (*polyuria*) and is therefore very thirsty and forced to drink unusually large amounts of liquid (*polydipsia*). Polyuria occurs only if cortisol (hydrocortisone) is present. Operative removal of the neurohypophysis produces no diabetes insipidus because the ADH-producing nuclei permit the hormone to enter the circulating blood directly. The *oxytocin* produced by the *paraventricular nucleus* initiates contractions of the pregnant uterus and has an influence on the secretion of milk by the breasts.

There is a second hypothalamus-pituitary connection via the *tuberoinfundibular (tuberohypophyseal)* tract. It is assumed that specific-action substances, called releasing hormones or factors, which are produced by certain hypothalamic nuclei, travel along this tract to the portal vascular network of the pituitary stalk (eminentia mediana). The substances reach the anterior pituitary lobe through these blood vessels and stimulate specific hormone-producing cells (Fig. 5.18).

The factors, the hormones and their actions are listed in Table 5.1. The cells responding to the factors are the *eosinophilic* or *alpha cells* and the *basophilic* or *beta cells*. The eosinophilic cells produce *growth hormone (GH)* or *STH (somatotropic hormone)* and *prolactin (PRL)* or *LTH (lactotropic hormone)*. The basophilic cells produce

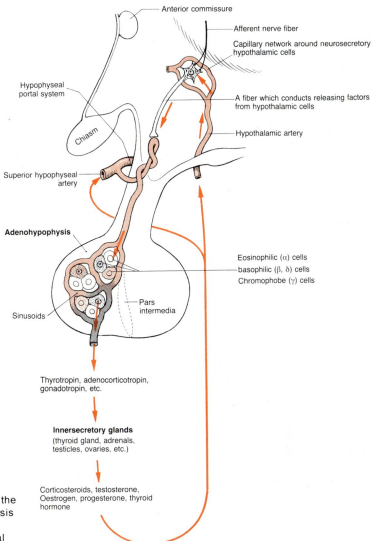

Fig. 5.18 Anterior lobe of hypophysis. Neurosecretory hormones from the hypothalamus passing through neurosecretory fibers reach the anterior lobe of the hypophysis (adenohypophysis) only indirectly through the arterial system.

thyroid-stimulating hormone (*TSH*) (*thyrotropic hormone*) and *adrenocorticotropic hormone* (*ACTH*). The *chromophobe* or *gamma cells* do not participate in the formation of hormones, except, perhaps, for ACTH.

The hormones produced by the cells enter the bloodstream and stimulate the various glands of internal secretion to produce their respective hormones. These hormones also enter the bloodstream and influence by their concentration within the blood the specific hypothalamic nuclei as well as the glandular cells and the anterior pituitary by a kind of feedback mechanism. As a result, the various cells of the adenohypophysis release only a limited amount of releasing factors or none at all. In this way the level of hormones within the blood is kept within rather narrow limits (see Fig. 5.18).

Function of Hypothalamus

Without doubt the hypothalamus possesses particular receptors, a sort of measuring sensors, that enable the central organ to control all autonomic functions of the body and to regulate them in such a way that factors in the internal environment are kept at the levels required for normal life (*homeostasis*).

It is of great significance for the hypothalamus as is serves this function that its neurons are surrounded by a particularly dense capillary network. This permits the hypothalamus to control neural as well as neurosecretory and humoral mechanisms.

The hypothalamic nuclei responsible for regulating water metabolism for the body and the interplay of functions of glands of internal secretion have already been mentioned. Similarly, the *heat metabolism* of the body is regulated by nuclei that have special temperature sensors. The rostral hypothalamus, the preoptic area in particular, plays a special role. As the temperature of the blood circulating through the hypothalamus increases, neurons in this region transmit impulses to a certain nuclear territory in the caudal portion of the hypothalamus that also receives information from cold sensors in the skin. This regulating center controls heat loss and heat production via descending pathways. If the body temperature decreases, vasoconstriction will occur in the skin in an attempt to prevent further heat loss. If this mechanism is not sufficient, the muscles begin to tremble (one shivers with cold) in an attempt to produce more warmth. Increased metabolism of energy-rich substances such as fats and carbohydrates produces heat. As the body temperature rises, heat is again given off through dilatation of the blood vessels of the skin and secretion of sweat. At the same time, the metabolic rate is reduced. Destruction of this temperature-regulating nuclear territory in the caudal portion of the hypothalamus results in *poikilothermy*, a condition in which the body temperature varies with the environmental temperature.

If the rostral portion of the hypothalamus is damaged, the patient may be unable to lose heat in a warm environment. The resulting high temperature is called *central fever*. Damage to the caudal portion of the hypothalamus causes an abnormally low body temperature in a cool environment.

The hypothalamus also regulates *food intake*. The lateral area of the tuber cinereum acts as a center for hunger or gluttony, whereas the feeling of satiation is centered in the area of the ventromedial nucleus. It has been determined in animal experiments that stimulation in the lateral tuber region produces voracity, which ends immediately if the area of the ventromedial nucleus is stimulated. If this area was destroyed by a lesion, the eating center prevailed and the animals displayed a voracious appetite. They ate much more than required and became obese in a short time. In contrast, a lesion in the lateral nucleus produced a total loss of appetite, leading to emaciation.

If the tuber cinereum is damaged in man, *adiposogenital dystrophy* (Fröhlich's syndrome) may be produced. Because the damage also involves cells that stimulate the release of gonadotropic substances, the obesity is associated with hypogenitalism. Just as the intake of food is believed to be controlled by the previously mentioned bipartite steering mechanism, it is suspected that such a mechanism exists for sexual functioning. Based on animal experiments, it is posited that a gonadotropic center is located in the infundibular nucleus or ventromedial nucleus and releases gonadotropic pituitary hormone. A sexual behavioral or inhibitory center is suspected to be located rostral to the ventromedial nucleus. Pubertas praecox has been observed in children in whom tumor or inflammation has destroyed the hypothalamus rostral to the infundibulum and ventromedial nucleus. A loss of the inhibitory center is considered the cause of the precocious puberty.

The hypothalamus is the primary center of the entire peripheral autonomic nervous system. Stimulation of the *rostral* hypothalamus, particularly the preoptic area, produces *increased parasympathetic (trophotropic) activity*, with sweating, vasodilatation, salivation, hypotonia, slowing of pulse rate, contraction of the urinary bladder, and an increase in peristalsis (indicating that the hypothalamus regulates even the function of the gastrointestinal tract). It is not rare for damage to the hypothalamus to lead to acute gastrointestinal bleeding (stress bleeding). Somatostatin depletion (see Table 5.1) appears to be a causative factor.

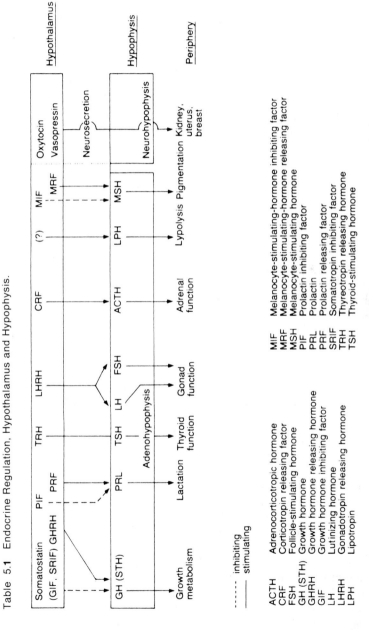

Table 5.1 Endocrine Regulation, Hypothalamus and Hypophysis.

Stimulation of the *caudal* hypothalamus, particularly the posterior nucleus and the area lateralis, produces *increased sympathetic (ergotropic) activity*, associated with mydriasis, hypertension, tachycardia, tachypnea, reduced peristalsis, and hyperglycemia.

Experimental stimulation of certain hypothalamic nuclei may produce an increase in sympathetic (ergotropic) activity, triggering a guarding reaction in the animal. It may turn into a defense, attack, or flight reaction. If the lateral segment of the hypothalamus next to the fornix is stimulated, a quietly sleeping cat suddenly wakes up. It becomes very tense, its hairs stand on end, its pupils widen, and it meows and spits and suddenly attacks or runs away. Bilateral coagulation of the ventromedial nucleus makes cats permanently aggressive and vicious.

A patient showing such aggressiveness or flight will also exhibit emotional expressions of anger, rage, or fear, all of which are linked to autonomic signs or symptoms. Such emotional reactions were noted in patients in whom the hypothalamus was the site of operation. When Foerster (1934) removed a tumor from the rostral hypothalamus under local anesthesia, pressure on adjacent rostral hypothalamic structures produced a change in the mood of the patient. He became euphoric and logorrheic and produced an unrestrained series of silly ideas. Operation in the caudal hypothalamus area produces stupor, akinesia, and possibly coma.

Every emotional exaltation is associated with numerous autonomic symptoms, such as palpitation, increase in systemic blood pressure, blushing, blanching, dry mouth, urge to urinate, and increased peristalsis. Such exaltations are often related to recollections of pleasant or disagreeable circumstances or emotional experiences or are caused by fear of unknown or seemingly threatening situations.

Such emotionally tinged modes of behavior are currently thought of as related to cortical, thalamic, and hypothalamic connections with the *limbic system*.

Limbic System

The cortex of each cerebral hemisphere has a line of origin or margin where it faces the corpus callosum and surrounds the midbrain. Next to these structures begins the cortex of the cingulate and hippocampal gyri, which are connected behind the splenium by the isthmus of the cingulate gyrus. Thus, one may think of both gyri as one arcuate, marginal lobe, as Broca did in 1878. Because *limbus* is the Latin word for "margin", Broca called it the "grand lobe limbique" (gyrus fornicatus of Arnold). This *limbic lobe* consists of archicortex (hippocampal and dentate gyrus), paleocortex (pyriform cortex of the anterior hippocampal gyrus), and juxtallocortex or mesocortex (cingulate gyrus).

The term **limbic system** encompasses the components of the limbic lobe and associated structures, among them the entorhinal and septal areas, indusium griseum, amygdaloid complex, and mamillary body (Fig. 5.**19a**). Because of the extensive fiber connections of these various components, Papez in 1937 proposed the theory that the circuit formed by the various units may very well be the anatomic substrate for the mechanism of emotions and their expression and for the affective components of instinctive drives (Papez circuit; Fig. 5.**20a**). Animal experiments by Klüver and Bucy have supported this theory (Klüver-Bucy syndrome). Based on rather precise anatomic and electrophysiologic investigations, MacLean introduced the term *limbic system*. It is still a subject of debate (Brodal, 1969).

The *Papez circuit* functions as follows: impulses originating in the horn of Ammon in the hippocampus are transmitted to the mamillary body via the arc of the fornix; from the mamillary body the mamillothalamic tract (the bundle of Vicq d'Azyr) transmits the impulses to the anterior thalamic nucleus; from there the thalamocingulate radiation projects the impulses into the cingulate gyrus; from the cingulate gyrus the cingulum, a subcortical bundle of association fibers partly encircling the corpus

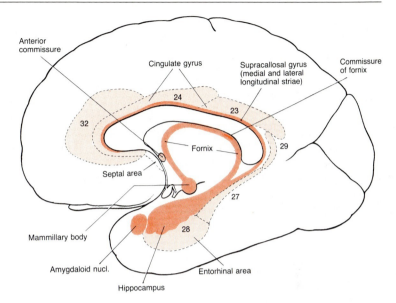

Fig. 5.**19a** Limbic cortex.

callosum, carries the impulses back to the hippocampal cortex, thus closing the neuronal circuit (see Fig. 8.**15a**).

The mamillary body occupies a key position in the system, because it connects it with the midbrain (Gudden's and Bechterew's nuclei) and the reticular formation. The mamillotegmental tract and the mamillary peduncle form their own feedback circuit (see Figs. 5.**15** and 5.**16**).

Impulses originating in the limbic system may be transmitted via the anterior thalamic nucleus not only to the cingulate gyrus but also to the neocortex by way of associating fibers. Impulses originating in the autonomic system may reach the orbitofrontal cortex via the hypothalamus and the medial dorsal nucleus. Emotional exaltations are accompanied by autonomic disorders (increase in systemic blood pressure, blushing, paleness, and so forth); conversely, autonomic disorders may produce emotional expressions (psychosomatics). What must occur in order to produce these reactions has not been elucidated so far, however. Therefore, we shall refrain from discussing further details.

Entorhinal Area

The entorhinal area is also part of the allocortex, and recent studies have shown it to be of particular significance. The entorhinal area is located lateral to the hippocampus near the parahippocampal gyrus (Brodmann's area 28), and rostrally it abuts the amygdaloid complex. The collateral fissure separates the entorhinal area from the temporal isocortex. Its allocortical afferent connections originate in the olfactory cortex while isocortical afferent connections come *from all neocortical association areas* to the entorhinal area. The most important efferent connections pass through the perforating tract to the hippocampus (Fig. 5.**19b**). Because of its many and diverse connections, the entorhinal area is believed to be an important center of association and integration. Olfactory, sensorisomatic, visual, auditory, and motor projections converge in the entorhinal area from where the partly processed information is passed on to the hippocampal function via the perforating tract. In this way, impressions that have been processed and stored in various association areas are transmitted to the limbic system.

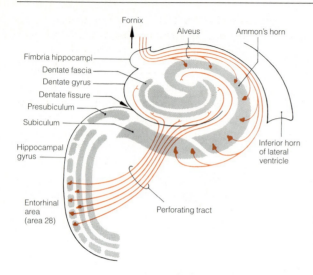

Fig. 5.**19b** Schematic diagram of the perforating tract, the most important connection between the entorhinal area and the hippocampal formation.

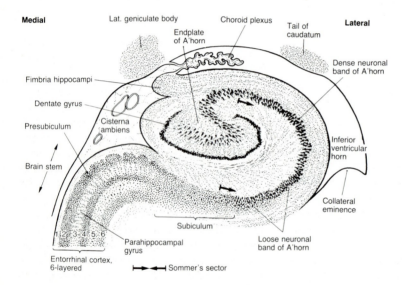

Fig. 5.**19c** The cytoarchitectural allocortex of the hippocampal formation with dentate gyrus (fascia dentata), Ammon's horn and parahippocampal cortex. Note that the fimbria hippocampi becomes caudally the fornix seen in Figs. 5.**19a** and 5.**20a**.

According to H. and E. Braak, the entorhinal cortex functions as a multimodal association center in the allocortex, providing the sole and—in terms of memory function—extremely important link between the isocortex and allocortex. Communication of the isocortex with the allocortex and limbic system is essential if something is to be retained in the memory (Braak and Braak 1989; also Rolls 1987 and Zilles 1985).

Amygdaloid Nuclear Complex

The gray mass of the amygdala is composed of various nuclei too numerous to be discussed here in detail. It will be mentioned only that this complex receives most afferent connections from the olfactory system. Its medial and central portions are related to the limbic system, and the stria terminalis originates there (see Fig. 5.**15**). It runs at first in a caudal direction, then turns around the posterior thalamus, extending some fibers to the habenular nucleus. Thereupon it runs anteriorly in a groove between caudate nucleus and thalamus. Upon reaching the interventricular foramen of Monro, its fibers divide, some running to the septal area and others to the rostral hypothalamus. The amygdaloid complex is believed to be connected also with midbrain and thalamus, more precisely with the dorsomedial nucleus of the thalamus, which projects to the orbitofrontal cortex. Furthermore, the two amygdaloid complexes are connected with each other.

Experimental stimulation of the limbic portion of the amygdala that gives rise to the stria terminalis produced pronounced emotional outbursts. Such reactions failed to occur when any of the other components of the limbic system were stimulated.

Hippocampus

The hippocampus, to which the Ammon's horn belongs is one of the important structures of the limbic system (Fig. 5.**19c**). Its cortex has three layers; the middle layer is characterized by a predominance of rather large pyramidal cells. The Ammon's horn is the most epileptogenic part of the entire brain. Lesions within or near its cortex, small tumors, areas of inflammation, scars, and other conditions that do not destroy the Ammon's horn often produce seizure-like conditions, referred to as *psychomotor attacks* or twilight states, and tend to produce synchronized discharges on the electroencephalograph. The attacks may comprise brief absence states or dreamy states, a seizure-like feeling of alienation, passing macropsia or micropsia, déjà-vu experiences, and transient depression, among other symptoms. These states may be associatied with olfactory hallucinations or other types of auras and with oral mechanisms such as chewing, swallowing, and smacking of lips. It is possible however for the epileptic discharges to spread over other parts of the brain causing a generalized epileptic seizure (page 300).

Limbic System as a Circuitry for Mechanisms of Expression, Formation of Emotions, Dispositions, and Instinctive Drives

Klüver and Bucy (1939) removed much of both temporal lobes, including the amygdaloid complexes, the hippocampal gyri, and the Ammon's horn in rhesus monkeys. The animals developed the following syndrome: inability to recognize objects optically (psychic blindness) or by touch (tactile agnosia); a compulsion to examine all objects, even if dangerous, by mouth; pronounced distractibility; hypersexuality; and change from wild and intractable behavior to docility with no evidence of fear or anger.

Both temporal lobes, including the Ammon's horn were also resected in patients who suffered from psychomotor epilepsy. They were cured from the attacks but had severe psychic changes with loss of drive, changes of personality with loss of instinct inhibition, and pathologic tractability and impressionableness.

Bilateral loss of the Ammon's horns causes disorders of consciousness, disorientation as to time and place, and loss of the ability to memorize (Milner and Penfield, 1955; Penfield and Milner, 1958; and others). Hassler (1964) considered the activity of the Ammon's horn to be a mechanism for the chronological registration and marking of perceptions and experiences. Unilateral damage to the Ammon's horn or a unilateral partial resection of the temporal lobe, including Ammon's horn, the uncus, and the amygdala, is said to produce no noticeable clinical deficits, provided that the other temporal lobe is intact.

Bilateral interruption of the fornix has been observed to cause an acute amnestic syndrome characterized by loss of ability to memorize new impressions.

Bilateral damage to the mamillary bodies produces an amnestic syndrome with confabulations (Korsakoff's syndrome). Old memories – already stored impressions – remain intact in this syndrome. An amnestic

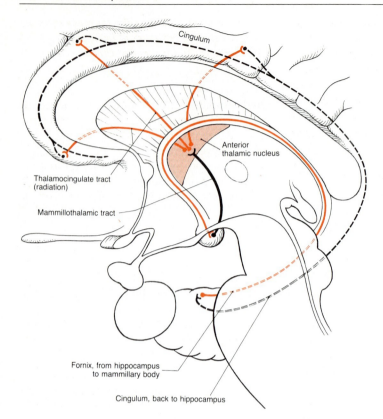

Fig. 5.**20 a** Papez circuit (hippocampus, fornix, mamillary body, anterior thalamic nucleus, cingulate gyrus, cingulum, hippocampus).

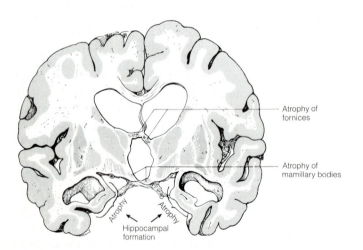

Fig. 5.**20 b** Limbic form of Alzheimer's disease. The cross-section of the brain of an 88-year-old woman at the level of the mamillary bodies shows severe symmetrical atrophy of the unci, hippocampi, and parahippocampal gyri with lateral widening of the interpeduncular cistern and expansion of the rostral inferior horns of the lateral ventricles. The cortex of the other gyri is not reduced. The mamillary bodies, fornices, and thalami show secondary atrophy with a widening of the third ventricle. The lateral ventricles are widened by diffuse secondary atrophy of the cerebral medulla (drawn from specimen).

syndrome may also follow a transient cerebral anoxemia or hypoxemia occurring during transient cardiac arrest, drowning, strangulation, acute edema of the glottis, or carbon monoxide poisoning. This amnestic condition is also attributed to damage of the mamillary bodies and Ammon's horns.

Damage to the same structures as a consequence of a degenerative process such as, e.g., the limbic form of Alzheimer's disease (Fig. 5.**20b**), results, among others, in a progressive loss of memory.

Bilateral extirpation of the cingulate gyri results in loss of initiative, emotional dullness, and loss of inhibition. The ability to memorize, however, remains intact.

These and similar observations suggest that the ability to memorize new impressions and to store them requires that the hippocampus-fornix-mamillary body system be intact. One must keep in mind, however, that in operative interventions not only these but also adjacent structures are removed or damaged. The following case report is presented to demonstrate that brain injury resulting from a transient lack of oxygen, in this case a carbon monoxide poisoning, may severely damage the ability to register new impressions (recent memory or ability to recall), whereas already stored impressions (old memory) remain intact.

Case report: A 28-year-old actor had taken a bath after a show and accidentally extinguished the pilot flame of the hot water boiler. One hour later he was found lying in the empty bathtub, unconscious from carbon monoxide poisoning. He slept throughout the night and the following day. When he awoke, it was noted that his behavior was strange. Contrary to his usual self, he was now very jolly, laughed a great deal, and appeared to be in a peculiar trance. His landlady informed the theater that his condition would not permit him to go on stage. The director, who had come to see him, found him in good spirits. When asked whether he felt well enough to play the same evening, the answer was, "Why? There is no reason that I cannot play." The director, however, became skeptical because the actor could not remember having been poisoned by gas and repeatedly asked which play he was to perform. "But, Mr. B." said the director, "you know it; you have so often presented it, this 'Head in the Noose.'" "Of course I can play it," the actor replied.

The director, although skeptical, had him picked up in the evening. B. was in an excellent mood, laughed constantly, and found everyone very charming. While changing, he asked the wardrobe master, "Well, what are we playing tonight?" When the wardrobe master told him the name of the play, he replied "Of course." Everyone worried about his extraordinary behavior and was convinced that the evening would end in a catastrophe. When the call came, B. went on stage and looked around happily. When his partner gave the cue, he answered with the appropriate dialogue, and the entire performance proceeded without incident.

Back in the dressing room between acts, he wanted to change and go home. The wardrobe master had to restrain him by telling him he had to perform another act. Thereupon B. asked again, "Well. what play is on tonight?" Back on stage he again spoke the correct lines on cue. Thereafter, however, he collapsed and had to be taken to the hospital, where he was treated for the following six weeks.

For the first two weeks, he was jolly and careless, disoriented as to time and place, and unable to retain what was said to him, repeatedly asking the same questions. Thereafter he noticed for the first time that he was sick and in a hospital. Very slowly he became able to retain memories again and to register them in chronological order. He did not become able to return to the theater until several weeks later. He could not remember the time of the carbon monoxide intoxication. Although he had regained recent memory, learning his roles by rote remained more difficult than it had been prior to the poisoning.

Such a severe amnestic syndrome is usually attributed to the cerebral hypoxemia incident of the carbon monoxide poisoning. It is doubtful, however, that oxygen deficiency per se is the cause of the various necrotic changes seen in cerebral and cerebellar cortex, including the Ammon's horns and in such structures as the pallida. According to Lindenberg (1955, 1963, 1971a, 1982), the alterations are caused by vascular compression, particularly compression of arteries in certain areas of predilection. In the absence of a space-occupying lesion, a swelling of the brain is responsible for this transient compression. The swelling develops very rapidly in sudden shock, in other words, if the output of the heart is suddenly decreased. The Ammon's horn is damaged so often because its arteries are vulnerable to compression where they cross, at a short distance, the sharp margin of the tentorium (see Fig. 8.38). Necrosis of the pallida is not specific for carbon monoxide poisoning; it is found with various other conditions in which swelling of the brain occurs. It is the result of compression of the pallidum branches of the anterior choroidal arteries.

Damage to the Hypothalamus

The hypothalamus may be damaged in various ways.

Trauma: If the base of the skull is fractured, there may be direct injury to the pituitary stalk. A longitudinal fracture may tear the chiasm and tuber cinereum apart, producing a direct communication between the third ventricle and basal cistern. In the presence of an extradural, subdural, or intracerebral traumatic hematoma, ventral displacement of the hypothalamus may result in local circulatory deficiencies that produce unilateral or bilateral focal areas of necrosis. The supraoptic nuclei may be deprived of sufficient circulation for some time, and this may result in transient or long-lasting diabetes insipidus associated with central fever and, if the patient is not unconscious, some psychic alterations.

Primary circulatory disorders: The hypothalamus receives blood via numerous small arteries, practically all branches of the arterial circle of Willis (Fig. 5.21). For this reason, infarcts are usually limited to small nuclear areas, if they occur at all, and may be asymptomatic if the lesion is unilateral.

Inflammatory changes: The hypothalamus is almost never the sole location of an encephalitic process. There may be encephalitis in other portions of the brain, such as a lethargic encephalitis in the midbrain, and this encephalitis may spread into the hypothalamus. The hypothalamus may be predominantly exposed to bacterial toxins, however, if leptomeningitis is concentrated in the basal cistern. If the basal meningitis is granu-

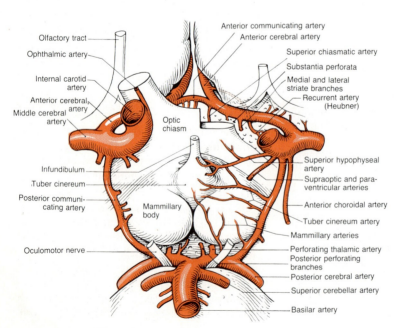

Fig. 5.21 Blood supply of hypothalamus.

lomatous (for example, in tuberculosis or syphilis), the blood vessels may be narrowed by vasculitis, and this may produce areas of circulatory deficiency within the hypothalamus. One of the inflammatory diseases is multiple sclerosis. Its first signs may be related to hypothalamic involvement.

Case Report: A 17-year-old girl gradually stopped menstruating. She consulted a gynecologist, who found a hypoplastic uterus. Thereafter, she experienced periods of unexplained anxiety associated with complaints of failing vision. The complaints were regarded as hysteric until retrobulbar neuritis was diagnosed. From then on the disease took a rather fast course, and the patient died at age 19. Postmortem examination revealed foci of multiple sclerosis involving, among other structures, the hypothalamus bilaterally (Lindenberg).

Wernicke's encephalopathy: This dysoric alteration, which is triggered by thiamine deficiency, usually occurs in alcoholics. It always symmetrically involves the same structures: the mamillary bodies and adjacent hypothalamic structures, the gray matter around the aqueduct, parts of the nuclei of III and IV, and the tegmentum of the medulla oblongata near the fourth ventricle, particularly the areas of the dorsal nuclei of X. The damage to the mamillary bodies results in *Korsakoff's syndrome*, mentioned earlier.

Tumors

Intrinsic tumors are pilocytic astrocytomas of the juvenile type in the region of the third ventricle and suprasellar germinomas or "ectopic" pinealomas, both occurring in the same region and most often in young persons. Ectopic pinealoma usually begins in the third ventricle and may produce polydipsia from diabetes insipidus before signs of visual pathway involvement appear. It may also grow by continuity into the sella turcica, expanding it as a pituitary tumor would and presenting a clinical picture of hyperpituitarism.

The most frequent *extrinsic tumors* damaging hypothalamus and optic chiasm by pressure are suprasellar meningiomas, craniopharyngiomas (epidermoids), and pituitary tumors. Occasionally an aneurysm of the circle of Willis, particularly one descending from the junction of the internal carotid and posterior communicating arteries, may be sufficiently large to involve the hypothalamus as a space-occupying alteration.

Extrinsic tumors may also produce diabetes insipidus, mental and emotional disorders, occasionally central fever, and perhaps adiposogenital dystrophy. Blocking of the third ventricle may be followed by an occlusive hydrocephalus of the lateral ventricle. There may be signs pointing to involvement of thalamus and basal ganglia. A visual field defect from pressure on chiasm and optic tract is common. When talking about pressure on these structures, one must keep in mind that they can tolerate a remarkable degree of displacement without developing dysfunction and that it is interference with capillary circulation in the displaced or compressed structures that is responsible for clinical deficits. Variations in the rate of capillary circulation may account for fluctuations in the degree of a clinical finding.

In order to demonstrate the diversity of the symptomatology that can be produced by the same type of tumor in this region, the hospital records of two patients with *craniopharyngiomas* of approximately the same size are reported. The two were patients at the Hospital of Nervous Diseases of the University of Frankfurt/Main in 1939 and 1940, respectively, long before the advent of computer tomography.

Case Report 1: A 51-year-old woman had a history of some loss of visual acuity and a slight protrusion of the left eye seven years prior to admission. At that time an abscess behind the left eye was found and repeatedly punctured. Improvement occurred after a nasal operation. One year prior to the patient's admission, diabetes mellitus was diagnosed and treated. Four months prior to admission, she developed a definite weakness in retaining fresh memories. Old events were recalled without hesitation, but new events were forgotten after five minutes. Her mood was depressed. Approximately $3\frac{1}{2}$ months prior to admission, she noticed a weakness in both legs that caused some insecurity of gait. At times she complained of headaches. On roentgenography a calcification the size of a small bean was noticed near the sella. A pneumoencephalogram revealed dilatation of the lateral ventricles. There was no papilledema. A craniopharyngioma was diagnosed and considered inoperable because of its size. On admission to the neurologic department, the patient exhibited an extreme alteration in her emotional behavior. She was agitated, used coarse language, thrashed about angrily and spat at the nurses. She was sexually excited, assumed shamelessly lewd positions, and seemed to enjoy making obscene comments and engaging in similar conversations about sexual matters. At times she wrangled, nagged, cried, and wailed. At other times she was exceedingly cheerful and happy, hyperkinetic and logomanic; she hummed and whistled and, in short, showed manic behavior. Because of her euphoria she had no physical complaints except that she was tormented by thirst day and night and continually asked for water. "Daddy, Daddy, please give me something to drink," she would say, "my whole mouth is dry, I want to drink a whole glass of water." Between requests she would fall asleep. She was rather obese. Blood pressure was 110/95 mm Hg; blood sugar was 270 mg/100ml.

Neurologic examination revealed sensitivity to tapping on the head; pain in trigeminal pressure points; hypersensitivity to painful stimuli in the face; slight protrusion of left eye; diabetic retinopathy; mild left facial weakness and tremor of tongue; slightly increased reflexes associated with positive Babinski's sign, more pronounced on the right; and total disorientation as to time and place. She believed she was in the city hall and did not know whether it was summer or winter. When asked questions she would shout, "How should I know that, you dumb cow! I am thirsty, that's all." During the examination she repeatedly fell asleep or shouted foul words. When somnolent she was incontinent. At other times she would be jolly again and sing and whistle, believing that she was in her own apartment and had to wake up her children and prepare their meal. In between, she would cry because she mistook another gravely ill patient for her own daughter. Despite increasing doses of insulin, her blood sugar climbed to high levels. Finally the patient developed a carbuncle and died in a high septic fever.

Postmortem examinations revealed the base of the brain to be occupied by a large craniopharyngioma that extended from the optic chiasm to the pons and bilaterally into the temporal lobes and showed cysts and areas of calcification. The mamillary bodies were totally destroyed, as was the floor of the third ventricle. The tumor almost filled the third ventricle with a huge cyst. The

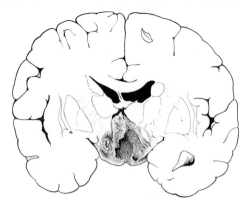

Fig. 5.22 Craniopharyngioma found in Case I (drawn from specimen).

periventricular hypothalamic gray matter was also destroyed, as were the anterior commissure and the parolfactory area. Pallida, putamina, and thalami were displaced. The lateral ventricles were somewhat enlarged (Fig. 5.22).

Some of the signs and symptoms in this patient are unequivocally hypothalamic in origin: the polydipsia caused by the diabetes insipidus, the vacillating mood with changes from depression to euphoria and mania, the instinctive outbursts of affective reactions with obscene and sex-dominated expressions, and the inability to retain recent memories, associated with disorientation as to time and place. This loss of memorizing faculty can be ascribed to the destruction of the mamillary bodies. The diabetes mellitus is not necessarily related to the hypothalamic damage, although it is not unusual to find this condition associated with diencephalic tumors. The same holds true for the obesity. The somnolence and the occasional inversion of sleep were probably caused by damage to the caudal portion of the hypothalamus in front of the periaqueductal gray matter that Hess called a dynamogenic zone. Together with the reticular formation of the midbrain, this area is believed to constitute a functional unit important for the activation of the cerebrum and responsible for the degree of alertness Because of the patient's condition, visual fields could not be measured. The postmortem findings, however, strongly suggested that field defects did exist.

The tumor was considered inoperable at the time because of its location and its size. Current microsurgical methods permit successful removal of such large tumors.

In the second patient the craniopharyngioma formed a large cyst that filled the entire third ventricle and produced early increased intracranial pressure caused by occlusive hydrocephalus of the lateral ventricles.

Case Report 2: A 51-year-old woman had never been ill until approximately 6 months prior to death, when she began complaining of severe fatigue and headaches. She was depressed at times, became somnolent, had difficulty concentrating, and complained of dizziness. Occasionally, she fell to the floor, vomited, and soiled. Gradually, she had become disoriented as to time and place and could not remember things.

On admission, she was slow, could not concentrate, and perseverated. She was totally disoriented, and the ability to deposit new memories was virtually absent. It was not possible to elicit a useful preadmission history. She was tall, obese, and somewhat bearded. Examinations revealed resting blood pressure of 140/80 mm Hg, anisocoria (right pupil wider than left), bilateral papilledema (2 diopters) with fresh hemorrhages, weakness of facial innervation of left side of mouth, slight decrease of power in arms and legs, increased tone on right side, intention tremor more pronounced on the right, tremor of both hands, bilateral grasping reflexes, tendon reflexes slightly exaggerated, Babinski's sign more pronounced on the left, and an inability to stand or walk without assistance. During the three weeks of hospitalization, the patient was akinetic, did not speak spontaneously, was stuporous at times, and soiled. She often was nauseated and vomited. There was a repeated tremor of the hands. Cerebral angiography indicated internal hydrocephalus. Somnolence eventually turned into coma, and death ensued after the patient developed a high fever.

At postmortem examination, a craniopharyngioma (epidermoid with stratified epithelium) was found to occupy the base of the brain between chiasm and mamillary bodies. The tumor was the size of a walnut, grew partially around the chiasm, and displaced the mamillary bodies in a caudal direction. On a coronal section through the tuber cinereum (Fig. 5.23), the rather firm tumor was partially cystic. One large cyst filled almost the entire third ventricle, obstructing the interventri-

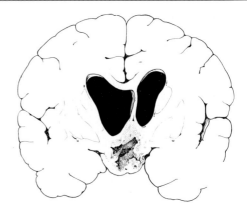

Fig. 5.23 Craniopharyngioma of Case II in the area of the hypothalamus between the optic chiasm and mamillary bodies, occluding the entire 3rd ventricle by a cyst (drawn from specimen).

cular foramina and producing an occlusive hydrocephalus of the lateral ventricles, more severe on the left. The tumor contained no areas of calcification.

Although the tumor was of the same type and location as that in the first patient, it produced a completely different clinical picture because of the early development of an occlusive hydrocephalus. It elevated the intracranial pressure to such a degree that papilledema developed. Usually these tumors press first on the optic chiasm and tracts, making primary optic atrophy the more common finding. It was mainly because of the increased intracranial pressure that the patient could not concentrate and was slow and drowsy. The patient's preadmission history remained scanty because of her disorientation and inability to remember. Only the amnestic syndrome, the depression, the somnolence, and perhaps the obesity may be attributed to disorders in hypothalamic function.

Both patients just discussed were already of advanced age and so ill at the time of admission that they were unable to provide detailed anamnestic data. In adults, early complaints are usually of visual disorders.

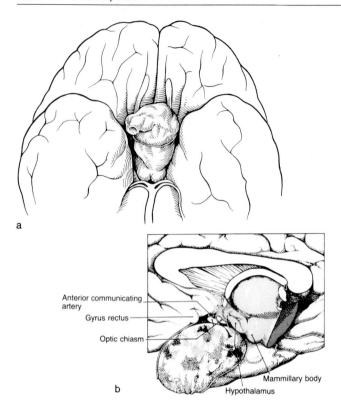

Fig. 5.24 Pituitary adenoma occupying basal cistern. **a** Basal view; **b** sagittal cut through center of tumor. (Drawn from specimen.)

The fundus shows an atrophy of the optic nerve heads, and the visual fields may reveal homonymous losses, often involving the upper temporal quadrants, or central scotomas. Bitemporal hemianopsias are not rare but are not seen as often as in cases of pituitary adenoma. In contrast to its incidence in children, papilledema is rare among adults. Frontal headaches and pain behind the eyes are frequent complaints and often lead to vomiting.

It is not unusual to find craniopharyngiomas in children and adolescents. Headaches, nausea, and vomiting are the most common complaints in children. Growth is often retarded. Some children tend to become obese, whereas others are frail and thin. Polyuria may be the cause of bedwetting.

Adolescents complain also of poor vision and sexual changes. Libido may decrease or disappear. The genitals are underdeveloped, and secondary hairiness is skimpy. Young woman become amenorrheal. Children, however, may develop pubertas praecox. A *neuronal hamartoma* (tumor-like hyperplasia) of the tuber cinereum may be its cause. This condition produces signs in small children up to the age of 6 years. There is premature growth of the genitals and of secondary sexual features, sometimes associated with an early onset of libido and adolescent behavior. If precocious puberty occurs in later childhood, its cause is most likely different and may be a tumor, such as a teratoma or craniopharyngioma. It may also be an inflammatory alteration, for example, a tuberculoma or an encephalitis.

As was mentioned earlier in the text, *pituitary tumors* often break through the diaphragm of the sella and grow toward the hypothalamus. This is common with chromophobe and rare with eosinophilic and basophilic adenomas. *Chromophobe adenoma* occurs most often in the fifth decade of life but may develop earlier or later. The initial symptom most frequently is frontal or bilateral headaches. They are believed to be caused by the stretching of the dural diaphragm of the sella and to lessen in intensity once the diaphragm has yielded to the pressure. Libido then decreases, and the genitals and the secondary sexual characteristics undergo atrophy to some extent. The pressure exerted by the tumor against the optic nerves, chiasm, and optic tracts leads to defects in the visual fields. A bitemporal hemianopsia is rather common. Visual acuity decreases as one or both optic nerves become atrophic. Figure 5.**24** demonstrates such a chromophobe adenoma and its topography. The sudden enlargement of the tumor by acute bleeding into its parenchyma is called *pituitary apoplexy*. It produces an acute deterioration of vision that requires immediate operative decompression.

Eosinophilic adenoma also produces frontal headaches initially and damage to optic nerves, chiasm, or tracts later, with corresponding visual field defects and optic atrophy. Characteristically, eosinophilic adenoma causes *gigantism* in young persons and *acromegaly* in older persons, because of the overproduction of somatotropic hormones (STH). *Basophilic adenoma* may produce *Cushing's syndrome*, consisting of obesity of face, neck, and trunk; abdominal striae distensae; hypertrichosis; hypertension; glucosuria; osteoporosis; sexual disorders; and mental changes. More often this syndrome is brought on by a tumor of the adrenal cortex. A balloon-like distention of the sella speaks in favor of a pituitary tumor. Such an enlargement may also result from a subarachnoid cyst within the sella, producing the so-called *empty sella*. An erosion of the sella is more indicative of a craniopharyngioma, a meningioma, or some other type of tumor in the area of the hypothalamus.

Peripheral Autonomic Nervous System

Control by the Hypothalamus

The hypothalamus, as mentioned earlier, represents a center of higher order for controlling or steering the entire peripheral autonomic nervous system. Stimulating its *rostral* portion results in greater *parasympathetic* (*trophotropic*) activity. There is decrease in minute volume, blood pressure, pulse rate, respiratory volume, basic metabolism, and delivery of epinephrine. The blood vessels dilate, and sweating and salivation, contraction of the urinary bladder, an increase in peristalsis, and a narrowing of the pupils occur. If the *caudal* hypothalamus is stimulated, the *sympathetic* (*ergotropic*) activity increases, characterized by increased delivery of epinephrine; increase in blood pressure, pulse rate, and volume of blood circulating through skeletal muscles and lungs; increase in blood glucose; emptying of blood depots, decreased respiratory volume; decreased circulation in viscera; inhibition of peristalsis; retention of urine; and dilatation of palpebral fissures and pupils. The word *ergotropic* means that these sympathetic reactions put the organism in a condition to perform and to withstand all assaults and stresses. The word *trophotropic* indicates that the parasympathetic reactions are oriented toward maintaining functions by rest and relaxation.

Function

The brain does not differentiate a sympathetic and a parasympathetic system as strictly as does the periphery. The hypothalamus regulates and steers the function of both systems by using three descending tracts: the *medial forebrain bundle*, the *mamillotegmental tract*, and the *dorsal longitudinal fascicle* (*Schütz's bundle*). These three pathways connect the hypothalamus with the descending reticular system of the midbrain, which conveys the central impulses to the various subdivisions of the parasympathetic and sympathetic systems. The hypothalamus also influences both systems via the pituitary, that is, via humoral action. The peripheral fibers given off by preganglionic and postganglionic neurons innervate the smooth musculature of all organs, the muscles of the heart, and all glands.

The autonomic nervous system regulates the vital functions that maintain the internal environment (homeostasis). It is assisted in this task by various nuclei of the brainstem (see Fig. 3.**51a**). These vital functions are, for example, respiration, circulation, metabolism, body temperature, water metabolism,

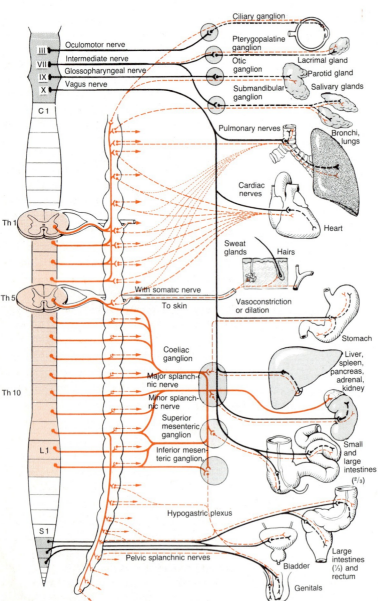

Fig. 5.**25** The peripheral autonomic nervous system and the organs innervated by it. The sympathetic system is shown in red; the parasympathetic system, in black. Only the left trunk is shown.

digestion, secretion, and procreation. They need not enter the level of awareness and are governed by their own laws; hence the term *autonomic nervous system*.

In the periphery the autonomic system consists of two functionally different components which act as antagonists by sending off either inhibitory or facilitory impulses. These components are called *sympathetic* and *parasympathetic* nerves. The sympathetic nerves use norepinephrine and the parasympathetic nerves acetylcholine as a transmitter substance; the two components are also referred to as *adrenergic* and *cholinergic* fibers.

The sympathetic fibers originate in the lateral horns of the thoracic and rostral lumbar cord (T1 through T12 and L1–L2); the parasympathetic fibers originate in nuclei of the brainstem (III, VII, IX, and X) and a distance away in the sacral cord (S2, S3, S4) (Fig. 5.25).

The fibers that leave together with cranial motor nerves and anterior motor roots of the spinal cord have visceral motor functions. The preganglionic neuron has its cell body within the central nervous system, and its axon is myelinated. It connects with a paravertebral or prevertebral ganglion, through which it relays its impulses to a second unmyelinated, postganglionic neuron, which sends its axon to the appropriate end-organ. Afferent fibers coming from the periphery connect with fibers of pseudounipolar neurons in ganglia at the base of the brain and along the spinal column. They continue centrally as part of an autonomic reflex arc and synapse, for example, with the visceromotor cells of the lateral horns (Fig. 5.26). Some of the afferent fibers from chest and abdominal cavities run centrally as part of the vagus nerve. The visceral receptors are located in the organs of chest and abdomen and in the walls of the blood vessels. They measure, for example, the pressure and degree of filling of the hollow organs, and transmit pain stimuli. These reflex arcs modify the visceromotor activity from the periphery.

Sympathetic Nervous System

Fig 5.25 demonstrates that the preganglionic sympathetic fibers (depicted in red) originate in the lateral horns of spinal cord segments T1 through L2 and accompany the anterior roots on their way through the intervertebral canals to the paravertebral ganglia of the sympathetic trunks. (Only the left trunk is shown.) Many of the fibers terminate at the paravertebral ganglia; others pass through the trunk and terminate at postganglionic

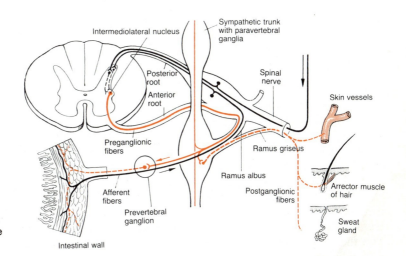

Fig. 5.26 Course of preganglionic and postganglionic sympathetic fibers, and the organization of the sympathetic trunk.

neurons in prevertebral ganglia. The axons of the postganglionic neurons terminate at the appropriate end-organs or effector organs.

Fig 5.26 shows in greater detail how the preganglionic neurons originate from the intermediolateral nucleus of the lateral horns and leave the spinal cord together with axons of the somatic motor neurons via the anterior roots. At the level of the spinal ganglia, they separate again from the somatic motor neurons and, being myelinated, form the *white communicating branches*, which enter the sympathetic trunk. Some of the fibers synapse there with postganglionic neurons; some run up and down within the trunk and synapse later at different levels. Still other fibers pass through the trunk and connect with postganglionic neurons in one of the prevertebral ganglia far outside the trunk. All postganglionic axons are unmyelinated. They leave the ganglia of the trunk and the other ganglia as *gray communicating rami* and join the spinal nerves on their way to the corresponding dermatomes of the skin. Here they innervate the blood vessels, the arrector muscles of hairs, and the sweat glands. The sympathetic nerve is the only regulator of the diameter of the arteries; increased sympathetic activity causes vasoconstriction, decreased activity a vasodilatation. The fibers innervating the sweat glands occupy a particular position in the sympathetic system. They act on the glands by releasing acetylcholine instead of norepinephrine; in other words, they are cholinergic at this point. (Sebaceous glands appear to have no innervation).

Many postganglionic fibers do not accompany the peripheral nerves but reach the effector organs via blood vessels and their branches. Because the cervical cord contains no nuclei from which sympathetic fibers originate, preganglionic fibers of the upper four to five thoracic segments spread rostrally within the paravertebral trunk to three ganglia in the cervical segments of the trunk. These are the *superior*, the *middle*, and the *inferior cervical ganglia*. The last is also called the *stellate ganglion*.

In these ganglia, impulses are relayed to those unmyelinated, postganglionic fibers that accompany the spinal nerves to their respective cervical dermatomes. Unmyelinated fibers of neurons in the superior cervical ganglion form the plexus of the external carotid artery, which supplies the sweat glands, the smooth muscles of the hair follicles, and the blood vessels of face and head. As the plexus of the internal carotid artery, these fibers innervate muscles of the eyes (dilator muscles of the pupils, orbital muscles, tarsal muscles) and lacrimal as well as salivatory glands (see Figs. 3.26, 3.27, and 5.25).

Postganglionic fibers of the cervical and upper 4 or 5 thoracic ganglia form the cardiac plexus innervating the heart and become pulmonary nerves for the sympathetic innervation of bronchi and lungs. Preganglionic fibers originating in spinal cord segments T5 through T12 travel over splanchnic nerves (greater, lesser, and lowest splanchnic nerves) to the prevertebral ganglia (celiac ganglia and superior and inferior mesenteric ganglia), where they connect with postganglionic fibers innervating the viscera in abdomen and pelvis. In contrast to the parasympathetic fibers, these postganglionic sympathetic fibers are rather long and form various plexuses prior to reaching their end-organs.

The adrenal glands occupy an exceptional position in the sympathetic system. They represent, so to speak, sympathetic ganglia. They receive directly preganglionic fibers that connect within the gland with modified postganglionic fibers (see Fig. 5.25). Sympathetic stimulation forces the adrenal medulla to release epinephrine and norepinephrine. These hormones enter the bloodstream, thus enhancing the effect of the sympathetic system. This is particularly important in stressful situations.

Unpaired prevertebral ganglia are located near the aorta and at branching points of individual larger arteries. They are named accordingly.

The preganglionic nerves originating in the lumbar segments run in lumbar and sacral splanchnic nerves to the inferior mesenteric ganglion. From there they transmit impulses to the postganglionic neurons that form extensive plexuses supplying the viscera of the pelvis. The preganglionic fibers for the cervical region run in the trunk cranially and those for the lumbosacral area caudally before they reach their relay stations. Because cervical, lower lumbar, and sacral segments of the cord thus carry no sympathetic neurons, there are considerably fewer preganglionic than postganglionic fibers.

The sympathetic fibers innervate the smooth muscles of vessels, viscera, bladder, rectum, hair follicles, pupils, heart, and the glands for sweating, lacrimation, salivation, and digestion. They have an inhibiting effect on the muscles of the viscera, including bladder and rectum, and on the glands of the digestive tract. They have a stimulating effect on all other end-organs.

It was mentioned in the discussion of cranial nerves (see Fig. 3.27) that injury to the ciliospinal center, sympathetic trunk, or cervical plexus produces an *ipsilateral Horner's syndrome*. The same syndrome results if the central sympathetic tract within the brainstem is damaged, for example, by the lesion that produces *Wallenberg's syndrome* (see Fig. 3.56). Concurrently, there is an absence of sweat secretion (anhidrosis) and a vasodilatation, causing the skin of the involved half of the face to be dry and reddened.

Because of the vasodilating effect of reduced sympathetic innervation, there has been an attempt to ameliorate headaches and various circulatory disorders by blocking the stellate ganglion, although this procedure may produce a transient Horner's syndrome. The vasodilating effect of sympathectomy has been used in the treatment of other circulatory disorders, such as Raynaud's disease. An interruption of the splanchnic nerves produces a considerable engorgement of the intestinal blood vessels (an internal exsanguination into the splanchnic area).

Parasympathetic Nervous System

The parasympathetic nervous system is effective only in particular areas and does not produce an overall, widespread reaction as the sympathetic system does. Its action is of rather short duration, because the acetylcholine acting at the nerve endings is soon degraded by cholinesterase.

In contrast to the sympathetic preganglionic fibers, those of the parasympathetic system are rather long. They originate in nuclei of the brainstem and in the sacral cord (S2, S3, S4). The parasympathetic fibers associated with cranial nerves III, VII (intermediate), IX, and X have been described in Chapter 3 and illustrated in Figs. 3.25, 3.26, 3.41, and 3.42. The postganglionic fibers are relatively short, because the ganglia from which they derive are located close to the end-organs. In the area of the head, for example, they are the ciliary, pterygopalatine, submandibular, and otic ganglia (see Fig. 5.25).

The parasympathetic portion of the vagus nerve originates in the dorsal nucleus of the nerve (see Fig. 3.42). Its preganglionic fibers travel to heart, lungs, and abdominal viscera with the exception of the distal third of the transverse colon and the sigmoid flexure and rectum. The neurons that give off the postganglionic fibers in this area are located in the immediately adjacent plexus or in the wall of the intestines (Auerbach's myenteric plexus and Meissner's submucosal plexus).

Stimulation of the parasympathetic system produces slowing of heart rate, lowering of systemic blood pressure, increase in secretion, and increase in peristalsis.

The Sacral Component

The sacral component of the parasympathetic system transmits impulses over the pelvic splanchnic nerves and the hypogastric, pudendal, and pelvic plexuses to the ganglia in the wall of the distal third of the transverse colon, of descending and sigmoid colon, rectum, bladder, and in genital organs. The parasympathetic nerves of the pelvis are mainly concerned with the emptying of these organs. They produce erection of the penis, whereas sympathetic fibers cause ejaculation by causing contraction of vas deferens and seminal vesicles.

The peripheral sympathetic and parasympathetic fibers are intermingled in the plexuses of the thoracic, abdominal, and pelvic cavities and act predominantly as antagonists in innervating the various organs (Table 5.2). Each system is relatively autonomous and functions by reflexes activated by numerous built-in regulatory feedback circuits. The systems are independent of voluntary motor actions.

Innervation of the urinary bladder

Control of the bladder musculature is predominantly parasympathetic. The pelvic splanchnic nerves originating in the sacral cord (S2–S4) terminate at ganglia in the wall of the bladder and in the internal sphincter muscle. Parasympathetic stimulation causes contraction of the pubovesical or detrusor muscle and relaxation of the internal sphincter muscle. The result is an emptying of the bladder (Fig. 5.27). Paralysis of the parasympathetic fibers produces an atonic bladder).

The sympathetic fibers innervating the bladder originate in the intermediolateral nuclei of the lateral horns of T12, L1, and L2. They pass through the caudal segments of the trunks and reach the inferior mesenteric ganglia by way of the inferior splanchnic nerves. Thereafter, the inferior hypogastric plexus transmits the impulses to the muscular wall of the bladder and to the smooth muscle of the internal sphincter. The precise function of the sympathetic stimuli is not known. Stimulation of the internal sphincter muscle may cause relaxation of the wall of the bladder. Damage to the sympathetic fibers has no noticeable effect on bladder function. The internal sphincter around the neck of the bladder is said to be present only in the male gender. It presumably prevents retrograde flow of the ejaculate and has little to do with maintaining continence. It opens only when the bladder is emptied.

The external sphincter muscle is striated and is under voluntary control. The somatomotor fibers belong to neurons in the anterior horns of the sacral cord (S2–S4). They accompany the pudendal nerves and supply the external sphincter muscle. Although it is under voluntary control, the muscle opens by reflex when urine passes through the internal sphincter and stays open until the bladder is empty.

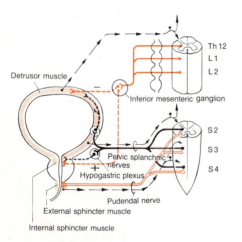
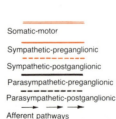

Fig. 5.27 Innervation of urinary bladder.

Afferent somatosensory fibers transmit stimuli from pain and proprioceptive receptors that are embedded in the wall of the bladder and respond to expansion. The greater the expansion, the stronger the tonic impulses sent by reflex from sacral segments S2–S4 via the pelvic splanchnic nerves to bladder and internal sphincter muscles. Increasing filling of the bladder is consciously perceived, since some of the impulses are transmitted in a central direction, via the posterior strands, to a detrusor center in the reticular formation near the locus ceruleus, continuing to the lobulus paracentralis on the median side of the brain. Impulses from the motor cortex of this lobulus permit the bladder to be emptied voluntarily. If this is not possible, for whatever reason, despite the bladder's being filled to capacity, an additional stimulus will finally bring about a reflex contraction of the detrusor muscle and a relaxation of the internal sphincter muscle, resulting in involuntary micturition.

It was mentioned in the section on spinal motor function (page 89) that a transverse paralysis at the level of the thoracic cord is followed by an "automatic bladder." The bladder cannot be emptied voluntarily; it empties automatically once it is expanded to a certain degree. Characteristically, there is always some retention of urine.

If the sensory portion of the sacral reflex arc is damaged, no desire to urinate is felt and reflex emptying of the bladder is lost. The bladder becomes atonic and fills beyond capacity. An overflow or paradoxical incontinence develops. This condition may be the result of a disease of the roots, as occurs in diabetes mellitus, or of the posterior tracts, as seen, for example, in tabes dorsalis. The urine must be drained with a catheter. A urinary infection is almost impossible to avoid. In rare instances (tabes dorsalis), the distention may lead to a rupture of the bladder.

Innervation of the rectum

The emptying mechanism for the rectum has much in common with that for the bladder (Fig. 5.28). Receptors sensitized by distention of the rectum send impulses through the pelvic plexus to sacral segments S2–S4. The external sphincter, consisting of striated muscles, is under voluntary control. Parasympathetic stimulation produces peristalsis of the rectum and relaxation of the internal sphincter muscle. Sympathetic stimulation inhibits peristalsis. Voluntary abdominal compression is essential for emptying the rectum.

A transverse injury of the spinal cord above the lumbosacral centers causes a retention of stool. Interruption of the afferent pathways means an absence of information on the state of filling of the rectum; interruption of the descending motor impulses paralyses abdominal compression. Sphincter

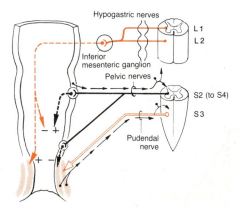

Fig. 5.28 Innervation of rectum.

Table 5.2 Sympathetic and Parasympathetic Nervous System.

Organ	Preganglionic Neuron	Sympathetic Postganglionic Neuron	Action	Preganglionic Neuron	Parasympathetic Postganglionic Neuron	Action
Eye	T1–T2	Superior cervical ganglion	Mydriasis	Edinger-Westphal nuclei (oculomotor nucleus)	Ciliary ganglion	Miosis: contraction of ciliary muscle (accommodation)
Lacrimal, sublingual, submandibular glands	T1–T2	Superior cervical ganglion	Vasoconstriction; viscous secretion	Superior salivatory nucleus	Pterygopalatine ganglion	Secretion of tears; secretion of watery saliva; vasodilatation
Parotid gland	T1–T2	Superior cervical ganglion	Vasoconstriction; secretion	Inferior salivatory nucleus	Otic ganglion	Secretion of saliva
Heart	T1–T4 (T5)	Superior, middle, inferior cervical and superior thoracic ganglia	Acceleration; dilatation of coronary arteries	Dorsal nucleus of vagus nerve	Cardiac plexus	Bradycardia; constriction of coronary arteries
Bronchi; lungs	T2–T7	Inferior cervical ganglion; superior thoracic ganglion	Dilatation of bronchi; Inhibition of secretion	Dorsal nucleus of vagus nerve	Bronchial and pulmonal plexus	Serous and mucous secretion; constriction of bronchi
Stomach	T6–T10; superior splanchnic nerve	Celiac ganglion	Inhibition of peristalsis and secretion; contraction of sphincter	Dorsal nucleus of vagus nerve	Gastric plexus	Peristalsis; relaxation of sphincter; evacuation
Small intestine and ascending colon	T6–T10	Celiac and superior mesenteric ganglia	Inhibition of peristalsis and secretion	Dorsal nucleus of vagus nerve	Myenteric plexus (Auerbach's plexus) and submucosal plexus (Meissner's plexus)	Peristalsis; secretion; vasodilatation

Table 5.2. (continued)

			Dorsal nucleus of vagus nerve	Periarterial plexus	Secretion
Pancreas	T6–T10	Celiac ganglion			
Colon descendens; rectum	L1–L2	Inferior mesenteric and hypogastric ganglia	Inhibition of peristalsis and secretion	S2–S4	Myenteric plexus (Auerbach's plexus); submucosal plexus (Meissner's plexus)	Secretion; peristalsis; evacuation
Kidney; bladder	L1–L2	Celiac ganglion; renal and hypogastric plexus	Stimulation of internal sphincter muscle; vasoconstriction	S2–S4	Hypogastric plexus (vesical plexus)	Relaxation of internal sphincter muscle; contraction of detrusor muscle; vasodilatation
Adrenal glands	T11–L1	Adrenal cells	Secretion (norepinephrine, epinephrine)	...	...	...
Male sexual organs	L1–L2; pelvic splanchnic nerves	Superior and inferior hypogastric plexus (pelvic plexus)	Ejaculation; vasoconstriction	S2–S4	Hypogastric plexus (pelvic plexus)	Erection; vasodilatation; secretion
Skin of head and neck	T2–T4	Superior and middle cervical ganglia		...	...	...
Arms	T3–T6	Inferior cervical and upper thoracic ganglia	Vasoconstriction; sweat secretion; piloerection	...	...	...
Legs	T10–L2	Lower lumbar and upper sacral ganglia		...	...	...

contraction is often insufficient because of reflex-induced spastic paresis. A lesion involving the sacral cord (S2–S4) causes loss of the anal reflex, resulting in rectal incontinence and discharge of stool if the fecal material is soft or liquid.

Innervation of genital organs

Efferent sympathetic fibers originating in the rostral lumbar cord reach the seminal duct, seminal vesicles, and prostate via the blood vessels of the hypogastric plexus. Stimulating this plexus causes ejaculation (Fig. 5.**29**). Stimulation of the parasympathetic fibers coming from segments S2–S4 causes erection. The pelvic splanchnic nerves (nervi erigentes) produce a vasodilatation in the genital cavernous bodies. The pudendal nerves innervate the sphincter muscle of the urethra and ischiocavernous as well as bulbocavernous muscles.

The genital centers are in part under neural influence by way of reticulospinal fibers and in part under humoral influence via centers of higher order in the hypothalamus.

According to Krücke (1948), the *dorsal longitudinal bundle* (Schütz's bundle) continues as the unmyelinated *parependymal fascicle*, descending on either side of the central canal down to the sacral cord. It is believed that this bundle connects the diencephalic sexual centers in the area of the nuclei of the tuber cinereum with the sexual center in the lumbosacral cord.

A transverse injury to the thoracic cord leads to impotence. It may be associated with reflex priapism and occasional ejaculation. Testicular atrophy has been observed. Impotence is also the result of injury in the area of S2–S4. In such injury erection and ejaculation are impossible.

Referred Pain

The afferent autonomic fibers form numerous autonomic visceral feedback circuits for the integration of impulses, but these impulses do not reach the level of awareness. A few impulses, however – those that signal the state of filling of organs and those related to pain – are consciously felt. Any irritation produces reflex spasm of the smooth muscles. This is what is felt as pain and is often called colic, such as hepatic or renal colic, caused, for example, by stones in the gallbladder or kidneys, respectively. Inflammatory swelling of organs or ischemia, for example, ischemia of the heart muscle, is felt as pain.

These pains from internal organs are usually diffuse and difficult to localize. Patients often feel them as "referred pain" in circumscribed areas of the surface of their bodies, in what are called *Head's zones* (Fig. 5.**30**). The afferent autonomic fibers have in common with the somatic afferent fibers that their neurons are situated in the spinal ganglia and that they take the path of the posterior roots for entering the spinal cord. The autonomic fibers from an internal organ and the somatic afferent fibers from corresponding myotomes and dermatomes then converge at their particular posterior horn and form a common pool. From there, the two types of impulses are transmitted centrally by the same fibers in the lateral spinothalamic tract (Fig. 5.**31**). At that point pain that originated in a certain organ is projected into the corresponding dermatome or myotome and is felt as **referred pain**.

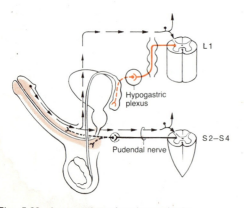

Fig. 5.**29** Innervation of male genitalia.

Peripheral Autonomic Nervous System

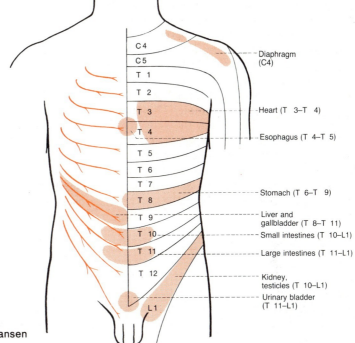

Fig. 5.30 Head's zones (after Hansen and Schliack).

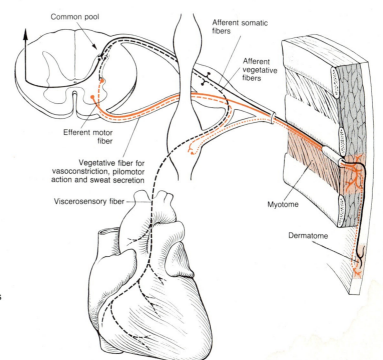

Fig. 5.31 Viscerocutaneous reflex arc with myotome, dermatome, and enterotome and somatic and autonomic connections for the explanation of referred pain.

Occasionally, there is a certain degree of hyperesthesia in such dermatomes or muscles. For example, those of the ventral abdominal wall may be tense. Various theories attempt to explain the mechanism leading to referred pain, but none has found unanimous approval. The rostral thoracic segmental roots may serve as an example. They carry afferent somatic fibers from the skin in the area of the left chest and left upper extremity and afferent visceral fibers coming from the heart. In coronary disease – for example, angina pectoris – the pain is often projected into the corresponding dermatome.

These cutaneous Head's zones are of diagnostic importance (see Fig. 5.**31**). Impulses deriving from the skin have an influence on the viscerally innervated organ related to the zone, as well as the reverse. Clearly, some connection must exist between afferent somatic fibers and visceral reflex arcs in the apparatus of the relay neurons of the spinal cord; otherwise, it is difficult to explain the therapeutic effect of hot or cold stimuli applied to the skin, packs of various sorts, liniments, production of wheals, and other treatments. Quite often they reduce pain originating in the autonomically innervated organs.

6 Basal Ganglia and Extrapyramidal System

Basal Ganglia

In general, the term *basal ganglia* is applied to the gray nuclear masses that derive from the telencephalic ganglionic hill of the embryo. These ganglia consist of the *caudate nucleus, putamen, claustrum* and *amygdaloid nuclear complex*. The latter structure has already been discussed in the section dealing with the limbic system.

The caudate nucleus and the putamen, although separated by the *internal capsule*, represent *one* nucleus and show the same histologic structure throughout (densely arranged small neurons and, in between, individual large multipolar neurons). The separation of these structures is not complete. They are connected by numerous gray bridges that extend through the fiber masses of the internal capsule and contain the same two types of neurons (Figs. 6.1, 6.2, 6.3). Rostroventrally, where almost no fibers enter the internal capsule, the nuclei are connected by a rather solid mass of nerve cells called the fundus of the striate body.

The term *striate body* or *striatum* is commonly used for both nuclei. The striae to which the name refers are the numerous white bundles of myelinated fibers that stand out in the pale gray matter (pale because of otherwise poor myelination) and converge toward the pallidum. The caudatum and putamen are also called *neostriatum*; the phylogenetically older globus pallidus or pallidum carries the name *paleostriatum*. The putamen and globus pallidus are commonly spoken of as one unit, using the term *lentiform nucleus* or *lenticular nucleus*, which lies like a wedge between the internal and external capsules (see Fig. 6.4). When using this term, one must be aware that the two components of the nucleus are different in their phylogenesis, structure, and function. The putamen develops from the matrix around the lateral ventricles, as does the caudatum, and is a relative of the neocortex. The *pallidum* belongs to the diencephalon, develops from the matrix of the third ventricle, and is a relative of the subthalamic nucleus (Richter, 1965).

The *caudate nucleus*, in its course, follows the lateral ventricle and forms an open ellipse (see Figs. 6.2 and 6.3). Head and body represent the convex ventrolateral wall of the anterior horn and cella media of the lateral ventricle (Figs. 6.5, 6.6, 6.7). The tail follows the roof of the inferior horn of the ventricle. On coronal sections (Figs. 6.3–6.8) it can be seen as a small round area of gray matter above the inferior ventricular horn (Fig. 6.7). Rostrally, the tail reaches almost the amygdaloid nucleus (see Fig. 6.2).

The *putamen* covers the lateral aspect of the pallidum like a shell (*putamen* is the Latin word for "shell"). It is separated from the pallidum by a layer of myelinated fibers, the pallidum's lateral medullary lamina. Laterally, the putamen is separated from the claustrum by the *external capsule*. In turn, the claustrum is separated from the deep cortex of the insula by the *extreme capsule* (Figs. 6.4 through 6.7). Some of the fibers contained in the latter capsule are association

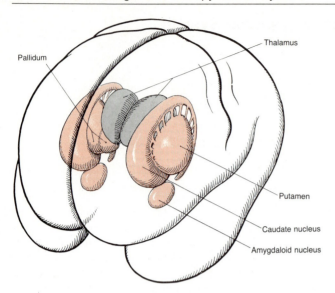

Fig. 6.1 Basal ganglia in their topographic relationships.

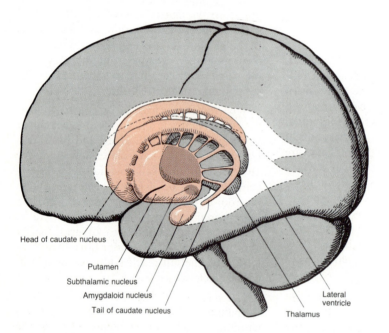

Fig. 6.2 Basal ganglia in relation to the ventricle system (lateral view).

fibers that connect, among other structures, the hearing area in the temporal lobe with the motor and premotor cortex.

Little is known about the function of the *claustrum*. It is only agreed that it is not part of the extrapyramidal system, and this holds true also for the amygdaloid nucleus. Therefore, these two grisea are not further discussed in this chapter.

Extrapyramidal System

The *extrapyramidal system* consists of the following gray structures: caudate nucleus,

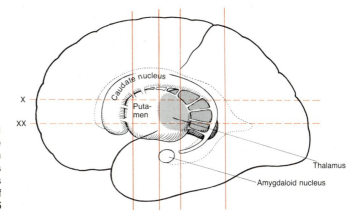

Fig. 6.3 Basal ganglia (lateral view). The X and XX indicate the level of the horizontal cuts through right (X) and left (XX) hemispheres shown in Fig. 6.4; the vertical lines 1 through 4 signify the planes of coronal sections shown in Figs. 6.5 through 6.8.

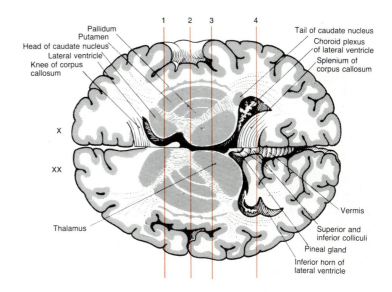

Fig. 6.4 Horizontal section through basal ganglia, showing levels of 4 coronal sections illustrated in Figs. 6.5 to 6.8.

putamen, pallidum, subthalamic nucleus, substantia nigra, and red nucleus. The term *extrapyramidal system* was briefly defined in the chapter on the motor system; the extrapyramidal pathways, which influence spinal motor activity, were mentioned there (page 32).

A brief discussion of the phylogenesis of the extrapyramidal system will aid an understanding of its functions.

The center of lowest order in the system is the spinal cord and the primitive apparatus of the reticular formation in the tegmentum of the midbrain. With further development in the animal kingdom, the paleostriatum (pallidum) became superimposed on these structures. Thereafter, in higher mammals and particularly in man, the neostriatum developed at the top. Its size corresponds to the degree to which the cerebral cortex has developed. As a rule, the higher centers dominate the lower centers. This means that in lower animals, lower centers can take care of the normal distribution of tone and the considerably automatic innervation of movements without great difficulty. But the higher an

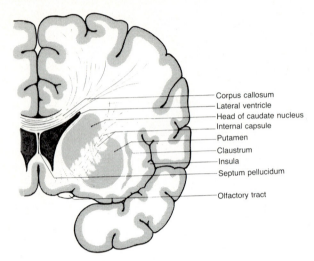

Fig. 6.5 Coronal section 1 through anterior striate body.

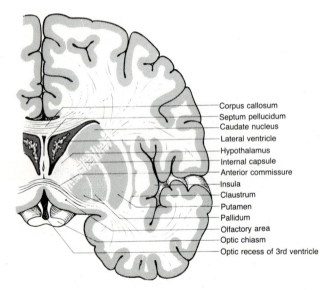

Fig. 6.6 Coronal section 2 through middle of pallidum.

animal ranks phylogenetically, the less able it is to compensate for dysfunction or loss of the higher centers.

As the formation of the cerebral cortex expands, the phylogenetically older motor centers (paleostriatum and neostriatum) become increasingly controlled by the new motor system, the system of the pyramidal tracts. Nevertheless, most mammals – for example, the cat – are still able to walk or run to some extent after the removal of the motor cortex. To man, however, an intact pyramidal system is crucial – even though a patient with a spastically paralyzed extremity may be able to perform certain involuntary, so-called *associated movements* with it. What is known about the fiber systems connecting the basal ganglia with one another and with other nuclear areas of the extrapyramidal system is

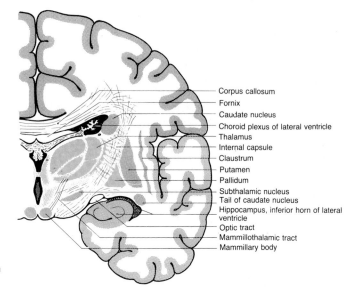

Fig. 6.7 Coronal section 3 through thalamus and mamillary bodies.

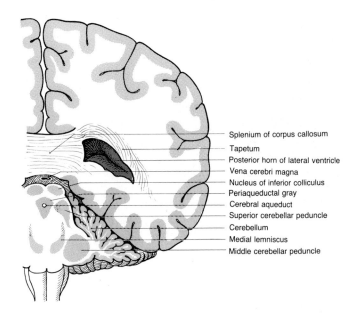

Fig. 6.8 Coronal section 4 through splenium of corpus callosum.

still incomplete. Consequently, only the essential afferent and efferent pathways will be discussed here.

The *striatum* is the center of higher order among the structures making up the extrapyramidal motor system. It receives impulses from numerous areas of the cerebral cortex, particularly from the frontal motor areas, including fields 4, 6aα and 6aβ. These afferent fibers are arranged in somatotopic order, run ipsilaterally, and are probably inhibitory in their action. Striocortical connections apparently do not exist. Another system of afferent fibers with point-to-point transmission of impulses reaches the striatum from the thalamic centromedian nucleus. Its action is probably facilitory. From both caudate nucleus and putamen, the main afferent fibers run to the lateral and medial segments of the pallidum, which are separated from each other by an internal medullary lamina. Apparently, there are no direct connections between the cortex and the pallidum. It is believed, however, that connections exist ipsilaterally from cortex to substantia nigra, red nucleus, subthalamic nucleus, and reticular formation (Fig. 6.9).

Aside from receiving afferent cortical fibers, which will be discussed further, the caudate nucleus and putamen have two-way connections with the substantia nigra.

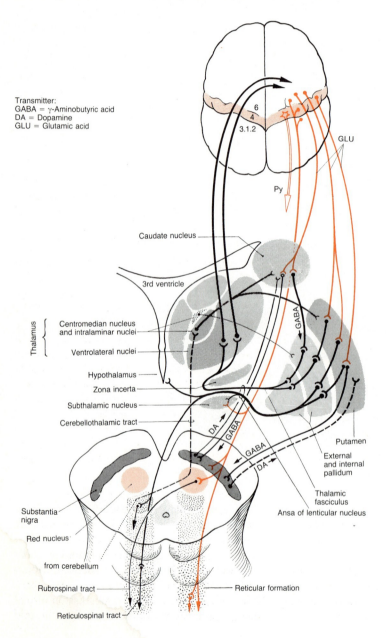

Fig. 6.9 Connections of the extrapyramidal system (after Hassler).

The afferent nigrostriatal fibers have been described to be *dopaminergic* and to reduce the inhibitory function of the striatum. On the other hand, the strionigral tract is *gamma-aminobutyric acid-* or *GABA-ergic* and has an inhibitory effect on the dopaminergic nigrostriatal neurons. This is a closed-loop feedback circuit (see Fig. 6.9). The GABA-ergic neurons of the strionigral fibers probably inhibit the descending, most likely dopaminergic, nigral neurons that control muscle tone via gamma neurons (Hassler).

All other efferent fibers of the striatum run through the medial sector of the pallidum. They form rather thick fiber bundles which have multiple terminal nuclei. One of these bundles is called the *ansa lenticularis*. Its fibers originate in the ventral portion of the medial sector of the pallidum and run ventromedially around the posterior limb of the internal capsule to the thalamus and hypothalamus and, reciprocally, to the subthalamic nucleus. After crossing, they connect with the reticular formation of the midbrain, from which a chain of neurons forms the reticulospinal tract (descending reticular system), which terminates at the anterior horn cells.

The main contingent of the efferent fibers of the pallidum goes to the thalamus as part of several regulating feedback circuits. This pallidothalamic bundle is also called the *fasciculus thalamicus* or *Forel's field H1*. Most of its fibers terminate in the ventroanterior nucleus (*VA*) and in the ventrooral anterior nucleus (*V.o.a.*) of the thalamus (shown in Fig. 5.5). The VA nucleus projects to cortical area 6aβ and the V.o.a. nuclear region to cortical area 6aα (see Fig. 5.5). Fibers originating in the dentate nucleus of the cerebellum terminate in the ventrooral posterior nucleus (*V.o.p.* in Fig. 5.5) of the thalamus, which projects into cortical area 4. All these thalamocortical connections transmit impulses in both directions. Within the cortex the thalamocortical pathways synapse with corticostriatal neurons and form various reverberating circuits.

The existence of the various reciprocal thalamocortical connections suggests by itself the operation of reverberating circuits that facilitate or inhibit the activity of the individual cortical motor fields.

Additional circuits are as follows:

1. putamen–pallidum–thalamus (V.o.a. nucleus)–area 6 aα-putamen
2. caudate nucleus–pallidum–thalamus (VA nucleus)–area 6 aβ–caudate nucleus
3. putamen–external sector of pallidum–reticular activating system–thalamic centromedian nucleus (receiving additional impulses from the emboliform nucleus)–striatum
4. external sector of pallidum–activating reticular system–thalamic intralaminar nuclei–external sector of pallidum (not demonstrated)
5. cerebellar dentate nucleus–thalamus (V.o.p. nucleus)–cortical area 4–pontine nuclei (or red nucleus–central tegmental tract–inferior olive)–cerebellar dentate nucleus (see Figs. 4.5 and 4.6).

The fibers of the basal ganglia, which descend in the direction of the spinal cord, are relatively small in number in contrast to the pallidothalamic fiber bundles and reach the spinal cord only via chains of neurons. This mode of connection suggests that the main task of the basal ganglia is probably to control and regulate the activities of the motor and premotor cortical fields via the various reverberating circuits so that voluntary movements can be performed smoothly and without interruption. The striate reverberating circuits are supported in this activity by those of the cerebellar, vestibular, and proprioceptive systems.

As mentioned in Chapter 2, the pyramidal tract originates in the sensomotor cortex (areas 4, 6, 3, 1, and 2). These are also the cortical areas where extrapyramidal motor pathways originate. These extrapyramidal pathways are, among others, the corticostriate, corticorubral, corticonigral, and corticoreticular pathways, which go to the motor nuclei of cranial nerves and to the spinal motor nerve cells via descending chains of neurons. Most of these projections of the motor cortex pass through the internal capsule. Consequently, lesions within the internal capsule usually interrupt not only the fibers of the pyramidal tract but also extrapyramidal fibers. *This interruption is the cause of spasticity.* A small contingent of these extrapyramidal fibers probably descends through the external capsule, perhaps explaining why in spastic hemiplegia stemming from a hematoma in the internal capsule, the paralyzed extremity is still able to perform certain voluntary movements.

The specific functions of the individual extrapyramidal grisea is not fully understood. Even new facts provided by sterotactic procedures resulted in only conditional clarification. The finding of specific deficits as a result of damage to one or another griseum does not permit us to conclude with certainty that the involved griseum constitutes a special center that is solely responsible for the lost function. It is more likely that a lesion in a griseum or in its fiber connections produces discord in the normally harmonious cooperation among the various components of the system and that the nature of the discord determines the nature of the clinical signs.

Signs Caused by Lesions in Extrapyramidal Grisea

The main signs of extrapyramidal lesions are disorders of muscle tone (*dystonia*) and involuntary movement disorders (*hyperkinesia, hypokinesia, akinesia*) absent during sleep. Two clinical syndromes can be differentiated. One is characterized by a combination of *hyperkinesia and hypotonia* and is caused by a disease of the neostriatum. The other presents as a combination of *hypokinesia and hypertonia or rigidity* and stems from a disease of the substantia nigra. It will be discussed first.

Hypokinesia-Hypertonia Syndrome

This syndrome is a classic finding in *paralysis agitans* or *Parkinson's disease* (shaking palsy). The tissue damage in this disease is degenerative and leads to a loss of melanin-containing neurons of the substantia nigra and of dopaminergic neurons that connect with the striatum. The disease process is usually bilateral. If the cell loss is unilateral, the clinical signs involve the contralateral half of the body.

In paralysis agitans the degenerative process is hereditary. A similar neuronal loss in the substantia nigra may have other causes. In that case the shaking palsy is referred to as *parkinsonian syndrome* or *parkinsonism*. If it is a late sequela of lethargic encephalitis, it is called *postencephalitic parkinsonism*. The syndrome includes, among other signs, autonomic disorders such as hypersalivation, facial seborrhea, oculogyric crises, and disorders of accommodation. Other conditions may also produce parkinsonism, among them cerebral arteriosclerosis, typhus, cerebral syphilis, primary or secondary involvement of midbrain by tumors or trauma, intoxication by carbon monoxide, manganese, phosgene, or other substances, and prolonged intake of phenothiazines or reserpine.

Paralysis agitans

Also known as Parkinson's disease, this condition is characterized by three cardinal signs: *akinesia, rigor,* and *tremor.*

Akinesia: In akinesia, the mobility of the patient slowly decreases. All mimetic and expressive movements and all associated movements gradually die. Starting a movement such as walking becomes very difficult. The patient first must take a few short, tripping steps. Once he is in motion, it is difficult for him to stop walking suddenly; before he can stop he has to take a few extra steps, because the counterinnervation is delayed. This continued activity is called *propulsion, retropulsion,* or *lateropulsion,* depending on the direction in which the final steps are taken. As the play of mimetic movements becomes frozen, the facial expression becomes that of a mask (*hypomimia, amimia*); only the eyes remain mobile. Instead of moving the head, the patient can move only the eyes in a given direction. Speech becomes monotonous and dysarthric, caused in part by rigor and tremor of the tongue. Finally, the entire body is held in a stiff, anteflexed position; all movements are extremely slow and are incomplete. The patient avoids any unnecessary movement. The arms do not swing during walking, and all mimetic and expressive concomitant movements, so characteristic of each individual, are absent.

Rigor: In contrast to spastic elevation of muscle tone, rigor can be felt in extensors as a sticky, waxy resistance to all passive movements. The muscles cannot be relaxed. In passive movements one can feel that the tone of the antagonist muscles decreases in steps and not in an even, continuous fashion (*cogwheel phenomenon*). The lifted head of a lying person, when suddenly released, does not fall down as usual but sinks gradually back onto the pillow (*head-dropping test*). In contrast to their behavior in a spastic condition, the proprioceptive reflexes are not increased, and no pathologic reflexes can be observed. Paresis is absent. If it is difficult to elicit reflexes, it is not possible to intensify the patellar reflex by *Jendrassik's maneuver*. (The patient hooks his hands together by the flexed fingers and tries to pull them apart as hard as he can while the patellar reflexes are checked). The result is an increase in the tonic stretching reflex, that is, an *activated rigidity*.

Tremor: Most patients show a passive tremor. If it is absent, the condition is called *paralysis agitans sine agitatione*. The passive tremor has a slow frequency of four to eight movements per second; it is rhythmic and results from a play between agonists and antagonists (*antagonist tremor*). In contrast to intention tremor, the antagonist tremor stops during intended movements. Pill-rolling or money-counting movements are characteristic of Parkinson tremor. The mechanism that causes the three signs just described is still not fully understood. The akinesia is probably caused by a lack of dopaminergic transmission that may occur in the striatum. It improves as the patient is treated with L-dopa. According to Hassler, the akinesia can be explained as follows: the damage inflicted on the neurons of the substantia nigra produces a loss of the inhibiting descending nigroreticulospinal impulses that normally exert an inhibiting influence also on the Renshaw cells (see Fig. 1.**9**). Recurrent collaterals of the large $alpha_1$ motoneurons connect with these Renshaw cells. If the impulses released by the $alpha_1$ cells are so strong that they endanger the innervated muscle fibers, the Renshaw cells, having a two-way connection with the same motor cells, reduce their activity by inhibiting actions. This inhibition is increased and renders the initiation of a voluntary movement more difficult if the nigroreticulospinal impulses with their inhibiting action on the Renshaw cells have been lost.

The *rigor* also can be explained as a result of the loss of substantia nigra neurons. Normally, these neurons have an inhibiting effect on the striate impulses, which in turn inhibit the pallidum. Their loss means that the efferent pallidal impulses become uninhibited. This has a facilitory effect on the spinal tonic stretching reflex (see Fig. 1.**10**) in two ways: (1) The descending tract of the pallidum crosses the midline into the midbrain and synapses in the reticular formation with reticulospinal neurons (see Fig. 6.**9**); these neurons bring about an increase in tone by facilitating the action of the interneurons in charge of the tonic stretching reflex. (2) The unimpeded impulses originating in the medial sector of the pallidum reach area $6a\alpha$ by way of the oroventral thalamic nucleus (V.o.a. nucleus). There, special neurons send off corticospinal fibers that have a facilitory effect on the interneurons for the tonic stretching reflex and in this way increase the tone to a level that is called rigor.

If the efferent cells and fibers of the pallidum are destroyed or interrupted by coagulation of the medial sector of the pallidum or the area of the ansa lenticularis or of the oroventral thalamic nucleus, much of the rigor disappears.

The *antagonist tremor* probably originates in the apparatus of relay cells of the spinal cord proper. In the resting state the neurons of this apparatus transmit rhythmical discharges to the motor neurons, which under normal conditions are suppressed by the desynchronizing influence of impulses from the substantia nigra. The unimpeded impulses, which originate in the medial sector of the pallidum and reach the cortex via the thalamus, facilitate the action of the corticospinal neurons. At the same time, the inhibitory impulses, originating in the striatum and transmitted via the substantia nigra, do not descend further to the relay apparatus of the spinal cord via the nigroreticulospinal tract. Thus, it is assumed that the tremor is the result of two factors: the facilitory effect of the synchronizing corticospinal pathway and the lack of the inhibitory, desynchronizing influence of the striatonigral complex (Hassler).

It is possible to reduce the tremor by stereotactically silencing the unimpeded impulses coming from the pallidum or by coagulating the medial pallidum, its pallidothalamic fibers, or the dentatothalamic fibers and their terminal thalamic nucleus (V.o.p.) (see Figs. 4.4 to 4.6). The results are not as satisfactory as those with rigor. In spite of coagulation, the tremor may appear again temporarily when the patient is emotionally agitated, indicating that the pyramidal tract receives facilitory impulses from still other sources. Attempts to eliminate the medial thalamic nucleus, which receives impulses from pallidum and hypothalamus and projects them to the cortex of the frontal lobes, resulted in further reduction of tremor. They produced concurrently, however, a *psychoorganic syndrome* characterized by dulling of emotional expression; this procedure therefore was discontinued.

A lesion in the medial pallidum and its efferent fibers connecting with the thalamus (V.o.a. nucleus) appears to reduce the rigor, whereas coagulation of the oroventral nucleus (V.o.p.) ameliorates the tremor more effectively.

Bilateral destruction of the pallidum supposedly produces severe disorder of consciousness and delirium or amentia.

Hyperkinesia-Hypotonia Syndrome

This syndrome develops if the neostriatum is damaged. Occasionally, such lesions are accompanied by others in the globus pallidus, thalamus, or cerebral cortex; in such cases the hyperkinesia is possibly caused by a loss of inhibitory neurons of the neostriatum that descend to pallidum and substantia nigra. In other words, a loss of a neuronal system of higher order has occurred, producing excessive excitation of the neurons of the next lower system. The resulting hyperkinesias are of different kinds: *athetosis, chorea, spasmodic torticollis, torsion dystonia, ballism,* and other conditions.

Athetosis

This kinetic disorder is usually caused by perinatal damage to the striate bodies. This damage takes the form of a circulatory loss of small neurons, resulting in irregular glial scars simulating veins in marble; hence the name *status marmoratus*. Involuntary movements ar slow and wormlike, with a tendency to overextend the peripheral portions of the extremities. In addition, there are irregular, spasmodic increases in muscle tensions between agonists and antagonists. As a result, postures and movements are rather bizarre. Voluntary movements are severely distorted by the spontaneous appearance of hyperkinetic movements that may include face and tongue and thus cause grimacing with abnormal tongue movements. There may be spasmodic outbursts of laughing or crying. The athetosis may be combined with a contralateral paresis; it may also be bilateral and is then called double athetosis, which usually occurs in association with spastic paraplegia (Little's disease, Vogt's syndrome). Intelligence may be preserved.

Chorea

The choreal syndrome is characterized by short, fast, involuntary jerks occurring in single muscles at random and producing various patterns of movements, some resembling voluntary movements. At first the peripheral portions of the extremities are involved; the proximal portions follow. Involuntary jerks of the facial muscles produce grimacing. In addition to the hyperkinesia, a decrease in the tone of the musculature is characteristic of chorea.

The choreal restlessness seen in children as *chorea minor* or Sydenham's chorea or St. Vitus's dance is an acute, usually self-limiting disorder that appears to be linked closely to rheumatic fever and has been called *chorea infectiosa*. The neuropathologic findings vary greatly. Some patients show no alterations at all. The same acute chorea may occur during early pregnancy and is referred to as *chorea gravidarum*.

Most important is *Huntington's chorea*, a dominant, hereditary, degenerative disease usually commencing in middle age. It may begin as early as adolescence with involuntary movements, which may be mistaken for parkinsonian hyperkinesia, or with mental changes, usually diagnosed as schizophrenia. The movements are generally not as jerky as those in chorea minor. They are more complex and sometimes slow like those seen in athetosis. They may be twisting, torque-like, and similar to those in torsion dystonia. The proximal extremities, the trunk, and the facial musculature are particularly involved, causing lively grimacing with forceful protrusion and retraction of the tongue. Speaking and swallowing are difficult. The early hypertonia changes later into rigor. Pathologic findings consist of an atrophy of the striate bodies associated with loss of the small neurons. Cortical neurons may also degenerate, and the disease may terminate in dementia. Choreal movements of similarly slow development may be a symptomatic condition, that is, secondary to another brain disease (such as encephalitis, carbon monoxide poisoning, vascular disease).

Spasmodic torticollis and torsion dystonia

These are the most important types of dystonia syndromes. In both diseases there are usually alterations within the putamen and the centromedian nucleus of the thalamus and in other extrapyramidal nuclei (pallidum, substantia nigra, and others).

Spasmodic torticollis, a tonic disorder, consists of spasmodic contractions of muscles in the neck region that result in slow, involuntary turning and bending movements of the head. The sternocleidomastoid and trapezius muscles are particularly often involved, in addition to other muscles of the neck. The causes vary. Occasionally, the spasmodic torticollis represents an abortive form of torsion dystonia or an early sign of another extrapyramidal disease, such as Huntington's chorea or Wilson's disease. Tonic spasms of the facial musculature have been considered psychogenic, as facial tics have been. After the epidemic of lethargic encephalitis in 1920, however, these hyperkinesias were very common, and postmortem studies revealed alterations, particularly in the striatum. We thus should be careful in attributing such movements to a psychogenic mechanism. Tic-like spasmodic contractions of the diaphragm are the cause of hiccups.

Torsion dystonia is characterized by rather extensive turning and twisting movements of trunk and proximal extremities. They can be so severe that the patient can neither stand nor walk without support. The disease may be idiopathic or symptomatic; in the latter case the cause may be birth injury, kernicterus, former encephalitis, early Huntington's chorea, Hallervorden-Spatz disease, or a hepatocerebral degeneration (Wilson's diease, Westphal-Strümpell disease).

Ballistic syndrome

This syndrome usually occurs as hemiballism. The involuntary movements are characterized by coarse outreaching and hurling movements, particularly of the muscles of shoulder and pelvis. This most dramatic of the extrapyramidal motor disorders is the result of acute damage to the *subthalamic nucleus of Luys* and its connections with the lateral sector of the pallidum. The hemiballism is contralateral to the lesion.

Myoclonic movements are usually indicative of damage in the area of the triangle of Guillain-Mollaret (see Fig. 4.6).

Stereotactic Treatment of Hyperkinesias

Because of the considerable improvement in rigor and tremor after stereotactic elimination of the various corresponding extrapyramidal areas, the same method has been used for treatment of hyperkinesias. One reason is that conservative therapy led only in exceptional cases to satisfactory or dramatic improvement. The stereotactic treatment is based on the premise that damage to the striatum produces a loss of its inhibitory effect on the next lower system of neurons – that is, on pallidum and substantia nigra – and that this produces an excess of stimulation in these nulcei. Hyperkinesias are supposedly produced by pathologic impulses permitted to travel over undisturbed pathways to the thalamus and further to areas of the motor cortex that transmit the impulses via efferent cortical neurons. It is therefore important that the fibers going to the cortical motor fields be interrupted. Coagulation of the medial sector of the pallidum has yielded rather good results, particularly with torsion dystonia and choreal hyperkinesia. In order to treat athetosis by this method, more widespread coagulations have been necessary and have had to involve in some cases an area of the internal capsule.

Other signs

In elderly persons with cerebral arteriosclerosis, it is not rare to encounter parkinson-like changes or hyperkinesias, particularly tremor, a tendency to repeat words or phrases (*palinphrasia*), spasmodic repetition of end-syllables of words (*logoclonia*), and iteration of movements (*palikinesia*). There may be a tendency to pseudospontaneous movements, but true choreiform or athetotic movements are relatively rare. In most cases the signs are caused by miliary and slightly larger necrotic lesions in striate bodies and, occasionally, in pallida. They can be identified postmortem as scars and tiny cysts. This condition is known as *status lacunaris*. The tendency to iterations and logoclonias has been attributed to such lesions in the caudate nucleus, and tremor to those in the putamen. Figs. 6.10 and 6.11 illustrate such circulatory cysts.

Case Report 1: Fig. 6.11 represents the finding in a 75-year-old man with generalized arteriosclerosis, hypertension, diabetes mellitus and diabetic

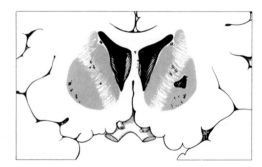

Fig. 6.10 Status lacunaris with larger cyst in left putamen (drawn from specimen).

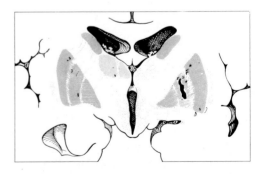

Fig. 6.11 Smaller and larger cysts in left pallidum (status lacunaris) (drawn from specimen seen from front). Case report 1.

polyneuropathy. The diabetes mellitus was diagnosed when he was 73 years of age. A four-day-old weakness of the legs was the reason for hospitalization. As sign of polyneuropathy, there was a decrease in reflexes and some weakness, particularly in the legs. Marked rigor with cogwheel phenomenon and tremor in the extremities and a tendency to perseverate in maintaining a posture were noted. Emotionally, the patient was depressed.

Case Report 2: A 61-year-old man had been mentally abnormal since childhood and had experienced several psychotic phases, diagnosed as catatonia and motility psychosis, in later life. Three months prior to hospital admission, he again had a psychotic episode. He did not wash himself or change his clothing. He became deceitful and committed senseless and criminal acts; for example, he tried to change an old, invalidated currency bill. Two months prior to admission he suddenly developed a left-sided paralysis, dizziness, visual disorders, pain in his ears, and paresthesias and numbness in hands and feet. His gait became wobbly, causing him to fall several times. His speech became monotonous.

Upon admission, he looked older than his age. His posture was rigid, and gait was stiff, short-stepped, and somewhat limping. All his movements were slow and ponderous. Facial expression was amimic. Speech was monotonous and fast with precipitous rhythm and a tendency to logoclonia. He gave the impression of being indifferent, dull, and suffering from an overall akinesia.

Neurologic examinations revealed the following: right pupil wider than left; slow reaction to light; slight horizontal nystagmus to both sides; weakness of left facial muscles; reduced strength in left arm and leg; increased left proprioceptive reflexes with positive Babinki's and Oppenheim's signs; bilateral rigor, left more than right; ataxia, left more than right; wobbly gait with tendency to fall; tendency to iterate movements and spoken words; no tremor; disorientation; difficulty in memorizing; considerable loss of old memory; very poor cognitive ability; questions often not answered at all; speech hardly understandable; low and monotonous voice; poor articulation of syllables. Some syllables or words were repeated rapidly several times (logoclonia). The patient appeared indifferent and dull. He was confused at times and complained of pain in the anterior left half of the body. Stupor later developed, and the patient died of pneumonia.

Postmortem study revealed brain edema. The area of the floor of the third ventricle bulged into the basal cistern, and the mamillary bodies had been transformed into a single pluglike structure. Coronal sections showed a small, elongated, compact tumor, gray-red in color, in the region of the right pallidum and hypothalamus, compressing the third ventricle to a thin slit and pushing it over the midline to the left. The right putamen was displaced laterally. The tumor extended caudally into the midbrain, involving the red nucleus and substantia nigra on both sides. The right ventral thalamus was infiltrated by the tumor, and the entire thalamus was displaced dorsally (Fig. 6.12).

Histologically, the tumor presented two different pictures. One part was sharply delineated and very cellular; the cells appeared to be of the same type. Deposits of calcium were detected within the tumor. The tissue outside this nodule showed a loose arrangement of tumor cells, with polymorphism and multiple small necroses. Calcium deposits involved particularly the right pallidum (possible oligodendrocytoma or spongioblastoma).

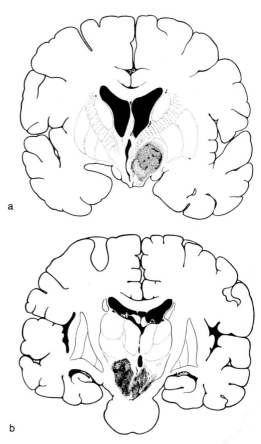

Fig. 6.**12 a** Small tumor (possibly oligodendroglioma or spongioblastoma) in the area of right pallidum. **b** Same tumor in the area of the substantia nigra. (Drawn from specimen.) Case report 2.

In retrospect, one can say that the early signs caused by the tumor were changes in the patient's personality. The patient became deceitful and committed illegal acts. This behavior led to the assumption that he was experiencing a recurrence of a former episodic psychosis. This time, however, he developed further signs of organic involvement in the form of left-sided hemiparesis and, in rapid sequence, signs indicative of involvement of extrapyramidal motor areas. The akinesia, amimia, rigid posture, and rigor in the extremities, left more than right, can be attributed to the involvement of the right pallidum and right and left substantia nigra. The growth of the tumor into the right cerebral peduncle and lower internal capsule explains the left-sided spastic hemiparesis. Involvement of the mamillary bodies can be regarded as the cause of the severe amnestic syndrome. The personality changes were probably related to damaged connections among hypothalamus, medial thalamus, and orbital lobe cortex.

7 Meninges, Ventricles and Cerebrospinal Fluid

Meninges

Brain and spinal cord are invested by three meningeal membranes: (1) dura mater or dura (pachymeninx), (2) arachnoid, and (3) pia mater or pia. Together, arachnoid and pia are called *leptomeninges*.

Dura mater

The dura consists of two layers of dense connective tissue. The outer layer serves as periosteum and is firmly attached to the bone. The inner layer is the actual meningeal layer and faces the very narrow subdural space. The dural or meningeal arteries run between the two layers. They are relatively large. They not only supply the cranial bone aside from the dura, but also act as temperature stabilizers protecting the brain against the changes in temperature to which the rather thin skull is exposed. The *middle meningeal artery* is the largest, spreading over the entire lateral convexity. It is a branch of the maxillary artery, which is in turn a branch of the external carotid artery. It enters the skull through the *foramen spinosum*. The *anterior meningeal artery* is rather small and supplies the medial portion of the frontal dura and anterior falx. It enters the skull in front of the lamina cribrosa as a branch of the anterior ethmoidal artery, which is a branch of the ophthalmic artery and therefore carries blood from the internal carotid artery. The *posterior meningeal artery* supplies the dura of the posterior fossa and enters the fossa through the foramen jugulare as a branch of the ascending pharyngeal artery, which originates from the external carotid artery. It is supported by a meningeal branch of the vertebral artery. It is important to know that the middle meningeal artery connects in the orbit with the lacrimal artery, a branch of the ophthalmic artery that descends from the internal carotid artery near the internal opening or the optic canal. Because of this anastomosis, it is possible for the retinal artery to receive blood even if the stem of the ophthalmic artery is obstructed.

The inner meningeal layer of the dura is separated from the outer layer at the sites where it forms the dural sinuses. Along the superior longitudinal and the transverse sinuses, the inner layer duplicates and partitions the cranial cavity as falx and tentorium (Fig. 7.**1**). It also forms the falx cerebelli, which extends between the cerebellar hemispheres, the diaphragm of the sella, and Meckel's cavity, which contains the gasserian ganglion. At the external margin of the foramen magnum, the dural layers separate completely. The outer layer continues as periosteum, and the meningeal layer forms the dural sleeve of the spinal cord (Fig. 7.**2**). The space between the two layers is called epidural or extradural but is, strictly speaking, an intradural space. It contains loose connective tissue, some fat tissue, and the *internal vertebral venous plexus*. Only where the roots of the spinal cord pass through the intervertebral foramina do the two dural sleeves rejoin. The dural sleeve terminates at the level of the 2nd sacral vertebra after sur-

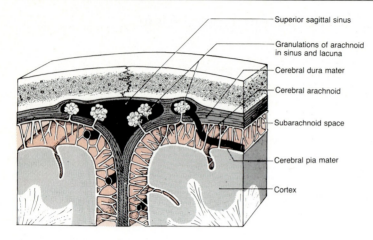

Fig. 7.1 Coronal section through superior longitudinal sinus demonstrating the meninges.

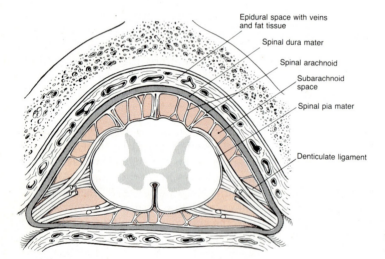

Fig. 7.2 Meninges of spinal cord.

rounding the cauda equina. At its caudal tip it continues as dural filum terminale, which is attached to the periosteum of the coccyx as the fibrous coccygeal ligament.

The dura above the tentorium is innervated by branches of the trigeminal nerve, whereas the infratentorial dura is supplied by the branches of the upper cervical spinal nerves and the vagus nerve. The sensory nerves of the spinal dura belong to the posterior roots of the spinal nerves. Dural nerves consist of myelinated and unmyelinated fibers that spread over the entire dura. Their terminal structures are apparently sensitive to stretching, because any pull on the dura is very painful. Particularly sensitive to pain are the sensory fibers of nerves accompanying the arteries. It is believed that headaches actually represent dural pain.

Arachnoid

This delicate, but tough structure consists of an outer cellular membrane and an inner connective tissue layer to which a loose meshwork of thin trabeculae is attached. This meshwork traverses the subarachnoid space like a spider web; hence the name *arachnoidea*

(Figs. 7.1, 7.2). The avascular arachnoid membrane is transparent and thin. It is strong and virtually impermeable to biologic substances. It has an outer layer of endothelium-like cells, the meningothelial or arachnoidal cells. The oval nuclei of these cells are tightly arranged in single, double, or multiple layers facing the subdural space. These cells give rise to the endotheliomatous or meningotheliomatous type of meningioma. The inner layer of the arachnoid and its subarachnoid trabeculae are covered by mesothelial cells able to respond to various pathogenic stimuli and to form, for example, phagocytes.

The arachnoid is not fastened to the dura except at the areas along the dural sinuses, to which it is attached by *pacchionian granulations* or *villi* (see Fig. 7.1). Because a small amount of clear fluid is always present in the subdural space, the arachnoid can glide relative to the dura without friction. Thus, an oscillation of the cerebral hemispheres within their intracranial compartments can be tolerated without damage to the extracerebral blood vessels or the brain tissue itself.

Wherever nerves leave the cranium or spinal canal, the dura and arachnoid accompany them for a short distance. This is best exemplified by the optic nerves, because there the distance is rather long. The dura lines the optic canal. When it reaches the orbit, its outer layer becomes the periosteum of the orbit and the meningeal layer follows the entire nerve, connecting ultimately with the sclera. Inside this dural sleeve is an arachnoidal sleeve with subdural and subarachnoidal spaces on either side that are extensions of the intracranial spaces. Because of this anatomical situation it is possible for intracranial subarachnoidal hemorrhage to extend anteriorly around the orbital segment of the nerve, and for an intracranial tumor, such as a meningioma, near the optic foramen, to grow freely into the subarachnoid space around the orbital portion of the optic nerve. A malignant tumor of the eye, such as a retinoblastoma or melanocytoma, may metastasize by continuity from the orbital into the intracranial subarachnoid space.

Pia mater

The pia consists of a thin, endothelium-like layer of mesodermal cells. In contrast to the arachnoid, this membrane covers all visible as well as hidden surfaces of the brain and spinal cord (see Fig. 7.2), except for the surface of the ventricles. It is attached in all places to an ectodermal membrane formed by marginal astrocytes. This piaglia membrane follows all blood vessels entering or leaving the nervous parenchyma and constitutes the peripheral border of the *Virchow-Robin perivascular spaces.*

Where the subarachnoid trabeculae are attached to the pia, they may form a dense, membrane-like network sometimes referred to as the epipial layer. This layer includes small blood vessels, and nerve fibers more numerous than those of the dura. In contrast to dural nerves, they are not sensitive to mechanical, thermic, or faradic stimulation. It is believed that they may respond to tensile stress or tonus changes in the walls of blood vessels.

Subarachnoid Space

This leptomeningeal space is filled with circulating cerebrospinal fluid (CSF). All blood vessels and nerves of brain and spinal cord pass through this fluid. Therefore, if the leptomeningeal space is infected, blood vessels and nerves may become involved by the inflammatory process. Arteritis and phlebitis are known to be potential causes of ischemic tissue necrosis.

The subarachnoid space is a continuum extending from the parietal areas of the cerebrum down to the end of the cauda equina in the region of the coccyx where the spinal-dural investment terminates. The subarachnoid space does not communicate with the subdural space. Therefore, leptomeningitis usually does not spread into the subdural space unless the infection is carried by septic thrombosis of cerebral veins that cross the subdural space (bridging veins). This is known to occur in *haemophilus influenzae* meningitis. The subarachnoid space is very narrow over those cerebral convolutions that rest on orbital roofs and tentorium during waking hours, when the head is held upright. Where the space is particularly wide, the areas are referred to as cisterns. Some cisterns are illustrated in Fig. 7.**3**. The unpaired *cerebellomedullary cistern*, or *cisterna magna* is located between the cerebellar tonsils and the dorsal aspect of the medulla oblongata. It receives practically all the intraventricular CSF through the foramen of Magendi. It is accessible by suboccipital puncture through the posterior atlantooccipital membrane. This procedure is sometimes used for collecting CSF and for injecting air into the ventricle system for pneumoencephalography.

The cisterna magna openly communicates with the spinal subarachnoid space, which is much wider over the dorsal than over the ventral aspect of the cord. Ventrally, the cisterna magna connects freely with the *pontomedullary cisterns* containing, among other structures, the vertebral arteries. The cisterns continue rostrally as the *pontine cistern*, extending over the entire base of the pons and accommodating the basilar artery, the trigeminal nerves, and, in part, the abducens. At the rostral border of the pons, the pontine cistern is followed by the large *basal cistern*. The latter structure is bordered laterally by the rostral hippocampal gyri, including their unci. Posteriorly, it includes the interpeduncular fossa, sometimes referred to as the *interpeduncular cistern*. Anteriorly, it reaches to the level of the optic chiasm. This anterior, chiasmatic part of the basal cistern encloses the intracranial segments of the internal carotid arteries. Where these arteries branch into anterior and middle cerebral arteries, the cisternal space accompanies the stems of these arteries and becomes the *interhemispheric* (anterior cerebral arteries) and

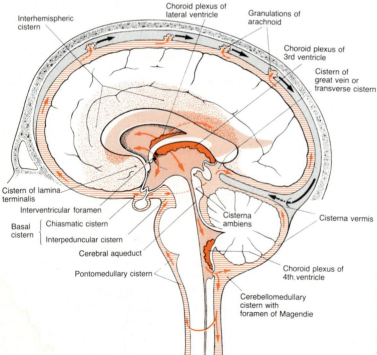

Fig. 7.**3** The cisterns of the brain. The circulation of cerebrospinal fluid is indicated by red arrows. The black arrows indicate the flow of blood in the superior longitudinal sinus.

lateral (middle cerebral arteries) *cisterns*, respectively.

The interhemispheric cistern is unpaired and follows in its course the outer surface of the corpus callosum as far caudally as to the splenium. There it connects with the relatively large *cistern of the great vein of Galen*, also called the *transverse cistern*. The pineal gland projects into it. The transverse cistern communicates with the cisterna magna via the *cisterna vermis* and with the basal cisterns via the *cisternae ambiens* which are situated on either side of the midbrain and accommodate the posterior cerebral arteries, the basal veins of Rosenthal and the trochlear nerves.

Ventricles and Cerebrospinal Fluid

Ventricles

The ventricle system of the brain is illustrated in Figs. 7.**4** and 7.**5**. It consists of *two lateral* and the *unpaired third and fourth ventricles*. Each lateral ventricle has an anterior horn, a cella media, a posterior horn, and an inferior or temporal horn. Both ventricles connect with the third ventricle via the *foramina* of Monro or interventricular foramina. The *aqueduct of* Sylvius connects the third and fourth ventricles. It is one of the landmarks of the midbrain. The fourth ventricle communicates with the subarachnoid space via three openings: two *foramina of Luschka* and one *foramen of Magendie*. The foramina of Luschka are located within the pontomedullary angles. They are the terminal outlets of the lateral recesses of the fourth ventricle and can usually be identified by the choroid plexus protruding to the outer surface of the angle (Bochdalek's *flower basket*). Far more important is the unpaired opening at the end of the fourth ventricle, the *foramen of Magendie*. This foramen lies behind the medulla and faces the cisterna magna.

Each of the four ventricles has a *choroid plexus*. The plexuses of the lateral ventricles are the largest. Where they curve from the cella media down to the inferior horn of each ventricle, they achieve their greatest size, an area referred to as the *glomus*. The stroma of these glomera is often the site of degenerative changes, including calcifications which can be seen, located symmetrically, on routine roentgenograms. Any change in this symmetry may be of diagnostic value. The plexuses of

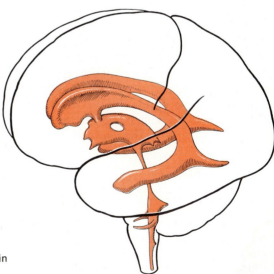

Fig. 7.**4** Topography of the ventricle system within the brain.

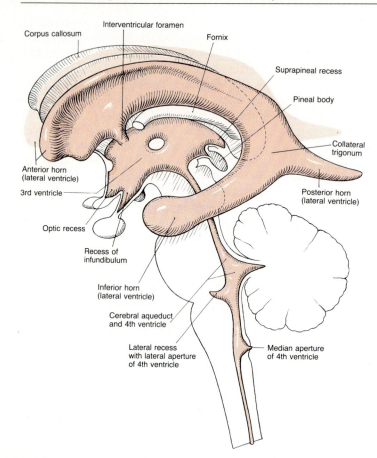

Fig. 7.5 The Ventricle system.

the lateral ventricles converge anteriorly, meet at the posterior margin of the foramina of Monro, and turn back to form the plexus of the third ventricle along its roof.

The choroid plexus of the fourth ventricle is independent. It is attached to the lower lateral walls of the ventricle and extends on either side into the lateral recesses of this ventricle at the level of the pontomedullary junction.

Cerebrospinal Fluid

The CSF is secreted by the choroid plexus, most of it by the plexus of the lateral ventricles. It enters the subarachnoid space through the foramina of Luschka and Magendie. Within the subarachnoid space, the CSF circulates up and around the brain and downward around the spinal cord. It is not an ultrafiltrate of the blood but essentially a secretion. It is clear like water, contains very few cells (about 2 per cubic millimeter) and little protein (25 to 40 mg/100 ml), and is in additional respects – for example, the composition of its ions – different from the blood (Table 7.1). The blood in the capillaries of the plexus is separated from the CSF in the ventricle by the *blood-CSF barrier*, which consists of the capillary endothelium, a basilar membrane, and the plexus epithelium. The barrier is permeable to water, oxygen, and carbondioxide and to a minor degree to electrolytes, but not at all to corpuscular constituents of the blood.

Table 7.1 Cerebrospinal fluid findings in Selected Diseases of the Central Nervous System

Disease	Appearance	Pressure in Recumbent position (mm H_2O)	Cell Content (per mm^3)	Protein (mg/100 ml)	Other Findings
Normal values of lumbar CSF	Clear, colorless	70–120	2; lymphocytes	20–45	Sugar 45–70 mg/100 ml; chloride 680–760 mg/100 ml
Brain tumor	Clear, colorless	Increased	Normal or increased	Increased (albumins)	Tumor cells (?)
Brain abscess	Clear, eventually cloudy	Considerably increased, 600–700	Normal or increased polymorphonuclear leukocytes	Increased (albumins)	Sugar lowered; Bacteriological examination
Encephalitis	Clear, colorless	Normal	Normal or increased; lymphocytes	Normal or somewhat increased	Sugar normal; virological examination
Acute purulent meningitis	Yellowish, cloudy, creamlike	Considerably increased, 250–700	Mostly above 3000; polymorphonuclear leukocytes	Increased (albumins); 100–1000	Chloride and sugar lowered; bacteriological examination
Tuberculous meningitis	Yellowish tinge	Moderately increased 200–450	10–500; mostly lymphocytes	Increased	Chloride and sugar lowered; cobweb coagulum

Table 7.1 (continued)

Disease	Appearance	Pressure in Recumbent position (mm H$_2$O)	Cell Content (per mm^3)	Protein (mg/100 ml)	Other Findings
Syphilitic meningitis	Clear to cloudy	Moderately increased; 200–300	100–1000; lymphocytes and some plasma cells	Somewhat increased (especially globulins)	VDRL +; rapid plasma reagin +
Multiple sclerosis	Clear, colorless	Normal	Normal or 50–300; lymphocytes	Normal or somewhat increased (relative increase in gamma-globulins)	Oligoclonal proteins +; myelin basic protein +
Brain trauma	Eventually bloody	Normal	Erythrocytes	Cannot be used; 4 per 1000 erythrocytes	Eventually bloody
Subdural hematoma	Occasionally yellowish	Mostly increased	Normal	Normal or somewhat increased	Not bloody
Subarachnoid hemorrhage	Bloody	Somewhat increased	Erythrocytes	Cannot be used; 4 per 1000 erythrocytes	Yellowish after centrifugation
Spinal tumor (Froin's syndrome)	Often yellowish	Normal or decreased	Normal or slightly increased	Considerably increased; 200–600	Eventually coagulation of CSF
Poliomyelitis	Clear or slightly yellowish	Somewhat increased	Somewhat increased, especially in 2nd phase	Somewhat increased	...
Polyradiculitis (Guillain–Barré syndrome)	Clear	Normal	Normal or only moderately	Distinctly increased (albumins)	Cytoalbumin dissociation

The *arachnoidal villi*, mentioned earlier in the text and shown in Figure 7.1, are essential for the resorption of the CSF into the venous bloodstream of the dural sinuses. Additional resorption probably takes place along the perineural sheaths of the exiting cranial and spinal nerves, along the ependyma of the ventricles, and via capillaries of the leptomeninges. Because of uninterrupted production of CSF by the choroid plexus and its resorption in peripheral portions of the subarachnoid spaces, CSF is continuously circulating through ventricles and over the external surface of brain and cord. The direction of the flow is indicated by red arrows in Fig. 7.3. The black arrows in that figure show the direction of the flow of venous blood in the superior longitudinal and transverse sinuses. The total volume of CSF in ventricles and subarachnoid spaces of the adult brain amounts to 130 to 150 ml. Approximately 400 to 500 ml are produced every twenty-four hours. Thus, all the CSF is exchanged several times during the course of a day. In the recumbent patient, CSF pressure is between 70 and 120 mm H_2O.

Blockages of Cerebrospinal Fluid Flow

In our discussion of diseases involving the brainstem, cerebellum, and diencephalon, hydrocephalus was repeatedly mentioned as a complication arising from the blockage of CSF flow by a primary lesion. Such distention of the ventricles is called *hypertensive internal hydrocephalus*. If the ventricular enlargement is caused by a lack of brain tissue stemming from malformation or atrophy, it is called *internal hydrocephalus ex vacuo*. In a degenerative condition, such as Pick's disease, the atrophy of convolutions produces an *external hydrocephalus ex vacuo*.

If the blockage is located within the ventricle system or involves the exits of the fourth ventricle, it is called an *occlusive* or *noncommunicating hydrocephalus*. A *communicating internal hydrocephalus* develops if the site of the blockage lies within the subarachnoid space. Occlusive internal hydrocephalus is limited to the lateral ventricles if both foramina of Monro are obliterated. An obstruction of the aqueduct produces in addition an enlargement of the third ventricle. All ventricles, including the aqueduct, are distended if the foramen of Magendie is blocked and the foramina of Luschka are not able to provide relief from the increased intraventricular pressure, as is often the case.

Selective obstruction of the foramina of Monro is most often the result of tumor-like alteration that occurs only in the roof of the third ventricle next to the foramina and is called a paraphyseal or colloid cyst of the third ventricle (Fig. 7.6a). Blockage of one foramen of Monro, resulting in distention of only one lateral ventricle, may be brought on by a glioma of the septum pellucidum or an ependymoma that may be pedunculated (Fig. 7.6b). For quite some time these lesions have a ball-valve action, producing intermittent, sudden increases in intraventricular pressure which are the cause of acute, severe headaches, often associated with nausea, vomiting, and autonomic signs. Characteristically, these headaches disappear just as suddenly when passage is restored spontaneously or by a change in the position of the head. A middle-aged executive who hoped to find relief from his attacks of severe "migraine" by being in the open air on the golf course noticed that not the open air but bending forward to pick up a golf ball terminated an attack rather rapidly. This observation led to the operative removal of a colloid cyst of the foramina of Monro.

An obliteration of the third ventricle by a tumor, such as a high-reaching craniopharyngioma (see Fig. 5.23), or compression of the ventricle by a lesion, such as a glioma of the thalamus (see Fig. 5.10), may be the cause of a hydrocephalus of both lateral ventricles.

Only one segment of a lateral ventricle may be enlarged. A tumor, an intracerebral hematoma, or an abscess in the deep centroparietal region may compress the cella media of a ventricle, causing hydrocephalic distention of its posterior and inferior horns. In the case of

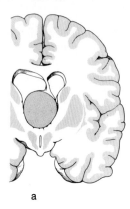

Fig. 7.**6a** Colloid cyst of foramen of Monro responsible for hydrocephalus of lateral ventricles (drawn from specimen).

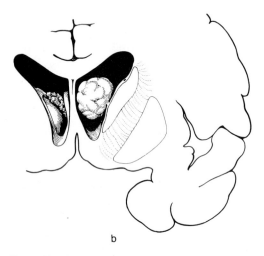

Fig. 7.**6b** Pedunculated ependymoma of the anterior horn of lateral ventricle, a potential cause of unilateral or bilateral hydrocephalus of lateral ventricles (drawn from specimen).

an abscess, the enlarged horns may be filled with pus, a condition called *pyocephalus*.

If the aqueduct is obstructed or stenosed, lateral and third ventricles distend. Aqueductal stenosis by ependymitis from former ventricular hemorrhage or infection is a frequent cause of hydrocephalus in early infancy. Because the sutures of the skull are still open at that age, the head may reach huge proportions.

Aqueductal stenosis from ependymitis is rare among adults. It is more likely that the aqueduct is compressed by a tumor, such as a pinealoma (see Fig. 3.**66**) or a periaqueductal astrocytoma, as mentioned earlier in the text (page 156).

If the fourth ventricle and its exits are the site of obstruction, all other parts of the ventricle system become expanded. Obliteration of the foramen of Magendie, the most important of the three exits, may be part of a malformation (Arnold-Chiari syndrome; basilar impression or platybasia; atlantooccipital fusion, sometimes part of Klippel-Feil syndrome; and others). An intraventricular tumor (ependymoma, epidermoid, or pearly tumor) may obstruct the lower portion of the fourth ventricle. The foramen of Magendie may be compressed by cerebellar tonsils that have herniated because of an intracerebellar tumor (medulloblastoma, cystic astrocytoma, or cystic angioblastoma). A granulomatous ependymitis (from tuberculosis, blastomycosis, or other conditions) may seal the exit of the fourth ventricle.

A *communicating internal hydrocephalus* develops if one of the important subarachnoid passageways, such as the pontine or basal cistern, is obstructed by blood, pus, or tumor (carcinomatous or gliomatous meningiosis) or by adhesions. In such a case, pneumoencephalography shows the ventricle system in all its details but shows no air in the cerebral subarachnoid space. The connection with the spinal subarachnoid space may remain open.

If the subarachnoid space is not blocked, it is possible that a severe retardation of resorption of CSF at the arachnoidal villi may be the cause of the internal hydrocephalus. The villi have been found to be packed with debris from subarachnoid hemorrhage in such cases. Inadequate resorption may produce a moderate enlargement of the ventricles after some time, without an increase in the intraventricular pressure. This is called *normal pressure hydrocephalus* (nonresorptive hydrocephalus).

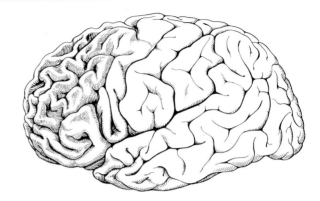

Fig. 7.6c Pick's disease. Severe atrophy of convolutions of frontal lobe and temporal pole with widening of sulci (external hydrocephalus). Preservation of anterior central and all other convolutions.

A moderately severe hydrocephalus is occasionally caused by an increase in CSF production stemming from an inflammatory irritation of the choroid plexus or a plexus papilloma (*hypersecretion hydrocephalus*).

Damage of the choroid plexus may, however, result in reduced production of CSF. Such *hypoliquorrhea* or *aliquorrhea* may occur after lumbar puncture, trauma, irradiation, or meningitis. It may be the cause of long-lasting, very obstinate headaches which may be dependent on the posture of the patient.

Internal hydrocephalus ex vacuo, mentioned earlier, is the result of cerebral atrophy and involves particularly the lateral ventricles, most severely those portions that are closest to the areas of more pronounced convolutional atrophy. Thus, in Pick's disease, in which the atrophy (external hydrocephalus) is limited to frontal, orbital, and anterior temporal convolutions, the internal hydrocephalus is most pronounced in the anterior and the rostral inferior horns of the lateral ventricles (Fig. 7.6c). Atrophy due to Alzheimer's disease likewise results in external hydrocephalus (Fig. 7.6d).

A widening of sulci similar to that shown in Fig. 7.6c, may be found at the convexity of one or both cerebral hemispheres in CT or MR scans of an elderly person not as a result of convolutional atrophy but of multiple *intra-arachnoidal cysts*. The cysts are formed

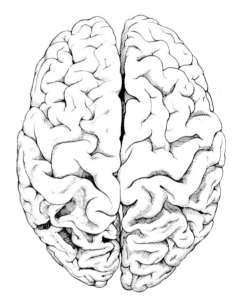

Fig. 7.6d Parieto-occipital form of Alzheimer's disease. The parietal and occipital gyri are severely atrophic. The central and frontal sulci are exposed because the meninges have been removed. The 67-year-old woman first showed symptoms at 56–58 years of age (drawn from specimen).

by a gradual separation of the outer layer of arachnoidal cells from its base, a tough connective tissue membrane. Clear fluid (not cerebrospinal fluid) accumulates within these spaces. This widens the sulci without leading to an atrophy of the convolutions. Best known is the solitary large intra-arachnoidal cyst, that develops over a temporal pole and leads to changes in the adjacent bones, which can be seen in routine X-rays. These cysts should not be confused with subarachnoid cysts which may have resulted from the organisation of local collections of blood or pus.

The cavum of the septum pellucidum present in most brains, has been called the fifth ventricle. If the two leaves of the septum remain intact, the cavum may develop into a space-occupying alteration that may interfere with CSF circulation through the foramina of Monro.

Whenever the circulation of CSF becomes impeded, intracranial pressure rises, producing headaches, dizziness, or nausea and vomiting. Headaches are probably caused by irritation of dural nerve endings responding to pressure and tension. Nausea and vomiting are probably caused by irritation of the vagus nerves. Fast-developing intracranial pressure may produce the objective signs of beginning or fully developed hemorrhagic papilledema. Longer-lasting papilledema leads to secondary atrophy of the optic nerve head, characterized by marked paleness of the papilla. This atrophy is often associated with deterioration of vision. If the third ventricle is part of a hypertensive internal hydrocephalus, its distended suprachiasmatic recess may press on the center of the chiasm, causing it to deform in the shape of an inverted horseshoe. The pressure may result in atrophy of crossing fibers and therefore in bitemporal hemianopic field defects. This may occur even if the tumor responsible for the internal hydrocephalus is far away in the cerebellum.

When hypertensive hydrocephalus develops, the lateral margins of the lateral ventricles become rounded from pressing into the white matter. Of all corticospinal fibers, only those innervating the lower extremities are exposed to this pressure. They originate in the dorsal and paramedial motor cortex and curve around the lateral ventricle on their way to the internal capsule. As a result the patient develops weakness of legs and lower trunk, making it difficult to stand up and to walk. This is illustrated by a case reported by Lindenberg, Walsh, and Sacks (1973).

Case report: A man, 60 years old at the time of report, had fallen on his head and had been briefly unconscious in early infancy. At age 4, he had pleurisy and was in bed for two months. Thereafter he had to relearn to walk, was emotionally irritable, and had a tendency to react with tantrums. He was intelligent and, when he grew up, became an editor. At age 36 he received an injury and stayed in bed for several days. After he recovered he had to learn to walk again but never lost some unsteadiness. At age 55 he became unable to walk without assistance. Occasionally, he lost control of his sphincters. At time of admission to a hospital, his legs and also his arms were held in a contracted position. Active movements were possible but were very slow. Reflexes were sluggish but not truly abnormal. The patient died from myocardial infarction.

On postmortem examination, the brain showed as the main finding a rather large communicating hydrocephalus of all ventricles. Both cerebellar tonsils revealed severe circulatory atrophy as a result of herniation that probably occurred in response to traumatic brain swelling in early infancy. By blocking the exit of the fourth ventricle, it became the cause of the hydrocephalus. The cerebral arteries showed only moderate arteriosclerosis.

An occlusive hydrocephalus can be relieved by one or the other of two operative procedures. A Thorkildsen drainage consists of creating a connection with a catheter between the hydrocephalic ventricle and the cisterna magna. If the blockage is located in the area of this cistern, the CSF can be drained by a catheter from one lateral ventricle through the jugular vein and the superior vena cava into the right auricle of the heart (ventriculoauriculostomy according to Spitz-Holter). If the block cannot be removed, herniation of the hippocampal gyri and the cerebellar tonsils will lead to impaction of the tentorium and foramen magnum, respectively (see Figs. 3.**66** and 3.**67**).

An internal hydrocephalus may originate during fetal life and enlarge further after birth. The cranium balloons more and more, the sutures open completely, and the enlarged fontanelles may bulge slightly. Tapping the cranium may produce a sound similar to that made by tapping a broken flowerpot. If the hydrocephalus develops after all sutures are closed, there is only moderate enlargement of the head, or none at all. The inner table of the skull will show a beaten-silver pattern, because of the chronic pressure exerted on it by the convolutions. The sella turcica, as well as the dorsum sellae and its posterior clinoid processes, becomes decalcified (pressure sella).

Diagnostic Considerations

It is possible for the intracranial and spinal subarachnoid spaces to become separated by tumor or inflammatory adhesions at the level of the lower medulla oblongata or upper cervical cord. In such a case the CSF below the blockage contains an abnormally large amount of protein without an appreciable increase in the number of cells (Froins's CSF loculation syndrome). The CSF above the blockage and gained by suboccipital puncture shows no increase in protein.

The following discussion of diagnostic techniques commonly used before the computerized era is justified on the basis of historical interest and also because the new diagnostic technologies are not always available.

The techniques of myelography and pneumocephalography have been largely superseded by cranial and spinal CT. Computed tomography and, in particular, MR imaging yield excellent results and can be carried out on an outpatient and practically risk-free basis.

The MR images (Fig. 7.7) demonstrate the excellent diagnostic results possible with this method. A careful analysis of the patient's case history and a thorough neurological examination precede and provide the indications for this expensive investigation method. The results are very good; taken in isolation, however, they do not communicate anything about the course of the illness and the neurological findings. The field of neurology is all the more interesting because it is possible—with the appropriate knowledge—to make at least a tentative diagnosis on the basis of the patient's medical history and a thorough neurological examination. Only then should the decision be made which technical diagnostic method is indicated for the case at hand.

Queckenstedt's test is usually sufficient for determining whether there is a partial or total blockage of the spinal CSF. This test is performed as follows: while the patient is lying on his side, a lumbar puncture is performed and the pressure of the CSF is measured by a manometer or ascension pipe attached to the needle. If the CSF column moves up and down in synchrony with pulse and respiration, the subarachnoid passage is free. Thereupon, pressure is exerted on the abdomen, or the patient is asked to apply abdominal pressure himself. This pressure causes an engorgement of the spinal veins and, in turn, a rather rapid increase in CSF pressure. When abdominal pressure returns to normal, CSF pressure falls rapidly to normal values. If increased intracranial pressure is not suspected, one may exert pressure on both external jugular veins. This produces passive venous engorgement within the cranium, causing an increase in CSF pressure which is transmitted to the CSF in the spinal leptomeningeal space. If there is a blockage in the spinal canal, the CSF pressure increase does not reach the manometer. If the CSF pressure in the manometer rises slowly and incompletely and returns slowly to normal values after pressure on the jugular veins is discontinued, one may assume that the blockage is incomplete.

Should Queckenstedt's test indicate a partial or total blockage, CT or MR scanning is indicated. If these methods are not available, *myelography* is recommended for further analysis. This method consists of injecting air, gas, or any other substance that provides contrast on roentgenography into the spinal subarachnoid space. Today innocuous, soluble contrast media are available for use in examination of the subarachnoid space below

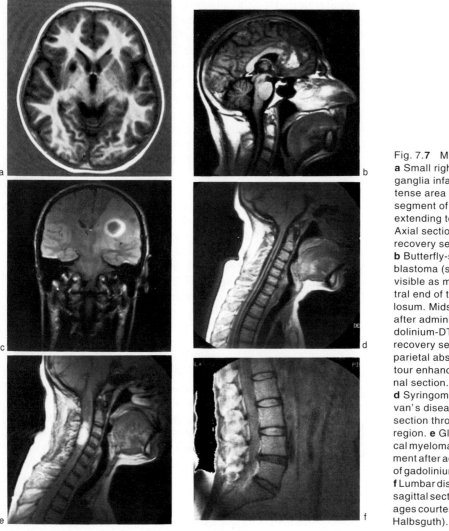

Fig. 7.7 MRI findings.
a Small right-sided basal ganglia infarct. Hypointense area in the rostral segment of the putamen extending to the pallidum. Axial section (inversion-recovery sequence).
b Butterfly-shaped glioblastoma (see Fig. 7.**8**) visible as mass at the rostral end of the corpus callosum. Midsagittal section after administration of gadolinium-DTPA, inversion-recovery sequence. **c** Left parietal abscess with contour enhancement. Coronal section.
d Syringomyelia (Morvan's disease). Sagittal section through cervical region. **e** Glioma of cervical myeloma with enhancement after administration of gadolinium-DTPA.
f Lumbar disk prolapse in sagittal section (MR images courtesy of Dr. A. Halbsguth).

the level of the spinal cord. There are also insoluble substances that are heavier than CSF and can be removed within the leptomeningeal space during fluoroscopy by tilting the table. In this way one can gain valuable information about the location and possible nature of the alteration obstructing the spinal canal. After the examination the contrast medium can easily be withdrawn with a syringe.

At this point it must be emphasized that in the presence of even a mild increase in intracranial pressure, the removal of CSF carries the danger of impaction of the tentorium or foramen magnum. In such a case a spinal tap should be performed only if facilities are available for immediate operative procedure.

Pneumoencephalography is now rarely used for visualizing the subarachnoid spaces and ventricles. In performing a lumbar or suboccipital puncture on the sitting patient, air or gas is exchanged for the CSF withdrawn. This exchange can be carried out only if there

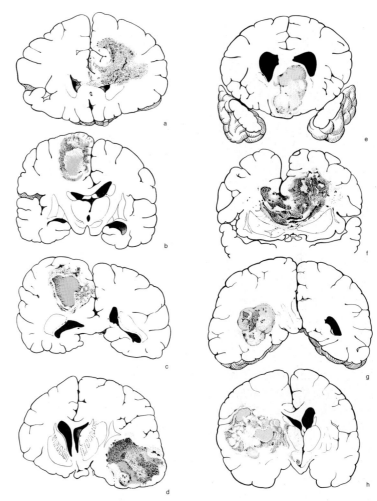

Fig. 7.8 Deformation and displacement of ventricles by cerebral tumors. **a** Glioblastoma multiforme in frontal lobe; **b** parasagittal meningioma of central region; **c** metastasis of carcinoma in parietal lobe; **d** glioblastoma multiforme in temporal lobe; **e** glioma in olfactory and subcallosal area; **f** glioblastome multiforme in frontal lobes and corpus callosum: **g** metastasis of carcinoma near posterior horn of lateral ventricle and occipital lobe; **h** metastasis of carcinoma in parietal and temporal lobes (drawn from specimens).

is no evidence of increased intracranial pressure. This method yields information not only about the width and configuration of the external and internal CSF spaces but also about the location of a space-occupying mass by revealing the patterns of distortion and displacement of the ventricles (Fig. 7.8).

Since the introduction of *computed tomography*, *NMR*, and *PET*, pneumoencephalography has been used only in selected cases. The new methods not only show CSF spaces, areas of atrophy, cysts, tumors, and other pathologic alterations very well, but they have the advantages of being painless, free of risk, and usable on ambulant patients. *Ventriculography* may be required for identification of a ventricular block. A needle is introduced into the anterior horn or into the

7 Meninges, Ventricles and Cerebrospinal Fluid

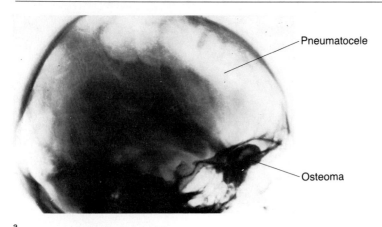

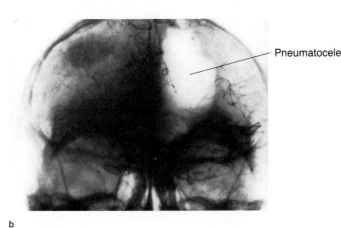

Fig. 7.**9** Osteoma of lamina cribrosa associated with pneumatocele.

posterior triangle of the lateral ventricle, and CSF is withdrawn and exchanged for air or a positive contrast medium. The need for both pneumoencephalography and ventriculography can often be avoided by using *serial angiography*. Digital subtraction angiography (DSA) is used instead of angiography in many cases, especially when the aim is to demonstrate the extracranial vessels.

Serial angiography has retained its importance as a diagnostic technique despite the introduction of the modern computerized techniques. It allows the diagnosis of arterial and venous stenoses or occlusions. The afferent and deferent blood vessels can be shown in the case of an angioma; similarly, it is possible to distinguish tumors (vascularization), abscesses, and extracerebral and intracerebral bleeding. When thromboses are present in several vessels, it is necessary to show all afferent vessels to determine the collateral supply. A vertebral angiography is necessary in many cases of vertebrobasilar insufficiency for confirmation.

Other diagnostic methods are *scientigraphy, electroencephalography, echoencephalography, sonography,* and *elective roentgenography* without contrast media. Routine roentgenograms often prove to be diagnostically valuable by showing, for example, displacement of a calcified pineal, an erosion of the sphenoid or petrous bone suggestive of a meningioma, calcifications at the base of the brain characteristic of a craniopharyngioma, an enlargement of the sella from pituitary tumor or intrasellar arachnoidal cyst (empty sella), or an enlargement of one optic canal suggesting an optic nerve glioma.

Fig. 7.**9** shows a spontaneous, collection of air within the cranium (*pneumocele*) related to an osteoma in the area of the lamina cribrosa. The tumor had eroded dura and arachnoid, permitting air from the nasopharyngeal space to enter the subarachnoid space. The case report follows.

Case Report: Ten days before admission to the hospital, a 32-year-old man noticed weakness and clumsiness in his right hand and right foot. He could still work, although his strength was reduced. Subtle movements, such as writing or handling knife and fork, became awkward. Because of weakness and some ataxia in the right leg, he experienced difficulty in walking. Three days prior to admission, he had fallen without losing consciousness. For the last ten days he had had headaches, particularly in the evening.

Neurologic findings included bilateral anosmia and mild right hemiparalysis, with increased reflexes and muscle tone. Being left-handed the patient had no speech disorder. Roentgenography revealed an osteoma in the area of the left lamina cribrosa, associated with a left-sided pneumocele. Recommended *therapy* consisted of covering the defect in the dura with a galeaperiosteum transplant.

A basal frontal fracture is a more frequent cause of a pneumocele. It is usually associated with *rhinal* or *nasal liquorrhea*. A fracture of the petrous bone may be the cause of *otic liquorrhea*.

8 Telencephalon or Cerebral Cortex

External Characteristics

Cerebral cortex and its white matter make up the largest portion of the telencephalon (endbrain). The striate bodies, a smaller part of it, have already been discussed.

The *cortex* faces the outer surface of the cerebrum and covers the *white matter* like a cloak, hence the alternate terms *mantle* and *pallium*. The cortex contains cell bodies, dendrites, and some axons of nerve cells, whereas the large mass of white matter consists only of myelinated axons. The internal surface of the white matter consists of the wall of the lateral ventricles.

Originally, the telencephalon is part of the round, monoventricular prosencephalic vesicle or forebrain (telencephalon plus diencephalon). During the fourth week of embryonic life, the rostral vesicle develops lateral pouches, which become the telencephalic hemispheres. At the end of the fourth month of intrauterine life, rostrocaudal development of the corpus callosum nears its completion. The hemispheres, separated by the interhemispheric fissure, are now connected by commissures; the phylogenetically old cortex of the olfactory-limbic system (*archipallium* plus *paleopallium*, also called *allocortex*) by the *anterior* and the still smaller *hippocampal commissures* (commissura fornicis), and the new cortex (*neocortex* or *neopallium* or *isocortex*) by the large *corpus callosum*. This commissure is of such great size because the new cortex by far outdistanced the old cortex in its growth during the phylogenetic development of the mammalian brain.

To achieve greater economy of space, the ever-enlarging cortex became more and more folded into gyri or convolutions, separated by fissures or sulci. The result is that in man the cortex visible from the outside of the convolutions (Figs. 8.1, 8.2, and 8.3) represents only one-third of the entire cortex, the other two-thirds being hidden within the sulci.

The pattern of the folding process of the cortex varies greatly among the various mammalian species, but it is always the same for all members of a given species and is in its basic design characteristic of the species. This holds true for the cerebral convolutions of man. Their basic pattern is so repetitive that each principal convolution has been given a separate name (Figs. 8.4 through 8.8).

Some of the sulci develop earlier in fetal life than others and are often referred to as fissures. The earliest are the collateral and rhinal fissures, which separate the hippocampal gyri from the other inferior temporal gyri (3rd month of intrauterine life). The lateral or sylvian, the central or rolandic, and the calcarine fissures also develop early. Most basic convolutions develop after the sixth fetal month. Development of subconvolutions—subdivisions of the basic convolutions by shallow sulci—follows as late as early infancy. They are a unique component of each brain and account for some convolutional differences between the two hemispheres of the same brain.

External Characteristics

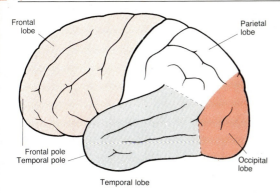

Fig. 8.1 The four cerebral lobes as seen at the convexity of the left hemisphere.

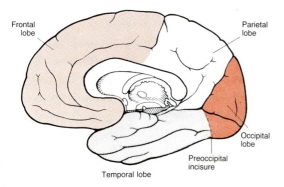

Fig. 8.2 The four lobes as seen at the medial aspect of the right hemisphere.

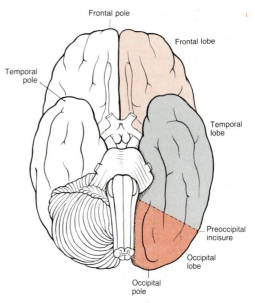

Fig. 8.3 Three lobes are seen at the base of the left cerebral hemisphere after removal of the left cerebellum. The orbital portion of the frontal lobe is often referred to as orbital lobe.

The central fissures at convexity and medial aspects of the hemispheres are anatomically and functionally most important. Anatomically, they represent the borders between *frontal* and *parietal lobes*. Functionally, they separate the *anterior somatomotor regions* from the *posterior somatosensory areas*, as will be described later.

Traditionally, each hemisphere has two additional lobes: the *occipital* and the *temporal lobes*. The occipital lobe has as natural boundaries only the parietooccipital fissure at the medial aspect of each hemisphere and the preoccipital incisure, a small notch at the end of the lower margin of the temporal lobes. The other borders with parietal and temporal lobes are somewhat arbitrary (see Figs. 8.1, 8.2, and 8.3). This reflects somewhat symbolically the fact that occipital and neopallial temporal lobes are also sensory, the occipital lobes subserving *vision* and most portions of the temporal lobes subserving *hearing*. Thus, all the neopallium located posterior to the central fissure is actually sensory, the posterior central cortex, the calcarine cortex, and the cortex of Heschl's transverse convolutions providing the primary receiving centers of somatic sensations, vision, and hearing, respectively. All cortex in between is responsible for higher integrated functions and intricate cooperations among these senses and for their connections with other parts of the brain.

As the cortical areas lying between the primary sensory centers enlarged in mass during phylogenesis and ontogenesis, the temporal lobes shifted anteriorly in an arcuate fashion. This development explains why some of the fibers of the optic radiation emerging from the lateral geniculate body

8 Telencephalon or Cerebral Cortex

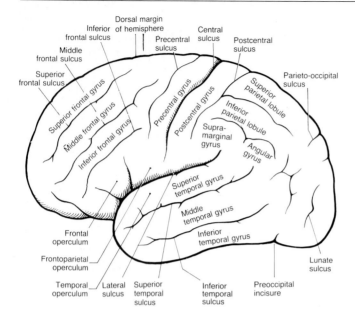

Fig. 8.4 Cerebral convolutions and sulci (lateral view).

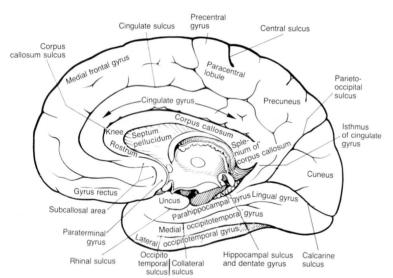

Fig. 8.5 Cerebral convolutions and sulci (medial view).

take a rostral course before turning around and proceeding caudally to the calcarine cortex. This phenomenon is known as *Meyer's loop*, as was mentioned earlier in the text (pages 84, 85).

More important, the anterior shifting of the temporal lobes gave rise to the lateral fissure and caused the *insula* to become totally covered by the temporal lobe. These deep-seated convolutions are confined by the semicircular fissure and are therefore referred to as the fifth lobe. In order to visualize them, the frontal and parietal convolutions serving as the dorsal lid or operculum of the lateral fissure must be resected and the temporal

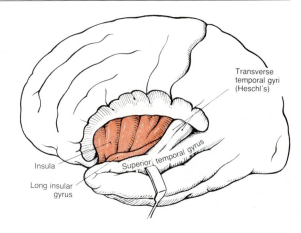

Fig. 8.6 Heschl's transverse convolutions and superior temporal gyrus.

lobe pulled downward, as was done in Figs. 8.6, and 8.7. This procedure is also necessary in order to visualize Heschl's *transverse convolutions* – the *primary hearing cortex* (see Fig. 8.6) – and the limen insulae, which connects the insula with the anterior third of the temporal lobe. It is unrelated to hearing.

The *limbic lobe* of Broca, discussed earlier in the text (page 202), may be considered the sixth lobe of the endbrain.

Finally, it will be shown that the basal part of the frontal lobe deserves to be separated as *orbital lobe*, the seventh lobe of the telencephalon.

Internal Characteristics

Cortex

The gray cortical band is of almost equal thickness throughout (approximately 4 mm). It is a little thicker over the crown of the convolutions than around the depths of sulci. Only a few segments of the cortex have specific gross features. The old cortex of the hippocampal formation is characterized by the curled, thin cortex of the Ammon's horn. In the neocortex the motor cortex of the anterior central convolution is the thickest of all, measuring approximately 5 mm in thickness.

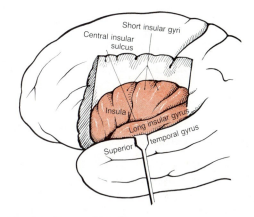

Fig. 8.7 Exposed insula.

It is also less sharply set off toward the white matter than the remainder of the cortex, because it has a relatively large number of neurons in the so-called seventh layer, which tapers off into the white matter. Adjacent to it is the sensory cortex of the posterior central convolution, which is, together with the calcarine cortex, the thinnest, measuring not much more than 1.5 mm in thickness. Sometimes, depending on the intensity of the gray color of the cortex, one can see two fine lines that run parallel to the outer surface as well as to each other through the center of the cortex. These are the *Baillarger's lines*. In the calcarine cortex only one line is distinctly visible. It is the *line of Gennari* and is equivalent to the outer Baillarger's line. Both types

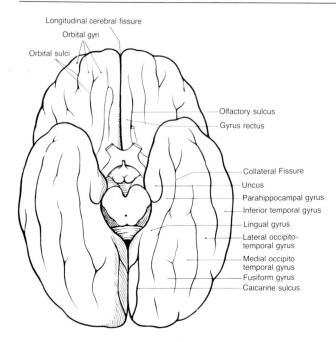

Fig. 8.8 Convolutions and sulci at base of brain.

of lines are white because they consist of myelinated fibers.

The cerebral cortex has been subdivided into numerous fields according to differences in the architectural arrangement of tissue components, such as nerve cells, myelinated fibers, and blood vessels; therefore, one speaks of cytoarchitecture, myeloarchitecture, and angioarchitecture. In recent years a chemoarchitecture has been added on the basis of histochemical investigations by Friede and others.

What is known about the *cytoarchitecture* of the cerebral cortex is tied to the names of Brodmann, Campbell, O. Vogt, von Economo, Koskinas, and von Bonin, to name only a few. Oscar and Cécile Vogt and their pupils have contributed much to *myeloachitecture*. R. A. Pfeiffer has been a leader in the field of *angioarchitecture*.

Fig. 8.9 demonstrates Brodmann's map of the cytoarchitectonic fields of the human brain. It should be mentioned that the fields were numbered in the order in which they were studied. The numbers bear no relation to the functional features of the areas.

The architecture of the phylogenetically old allocortex shows little differentiation when compared with the neopallial isocortex. This can be seen in Fig. 8.10, showing the Ammon's horn of the hippocampus and the very small cortical band of the dentate gyrus, consisting of densely arranged, very small neurons. This cortex follows the curved but obliterated hippocampal fissure and encircles the end-plate of the cortex of the Ammon's horn which continues in a semicircle around the other side of the hippocampal fissure. This cortex consists of other equally large pyramidal as well as double pyramidal cells. The cortex of the horn becomes wider and continues toward the subiculum, the cortex of which consists in places of four layers. The second layer consists of numerous islands of neurons, reminiscent of similar islands in the equally old area olfactoria. The cortex of the subiculum gradually changes into a modified, six-layer cortex (parahippocampal gyrus). At about the level of the collateral fissure the

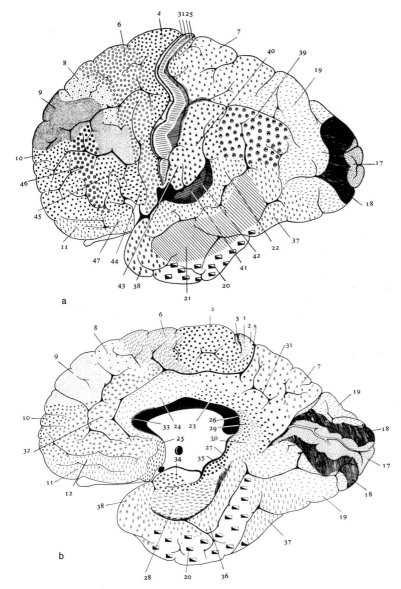

Fig. 8.9 Cytoarchitectonic fields of the human cortex. **a** Convexity of left and **b** medial side of right hemisphere. Numbers denote cortical fields. (After Brodmann; from Bargmann, W. Histologie und mikroskopische Anatomie des Menschen, 6th edition, Thieme, Stuttgart, 1967.)

cortex demonstrates the typical six layers of the isocortex of the neopallium.

The architecture of this cortex is illustrated in Fig. 8.**11**. It demonstrates side-by-side cytoarchitecture in a preparation impregnated with silver and another stained with the Nissl technique. The third column in this figure demonstrates the rich pattern of myeloarchitectonics. One can differentiate among the neurons the following layers, starting with the layer next to the surface of the cortex.

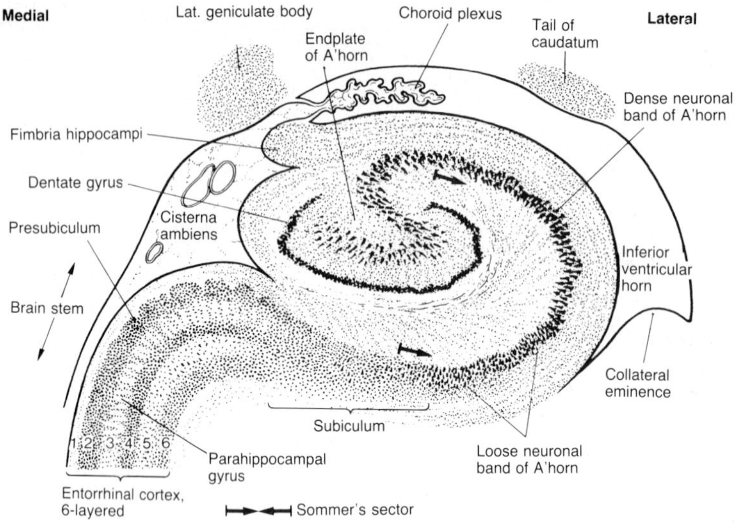

262 8 Telencephalon or Cerebral Cortex

Fig. 8.10 Cytoarchitecture of allocortex of hippocampal formation with Ammon's horn. Hippocampos, Greek, means sea horse. When viewing the Figure from the right, the parahippocampal gyrus forms the neck and the Ammon's horn (ramshorn of Egyptian God Ammon) the curled tail of the sea horse.

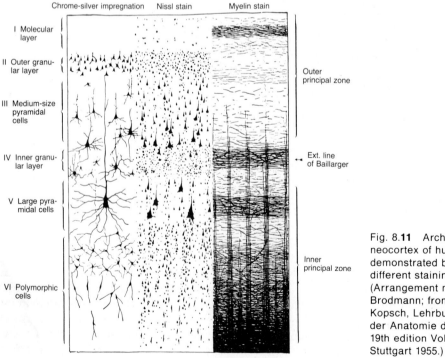

Fig. 8.11 Architecture of neocortex of human brain, demonstrated by three different staining procedures. (Arrangement made by Brodmann; from Rauber-Kopsch, Lehrbuch und Atlas der Anatomie des Menschen, 19th edition Vol. II, Thieme Stuttgart 1955.)

First or molecular layer: This layer contains only a limited number of rather small neurons (Cajal cells). The dendrites of these cells run tangentially within the first layer, whereas the axons proceed toward the white matter. These cells receive impulses from pyramidal and fusiform cells in other cortical areas of the hemisphere, explaining why the molecular layer has rather numerous tangentially running fibers.

Second or external granular layer: Neurons in this layer are small and granular. A few small pyramidal cells are seen in between. The dendritic connections occur in the same layer.

Third or external pyramidal layer: This layer consists of pyramidal cells that become larger toward its base. The axons of these pyramidal cells are directed toward the white matter and are already myelinated within the layer. Within the white matter they run as projection, association, or commissural fibers. Dendrites leaving the tips of the cells extend into the first molecular layer. All other dendrites branch predominantly within the pyramidal cell layer.

Fourth or internal granular layer: This layer corresponds to the outer granular layer. The granule cells receive stimuli predominantly via thalamocortical pathways. Like the outer granular layer, this layer contains numerous relay stations with internuncial neurons and controlling feedback circuits. Whereas the fibers in the outer pyramidal layer are basically arranged in radial order, the fibers of the internal granular layer run essentially tangentially, forming the external Baillarger's line. Most of the fibers belong to thalamic neurons, probably to neurons of specific thalamic nuclei.

Fifth or internal pyramidal layer: The pyramidal cells of this layer are of medium or large size. In the precentral gyrus this layer contains the giant pyramidal (Betz's) cells. The axons of these cells are surrounded by particularly thick myelin sheaths. They form the corticonuclear as well as the corticospinal tracts. This layer also contains the tangentially oriented myelinated fibers that form the internal Baillarger's line.

Sixth or multiform cell layer: These cells are in part modified pyramidal cells, in part triangular or spindle cells. The cells are usually smaller toward the fifth layer and larger toward the white matter. This cell layer gives off fibers that connect with other cortical areas as well as with subcortical nuclei.

In general, one can say that the cortex contains two main groups of cells: (1) pyramidal and fusiform cells that are corticofugal and efferent, and (2) granule cells that receive afferent impulses. Fig. 8.**12** shows the afferent fibers in back in a simplified manner. They come from the thalamus as projection fibers (indicated in the figure as (*1*), and from other areas of the cerebral cortex as association fibers (*2*) and terminate within the cortex at the granule cells of the second and fourth layer. The efferent fibers are shown in red. The axons of the pyramidal cells of the fifth layer go via the internal capsule to thalamus, corpus striatum, brainstem nuclei and spinal cord (*3*) ; others act as association and commissural fibers and connect with other cortical areas (*4*).

The 6-layer cortex shown in Fig. 8.**11** is referred to as *homotypic*. There are cortical fields in the adult brain in which it is difficult to differentiate the six layers; these fields are called *heterotypic*.

In the primary sensory fields receiving impulses from body sensations, vision, and hearing, granule cells predominate over pyramidal cells. Therefore, one speaks of a *granular cortex*.

In contrast, pyramidal cells predominate over granule cells in motor fields, which for this reason are called *agranular cortex*.

Brodmann's receptive fields 3, 1, 2, 41, and particularly 17 (area striata or visual cortex) are representatives of the *granular cortex* or *koniocortex*, whereas fields 4 and 6 are typical agranular fields. Brodmann identified a few more than 50 different architectonic fields.

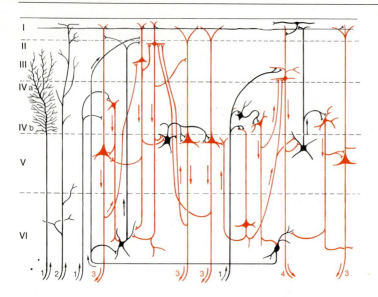

Fig. 8.12 Simplified model of some intracortical neuronal chains (after Lorente de Nó and Larsell).

His map is generally used because it is simpler than that of von Economo, who counted twice as many fields. Some observers have identified over two hundred. Von Economo (1925) found that the various architectonic fields have one or another feature in common and can be reduced to five basic types, illustrated in Fig. 8.13. As can be recognized in Fig. 8.9, the cytoarchitectonic fields do not correspond exactly to the course of the convolutions; they overlap in part and also show individual variations in extent (Filimonoff, 1929; Sarkissow and co-workers, 1967).

Many attempts have been made to correlate various rather detailed brain functions with the various cytoarchitectonic fields, particularly because it was determined rather early that areas 4 and 6 subserve motor functions and that areas 3, 1, 2, 41, and 17 are the primary receiving areas of somatic sensations, hearing, and vision.

Before we present what has become known about the functional organization of the cerebral cortex, its fiber connections must be discussed.

White Matter

The cerebral white matter may be likened to a huge, complex aggregation of two-way wires connecting as *projection fibers* the cortex with subcortical centers, as *association fibers* cortical areas of the same hemisphere, and as *commissural fibers* centers of the two hemispheres.

Projection Fibers

The *efferent* corticofugal fibers enter the internal capsule, as described in the chapters on motor function and on the extrapyramidal system. These are the fibers of corticonuclear, corticospinal, and corticopontine pathways and also of the fascicles that connect the cortex with the thalamus, striatum, reticular formation, substantia nigra, subthalamic nucleus, quadrigeminal plate, and red nucleus (see Fig. 6.9). The longest are the corticospinal fibers, which originate in Brodmann's areas 4, 3, 1, 2, and 6. Other efferents, such as the corticopontine and corticothalamic fibers, derive from larger association areas.

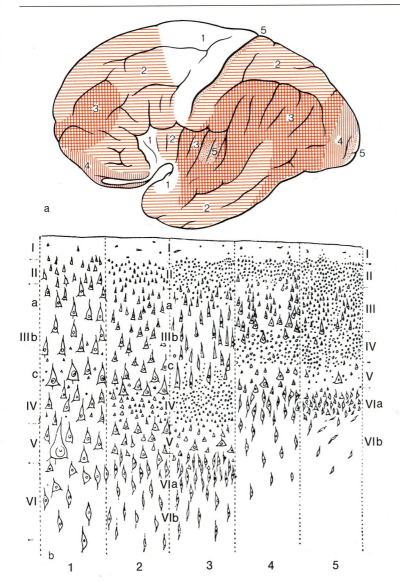

Fig. 8.13 The five basic types of the cerebral cortex (after von Economo): 1 = agranular; 2 = frontal type; 3 = parietal type; 4 = polar type; 5 = granular (koniocortex). **a** Their distribution at the convexity; **b** their cytoarchitectural patterns. (From von Economo, C., Zellaufbau der Grosshirnrinde des Menschen. Springer Berlin, 1927.)

Practically all *afferent* fibers come from the thalamus and go to widely distributed areas of the cerebral cortex. More specifically, they include all somatosensory pathways that connect with areas 3, 1, 2, and 4. Other afferent impulses come from cerebellum, pallidum, and mamillary bodies and go via the thalamus to the cortex. Only olfactory fibers do not use the thalamus; they go directly to the cortex.

Between cortex and internal capsule the projection fibers form the *corona radiata*. The optic radiation, connecting the lateral geniculate body with area 17, and the acoustic radiation, connecting the medial geniculate body with area 41, are also part of the projection system (see Figs. 1.20, 2.2, 3.12, 3.37, 8.14, and 8.15).

Association Fibers

These fibers account for most of the white matter. They interconnect adjacent as well as remote cortical areas. In this way all functionally important cortical areas can cooperate intimately, putting the cerebral cortex in a position to fulfill its associative and integrative functions. The extensive fiber connections among the individual cortical areas probably explain the fact that brain function loss caused by a lesion is not always permanent. Perhaps some fibers remain intact and are able to restore some of the lost function after exercise is provided for a time.

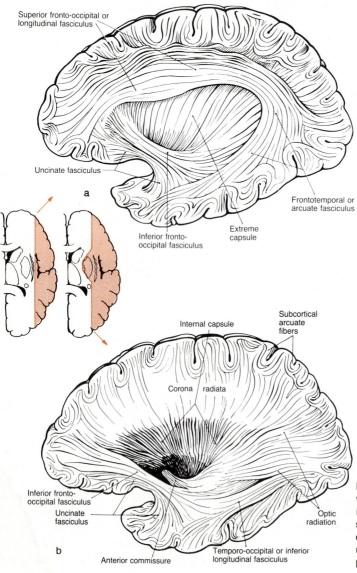

Fig. 8.14 Association fibers of white matter seen when looking in mediolateral direction (see insert). **a** Section through extreme capsule; **b** section through internal capsule after removal of putamen.

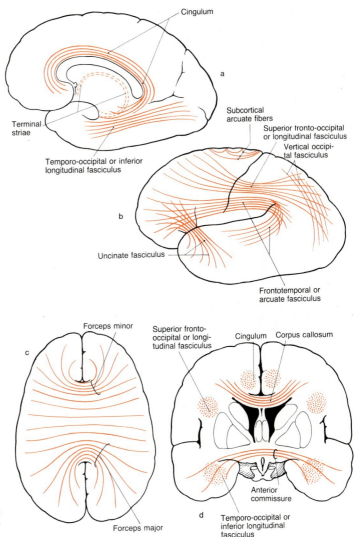

Fig. 8.15 The most important associaion and commissural fiber bundles.

The most important association fiber bundles are illustrated in Figs. 8.14, and 8.15. A few deserve special comments.

The *arcuate fibers* are also called U-fibers. They occupy the immediate subcortical white matter, form U-shaped layers around the deep projections of the cortex, and interconnect adjacent cortical fields. They are known to be resistant in some demyelinating leucoencephalopathies.

The *superior longitudinal fascicle* passes dorsal to the level of the insula in an anterior-posterior direction and connects the frontal lobes with large portions of the parietooccipital and temporal convolutions. Its frontotemporal portion circles around the posterior end of the sylvian fissure and is called the *arcuate fascicle*. It is believed that his fascicle connects temporal (Wernicke) and frontal (Broca) areas of speech. The *inferior longitudinal fascicle* connects the temporal and occipital lobes. The *uncinate fascicle* runs around the anterior portion of the sylvian fissure as it connects the orbital lobe with the temporal pole. The *cingulum* is one of the association bundles of the limbic system and connects the subcallosal area with the parahippocampal gyrus circling all along the corpus callosum. Very important association bundles are the *superior* and *inferior occipitofrontal fascicles* and the *vertical occipital fascicle*.

Commissural Fibers

The *corpus callosum* is the largest commissure and is the commissure of the neopallium. Fibers pass through the commissure to either hemisphere and radiate thereafter into various directions, connecting all homotopic cortical areas except the primary visual cortex (area 17) and the hand and foot areas in the somatosensory cortex. Fibers of the callosal radiation cross the fibers of the corona radiata and also other association bundles. Because the corpus callosum is shorter than the hemispheres, fibers crossing through rostrum and knee and through the splenium must take arcuate courses to the frontal and occipital poles, respectively. These arcuate fiber bundles are referred to as anterior (minor) and posterior (major) forceps of the callosal radiation (see Fig. 8.**15c**). The *anterior commissure* is the commissure of the olfactory brain, of the temporal lobes and, to a small extent, of some suprarostral frontal cortex. The *hippocampal commissure* essentially connects the posterior columns of the fornix (crura fornicis).

Functional Organization of the Cortex

Until 1861, the cerebral cortex was held to be functionally homogeneous and omnivalent. Being the seat of "soul" and "mind" and the two being in unity, the functions of the cortex had to be undivided. This theory had been considered valid ever since Pierre Flourens, comparative anatomist and physiologist at the University of Paris, had published it in 1824 as a result of his animal experiments (mainly on birds).

In 1861 it was again in Paris that Pierre Paul Broca addressed the Société d'Anthropologie and demonstrated on a human brain that the cerebral cortex has localized functions. He had found that the aphasia in one of his patients had been caused by a lesion that had destroyed the posterior third of the left third frontal convolution – "Broca's convolution", as it was later called. Soon more evidence was presented by both clinicians and physiologists in favor of the localization of various functions in the cerebral cortex.

Hughlings Jackson (1864) studied patients with focal epilepsy and attributed its cause to irritations in the precentral cortex. Carl Wernicke (1874) described for the first time sensory aphasia and its localization in the posterior part of the first temporal convolution. He also provided a convincing demonstration of unilateral cerebral dominance. In the United States, Weir Mitchell of Philadelphia (1860) had expressed the notion that the muscles of one side of the body are innervated by the cortex of the contralateral cerebral hemisphere. The Civil War brought an end to his studies. Robert Bartholow of Cincinnati (1874) had a patient whose skull had been destroyed by a malignancy. He used this opportunity to apply electrodes to the cortex and found that faradization of a circumscribed area produced contraction of the limbs of the opposite side of the body and ipsilateral turning of the head. When these findings were published, the humanitarian and religious citizens of Cincinnati forced him to leave town.

Fritsch and Hitzig (1870) were the first to identify the motor cortex in dogs by electrical stimulation and to demonstrate the somatotopic order of the cortex for contralateral movements. They were followed by equally outstanding physiologists, among them Ferrier (1876), Beevor and Horsley (1890), Grünbaum (1901), and Sherrington (1906).

Regarding sensory cortical representation, von Gudden (1870) demonstrated that the removal of both eyes in a young animal impeded the development of the occipital lobes. Munk (1879) announced that dogs without occipital lobes are blind and that damage limited to the cortex adjacent to the occipital convexity produces "Seelenblindheit," now called *optic agnosia*. Ferrier in 1879 and 1892 observed animals to raise their ears when certain areas of the temporal lobes were stimulated. Dusser de Barenne (1916) used strychnine instead of electrical current to stimulate the cortex. Applying it to circumscribed areas of the postcentral gyrus, he found that stimulating different portions of the gyrus caused the animal to scratch different portions of its body. In this way it was possible to subdivide also the sensory postcentral gyrus into somatotopic units.

In this attempt to identify and localize cortical functions, true progress evolved slowly over many years of controversy. The visual cortex may be mentioned as an example. What is known today about its function and relation to retina and lateral geniculate bodies was a matter of dramatic controversy. The last issues of the debate were not resolved until after World War I (Polyak, 1957; Lindenberg, 1977).

At that time, *Karl Kleist*, a pupil of *Wernicke*, wrote his comprehensive Hirnpathologie (Brain Pathology), published in 1934. He analyzed the clinical and neuropathologic observations he had made on almost 300 brain-injured soldiers during World War I and on 106 hospital patients with focal, mostly circulatory cerebral lesions for the purpose of gaining further insight into the functional organization of the cerebrum, including the localization of basic psychic functions.

Much useful information had accumulated after Wernicke's death (1905). Most important for Kleist was the discovery that the gray mass of the cerebral cortex represents a composite of numerous individual units, each of them identifiable by the pattern of its cytoarchitecture and of a corresponding myeloarchitecture (Campbell, 1905; E. Smith, 1907; Brodmann, 1909; O. Vogt, 1910; v.Economo and Koskinas, 1925; Beck, 1925; Rose, 1928). It also intrigued him that the cellular layers forming the cortex were shown to have different functional significance (Nissl, 1908; Cajal, 1911; Kappers, 1920; and many others).

Ultimately, Kleist concluded that the cerebral cortex as a whole is made up of groups of architectonic fields representing predominantly sensory spheres, and that each sphere is composed of the actual sensory zone and two more or less prevailing zones, one for motor and the other for psychic functions. He listed the following spheres: a visual sphere in the occipital area, a hearing sphere in the temporal lobe, a touch sphere in the centroparietal lobe (including the motor area), a gustatory sphere in the subcentral opercular region, a labyrinthine-myesthenic sphere in the frontal convolutions, a sphere for internal feelings (ego area) in orbital and cingulate gyri, and an olfactory sphere in the piriforme lobe and the hippocampal formation.

Kleist's map of the cerebral cortex is reproduced in Fig. 8.**16** and 8.**17** for historical reasons. It shows the various functions he attributed to the numbered cytoarchitectonic fields of Brodmann, revised, in a few places, by v.Economo and O. Vogt. As soon as the map was published, Kleist was severely criticized, particularly for correlating individual psychic functions to small architectonic fields. Attaching "egos" (not to be confused with Freud's Ego) to circumscribed cortical territories was called brain mythology.

In the following years the psychological concepts of *holism* and *gestaltism* gained much interest. Some believed it to be impossible to localize individual functions. This did not, however, discourage clinicians, neuropathologists, and physiologists.

There is no doubt that it is possible to localize a number of functional deficits. What had been learned regarding localization of function in animal experiments was found by

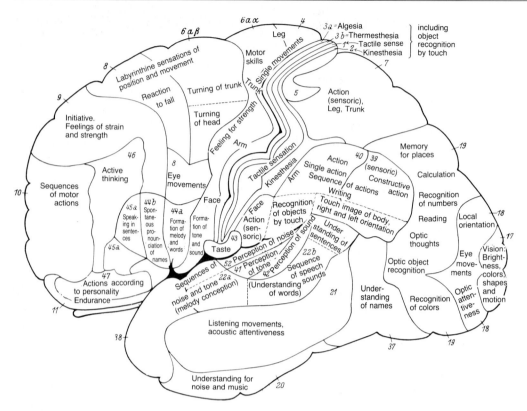

Fig. 8.16 Localization of functions of the cerebral cortex on a cytoarchitectonic basis (after K. Kleist). Convexity of left hemisphere.

neurosurgeons to exist also in man (Cushing, 1932; Foerster, 1936; Penfield, 1950; and others). By stimulating the cortex of patients whose brains had been exposed for surgical reasons under local anesthesia, new findings could be added (Figs. 8.**18**, 8.**19**, 8.**20**, and 8.**21**). By ablation of circumscribed portions of the cortex in animals and human patients, additional facts became known (Minkowski, 1917; and others). Unfortunately, stimulation and ablation of the cerebral cortex are not physiological methods. Therefore, movements produced by electrical stimulation of the cortex do not correspond to natural voluntary movements. This was one of the impetuses for the still ongoing search for better methods to gain insight into the functions of the cerebral cortex.

Electroencephalography has brought about considerable progress in this respect. It was found that natural or experimental stimulation of peripheral receptors, such as eyes, and ears, produces recordable changes in the potentials of the cerebral cortex. These *evoked potentials* permitted rather exact localization of the area of the cerebral cortex receiving the stimuli (Adrian, 1941; Woolsey, 1964; and others). Such evoked potentials were recorded not only from the cortex but also from deeper structures of the brain through implanted microelectrodes.

It can now be stated with certainty that cytoarchitectonic areas 3, 2, and 1 constitute the region of primary somatosensory projection and that area 17 receives visual im-

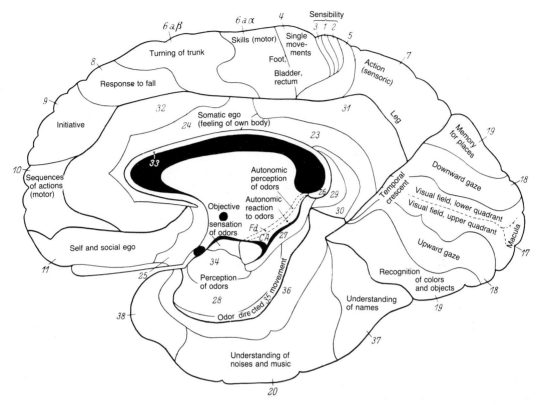

Fig. 8.17 Localization of functions of the cerebral cortex on a cytoarchitectonic basis (after K. Kleist). Medial aspect of right hemisphere. (Figs. 8.16 and 8.17 from Kleist, K., Gehirnpathologie. In Handbuch der ärztlichen Erfahrungen im Weltkrieg 1914/18, Vol. IV, Barth, Leipzig, 1922–1934.)

pulses, area 41 acoustic stimuli, and area 43 gustatory or taste sensations. In addition, it can be accepted as fact that stimuli arrive in several primary projection areas of the cortex in a point-to-point order, that is, in somatotopic, retinotopic, and tonotopic order.

The introduction of *stereotactic methods* has greatly advanced our knowledge. These methods permit us to stimulate or paralyze all deep-seated structures of the brain and to record evoked potentials from distinct nuclear areas through implanted microelectrodes.

Psychosurgical operations, such as *lobotomy, leucotomy,* and *cingulotomy,* in patients with certain mental disorders (such as schizophrenia and compulsion neurosis) contributed much insight into the importance of the anterior frontal lobes (prefrontal region) for certain psychological behavior patterns.

In recent years diverse new tools, such as *electron microscopy, fluorescence microscopy, autoradiography,* and *histochemistry,* have yielded new insight into structure, metabolism, and function of neurons. The introduction of *microelectrodes* for recording potentials from single nerve fibers and cells proved to be extremely important. This method, sometimes amplified by one or two other new techniques, has enabled physiologists to map the cerebral cortex according to neuronal functions. Initially, they were skeptical of the great number of fields that Brodmann, von Economo, and others had

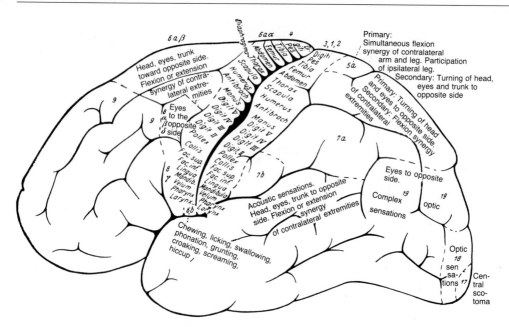

Fig. 8.18 Pattern of motor reactions produced by electrical stimulation of individual cortical motor fields. (Figs. 8.18 and 8.19 from O. Foerster, Grosshirn. In Bumke, O. and Foerster, O., [eds.], Handbuch der Neurologie, Vol. VI, Springer, Berlin, 1936.)

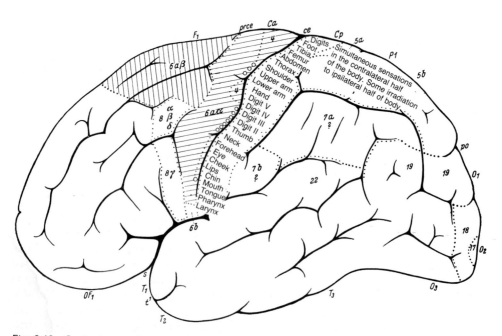

Fig. 8.19 Cortical areas for somesthesia in the human brain.

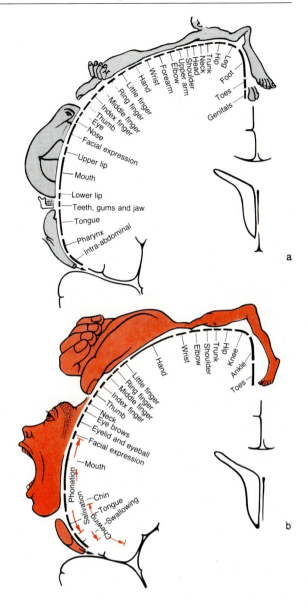

Fig. 8.20 Representation of the body in **a** primary sensory and **b** primary motor fields of the human cerebral cortex. (From Penfield, W. and Rasmussen, T., The Cerebral Cortex of Man, Macmillan, New York, 1950.)

described as separate cytoarchitectonic entities. It is now anticipated that the number of areas that can be differentiated may indeed lie between 50 and 100, according to Hubel and Wiesel (1977).

These two authors have been recognized as leaders in this immensely intricate and exciting field. They have concentrated on the visual cortex (Brodmann's field 17) in the macaque monkey; their findings can be summarized as follows: The granule cells of the lower third of layer IV of the visual cortex receive impulses coming from the lateral geniculate body and react best to small, *circular* stimuli, as do the ganglion cells of the retina and the neurons of the geniculate body. The circular, symmetrical fields of information in

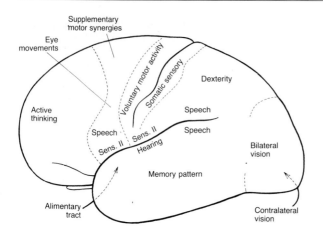

Fig. 8.21 Overall functions of cortical areas determined by electrical stimulation of the cortex during operation. (Penfield, W. and Rasmussen, T., The Cerebral Cortex of Man, Macmillan, New York, 1950.)

the lower granular layer must be rearranged, however, because all cells outside layer IV respond best to specifically oriented segments of *linear* stimuli. The cells preferring the same orientation of linear stimulus are packed in roughly parallel, vertical slabs of cortical tissue, each representing an "orientation slab." Cells responding to stimuli coming from only one eye occupy a vertical slab adjacent to another slabs of cells, which respond to stimuli from the other eye. One set of these "ocular dominance" slabs subserves both eyes. The combination of one set of slabs subserving all orientations and one set of ocular dominance slabs constitutes what the authors consider an elementary unit of the primary visual cortex. Each such vertical column measures about 1 mm² and is 2 mm deep. Such functional partitioning in vertical columns has been found to be present also in other cortical fields. It was first described in the primary somatosensory area by Mountcastle in 1957.

Primary Receptive Fields of Parietal, Occipital, and Temporal Cortex

In discussing the clinical functions of the neocortex, it appears best to start with those of the primary receptive cortex, where somatosensory, visual, and acoustic stimuli first arrive. This description will be followed by a discussion of the frontal lobes and the secondary receptive cortical areas in parietal, occipital, and temporal lobes.

The primary sensory areas of the cortex are projection areas of specific sensory thalamic nuclei (Fig. 8.22). The somatosensory cortex, occupying Brodmann's areas 3, 1, and 2 of the postcentral gyrus, receives afferent fibers from the posterolateral and posteromedial ventral nuclei. The primary visual cortex of Brodmann's area 17 around the occipital calcarine fissure receives its impulses from the lateral geniculate body, and the primary acoustic cortex, Brodmann's area 41 of the temporal transverse (Heschl's) convolutions, receives those from the medial geniculate body. The specific thalamic projections rather than the course of convolutions determine the territory of each of the primary sensory areas.

Primary Somatosensory Cortex

The primary somatosensory cortex corresponds roughly to the postcentral gyrus and a portion of the precentral gyrus. It turns around the upper margin of the hemisphere and occupies the posterior portion of the paracentral lobule at the medial aspect of the hemisphere. The cortex of area 3 is granular and heterotypical. Most of it occupies the posterior wall of the central fissure. The axons that conduct pain impulses terminate there. Most portions of areas 1 and 2 occupy

Functional Organization of the Cortex

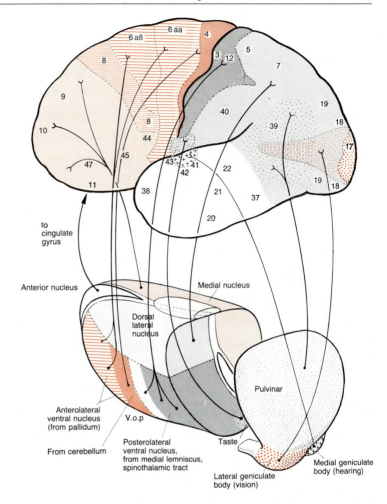

Fig. 8.22 The most important thalamocortical connections and the relationship of individual cortical fields to thalamic nuclei.

the crest of the posterior central convolution and have a slightly thicker, homotypical cortex. The axons originating in the posterior lateral and posterior medial ventral nuclei of the thalamus and transmitting surface sensibility terminate mainly in area 1, whereas those conducting deep sensitivity go to area 2 (see Fig. 5.**5**). The stimuli arrive in somatotopic order, as illustrated in Fig. 8.**20a**. Sensory stimuli, particularly those pertaining to pain, are already felt in some coarse manner at the level of the thalamus. In the somatosensory cortex, however, they are more precisely differentiated in localization, intensity, and manner of irritation. The cortex is always involved in vibration perception, position sensation, and discrimination of stimuli.

Lesions in this cortex produce a marked decrease in the perception of pain, temperature, pressure, and touch, and a loss of sensation for discrimination and position in the corresponding contralateral portion of the body. If this cortex is stimulated during an operation performed under local anesthesia, the patient feels only a pricking, formication, or numbness but no pain.

Primary Visual Cortex

The primary visual cortex extends bilaterally along the calcarine fissure at the medial aspect of the occipital lobe and spreads over the convexity of the occipital pole. The cortical band is only 1.5 mm thick. Histologically, it is

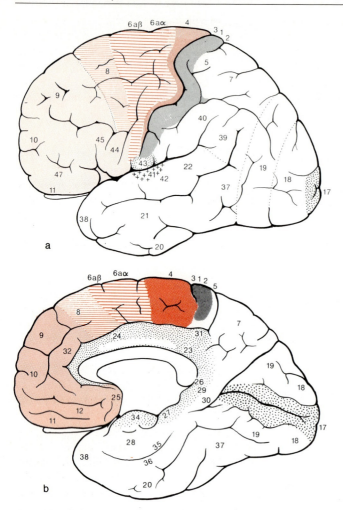

Fig. 8.23 Sites and sizes of primary motor, sensory, visual, gustatory, and auditory fields and those of premotor, prefrontal, including orbital, and limbic cortical areas as seen at the cerebral convexity **a** and at the medial hemispheral aspect **b**.

granular and heterotypical and corresponds to Brodmann's area 17 (Figs. 8.**23a** and **b**; see Fig. 8.**22**). Neighboring areas 18 and 19 are homotypical. Area 17 can easily be recognized on coronal section by the line of Gennari. Because of this line, the visual cortex is also referred to as the area striata. It receives its impulses from the lateral geniculate body via the optic radiation of Gratiolet (see Fig. 3.**12**) in strict retinotopic order (see Fig. 3.**11**).

The axons coming from the lateral geniculate body carry impulses from the ipsilateral (temporal) and the contralateral (nasal) halves of the retina. For this reason the left visual fields are represented in the right and, vice versa, the right visual fields in the left visual cortex (see Fig. 3.**10**). Impulses coming from the macula terminate in the caudal portion of area 17, including the cortex at the convexity of the occipital pole. Impulses from other parts of the retina terminate in the rostral portion of area 17. Stimulation of the visual cortex in patients under local anesthesia produces only sensations of lightning-like flashes, bright lines, and colors.

A lesion in area 17 produces a homonymous hemianopsia toward the opposite side.

If the cortex of the upper lip of the calcarine cortex is involved, the hemianopsia is limited to the inferior quadrants of the visual fields. Conversely, a lesion destroying the lower lip of the calcarine cortex produces upper quadratic homonymous hemianopsia. If the lesion is large but limited to the cortical band, central vision often remains intact, because its cortex over the convexity of the occipital lobe is usually saved from infarction by collaterals between middle and posterior cerebral arteries in this area. Bilateral infarction of the entire primary visual cortex, occurring, for example, as a result of transient cardiac arrest, produces cortical blindness (see page 315).

Primary Auditory Cortex

The primary auditory cortex corresponds to area 41 and occupies Heschl's transverse convolutions, which belong to the superior temporal lobe and are hidden in the sylvian fissure (see Fig. 8.6). Histologically, the cortex is granular and heterotypical. It receives its impulses from the medial geniculate body in tonotopic order (see Fig. 3.36). Low frequencies are located in the anterolateral, and high frequencies in the posteromedial, segments of the cortex. The medial geniculate body receives its impulses from both organs of Corti via the lateral lemniscus. Therefore, a lesion destroying the lateral lemniscus on one side produces only a minor reduction in hearing acuity, more noticeable contralaterally. A unilateral destruction of the auditory cortex produces a decrease in the perception of sound direction. During stimulation of the primary auditory cortex, simple sounds of low or high frequency, but no words, are heard.

Primary Gustatory Cortex

A primary cortex for taste has been found that corresponds to Brodmann's area 43 in the frontoparietal operculum, ventral to the somatosensory cortex and just above the sylvian fissure. The cortex of the insula also subserves taste.

The afferent fibers of the primary gustatory cortex come from the rostral portion of the solitary nucleus (see Fig. 3.33). They probably use the medial portion of the ventrocaudal internal parvocellular nucleus of the thalamus as a relay station (Hassler) (see Fig. 8.22).

Primary Vestibular Cortex

Based on the analysis of evoked potentials, it is suspected that the lower portion of the postcentral gyrus posterior to the somatosensory head region contains a primary vestibular area. Pathways connecting the vestibular apparatus with the cortex have not yet been verified.

As mentioned earlier, impulses reaching the primary sensory cortex produce excitation of columns of neurons that are arranged in vertical order. There the impulses are modified and rearranged in a complex fashion before being transmitted to other cortical areas (association areas), where they can be compared with earlier information and their significance is finally recognized. It is still not known how the various neuronal collectives in the primary cortical areas and in the secondary and tertiary areas of association cooperate. Also, nothing is known about how the brain is able to select the innumerable pieces of information processed daily and stores them so that they can be recalled at any time. A melody, a picture, even a faint scent of a flower may induce recall of entire memory complexes in their full vividness, although they may date back many years.

Figs. 8.23 and 8.24 demonstrate that the primary sensory cortical fields and the primary motor areas make up not more than 20 percent of the total surface of the cortex. The far greater remaining surface is occupied by association areas (see Fig. 8.26).

Frontal Lobe

The frontal lobe includes all cortical territories in front of the central fissure, in other words, the primary somatomotor cortex of the precentral gyrus (area 4), the premotor areas (areas 6aα, 6aβ, and 8), the prefrontal areas (areas 9, 10, 11, 12, 45, 46, and 47), and the motor speech area (area 44) (see Figs. 8.**23** and 8.**24**).

Primary Somatomotor Cortex (Precentral Gyrus)

The precentral gyrus or area 4 initiates all voluntary movements. This voluntary motor system matures rather slowly in primates and man. The first movements of an infant are mass movements of arms and legs, controlled by the extrapyramidal system. Gradually, the movements become more directed. Once the pyramidal tract system has matured, movements are performed with precision and dexterity. To perform complicated movements with precision, it is necessary that they be practiced over and over again and that the particular pattern of movements be learned and become a motor engram.

The primary motor cortex starts along the bottom of the central fissure and occupies much of the anterior central convolution, including the anterior portion of the paracentral lobule at the medial aspect of the hemisphere (area 4 in Figs. 8.**23a** and **b**). It is approximately 4.5 mm thick and is histologically agranular and heterotypical. The fifth layer contains the giant pyramidal cells (Betz's cells), which give rise to the heavily myelinated and fast-conducting fibers of the pyramidal tract.

Afferent stimuli entering area 4 come from the posterior ventrooral nucleus of the thalamus (see Fig. 5.**5**), from the premotor areas 6 and 8, and from the somatosensory area. Approximately 40 percent of all fibers of the pyramidal tract originate in area 4, approximately 20% in the postcentral gyrus, and the remainder probably in the premotor area. Only 3 to 4% of the fibers coming from area 4 are axons of the giant pyramidal cells. Stimuli applied to area 4 produce muscle contractions in the contralateral portion of the body but also in some ipsilateral areas, such as face and trunk.

Figure 8.**20b** illustrates the somatotopic arrangement of motor functions in area 4. The body is represented in an inverted position, as it is in the somatosensory areas 3, 1, and 2 (see Fig. 8.**20a**). Those portions of the body that perform highly differentiated movements, such as the fingers, are represented by correspondingly larger territories. In area 4 the weakest stimuli already produce contralateral muscle contractions. Destruction in area 4 causes a *flaccid* paralysis in the corresponding contralateral part of the body. If the adjacent premotor area 6 is also damaged, extrapyramidal fibers will be interrupted, and the result is a *spastic* paralysis. Paralysis caused by a lesion in area 4 is usually followed by some recovery of movement except in the very distal portions of the extremities; there the paralysis is permanent. In primates a secondary cortical motor area has been identified at the medial aspect of the hemisphere. It is probably also present in man but appears to have no clinical importance.

Premotor Cortex

The premotor areas 6aα, 6aβ, and 8 represent the cortical centers of the extrapyramidal system. The cytoarchitecture of this region is similar to that of area 4, except that giant pyramidal cells are almost totally absent. These cortical fields have two-way connections with the anterolateral ventral thalamic nucleus, which in turn is connected with pallidum and cerebellum (see Fig. 5.**5**).

The primary motor area, the premotor cortex, and the cerebellum are interconnected by a feedback circuit consisting of the frontopontocerebellar tract, dentate nucleus, thalamus, and motor cortex (see Figs. 4.**5** and 5.**5**). This is the reason destructive lesions in the premotor cortex produce disorders of equilibrium and a tendency to fall. Before angiography was introduced as a diagnostic tool, a frontal lobe tumor was occasionally misdiagnosed as being located in the cerebellum. The premotor cortex receives impulses also from other brain regions via association and commissural fibers.

Area 6 requires stronger stimulation than does area 4 in order to produce muscle contractions. In general, contractions involve *synergic muscle groups*; antagonistic muscles become relaxed. If area 4 has been ablated or separated by a cut from area 6, stimulation of area 6 produces unintentional stereotypic movements in the form of mass movements of the extremities or torsion movements of body, head, and eyes. This indicates that *area 6 is a frontal adversive field*. The impulses originating in the premotor cortex run mainly through area 4 but also directly to the spinal cord as part of the pyramidal tract or the extrapyramidal pathways. As mentioned earlier, feedback circuits exist between areas 4 and 6 and the basal ganglia (see Fig. 6.9) and influence pyramidal motor activity. If the premotor cortex is damaged, contralateral spasticity results. Apparently, the premotor cortex inhibits the spinal stretching reflex under normal circumstances. An irritative alteration in areas 6 or 8 produces attacks of eye, head, and trunk turning to the opposite side (*adversive attacks*).

At the medial aspects of the hemispheres, there is supposedly a supplementary motor area in front of the region responsible for the leg and above the cingulate gyrus. Damage to this area is supposed to produce a grasp reflex or forced grasping.

Clinical observations suggest that formerly learned motor engrams are stored in the premotor cortex in cooperation with cerebellum and basal ganglia, a process similar to the storage of somatosensory, visual, and auditory memories in the association area of the primary centers. For example, a lesion in the premotor cortex in front of the territory of the hand in area 4 produces a loss of stored motor engrams concerning the hand and therefore a loss of more refined and complex hand movements. This *limb-kinetic apraxia* may lead, for example, to agraphia without voluntary movement being curtailed by paresis or paralysis. The patient has to practice for the movements to become as automatic as they were before.

Many of the movements are seemingly voluntary but in reality involuntary. They represent reflexes that are activated with automatic ease because they have been programmed in the cortex. Such programming is usually the result of a particular stimulus being repeated over and over. For example, while driving an automobile one immediately and automatically applies the brakes if one sees an unexpected obstacle in the road. This reflex originates in the retina, passes through areas 17, 18, and 19, where the significance of the obstacle is realized, and continues over association pathways to the motor cortex on both sides. From there the impulses travel to the spinal cord, where the muscles needed to operate the brakes are innervated according to the stored program.

The precentral area 8 contains the motor eye field. Here *voluntary eye movements* originate (see Fig. 3.21). An irritation of this eye field produces a conjugate deviation toward the opposite side. A paralyzing lesion of this field causes a conjugate movement to the same side because of the predominance of the still functioning contralateral area 8 (see Fig. 3.22).

Motor Speech Cortex (Broca)

Damage to the left area 44 in a right-handed person (see Fig. 8.26) produces a motor aphasia, as was first demonstrated by Broca in 1861. The patient is able to understand spoken words but is not able to speak, because the motor engrams of the movements necessary for speech are absent. The muscles needed for speaking are not paralyzed, but the patient is unable to innervate them in the proper intensity and sequence. If only the cortex of area 4 is damaged, a *cortical motor aphasia* occurs. If the fibers connecting area 44 with the motor area for vocalization (see

Fig. 8.**20b**) are interrupted, the resulting condition is called a *subcortical motor aphasia* or pure motor aphasia or, as Broca called it, an *aphemia*.

A *subcortical motor aphasia* will be described in a man whose brain revealed a circumscribed embolic infarct, approximately 0.5×1 cm in size, in the left hemisphere be-

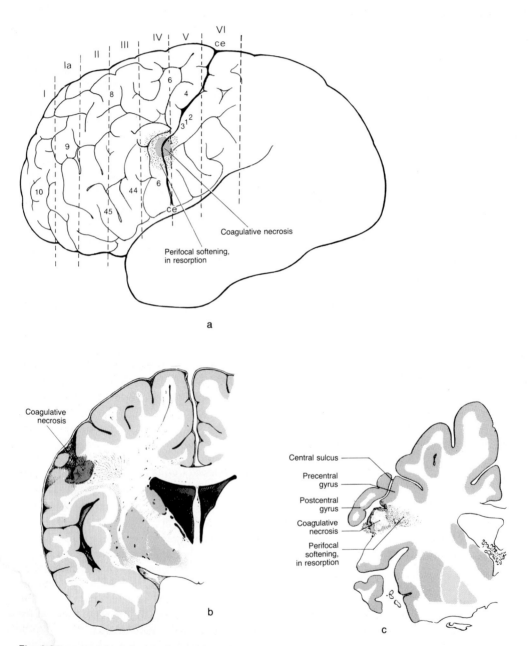

Fig. 8.24 **a** and **b** A focus of an older coagulative necrosis from embolism in the lower third of the precentral gyrus (areas 6 and 4) and extending into the postcentral gyrus (areas 3, 1, and 2). **c** Microscopic section. Gray = cortical necrosis; dotted area = perifocal white matter defect. (Drawn from specimens.)

tween the intact area 44 and the primary motor cortex (Figs. 8.**24a, b,** and **c**).

Case Report: A 49-year-old, right-handed man felt ill for several months. He was always tired and experienced sporadic temperature elevations, coughing, much night sweating, headaches, and stabbing pains in the heart region.

One morning he awoke with pain in parietal and temporal regions and found that the right side of his face was paralyzed and that he was unable to speak. When eating his breakfast, he could not move food to the back of his mouth, although he had no difficulty swallowing. His tongue was apractic. He could drink liquids only with a straw. He had no other complaints. There was no paralysis of arms or legs.

When seen by his physician, he was unable to speak but understood everything and was also able to read. He answered questions by moving his head. He was unable to hold a pencil in his right hand. There was a right-sided central facial paralysis. Whistling was impossible. The tongue deviated partly to the right. Otherwise, cranial nerves were normal. Muscle power and tone were normal in both hands; there was, however, mild apraxia of finger movements on the right. During a finger-to-nose test a mild tremor was noted, on the left side more than the right. Abdominal reflexes and all reflexes of the extremities were normal. No spastic reflexes could be found. The patient was admitted to the University Hospital in Frankfurt/Main with the diagnosis of subacute bacterial endocarditis associated with brain embolism and aphasia.

The next day the patient could eat again without difficulty but could still utter only unintelligible sounds. On the third day a few transient Jacksonian attacks occurred, involving the right arm and right half of the face. Numbness of the right hand disappeared, and the patient was able to write without difficulty. He continually attempted to speak, but what he said remained unintelligible. It was clear that he was making a great effort to form single words by concentrating on the innervation of necessary muscles in the proper sequence and strength. After about 3 weeks the facial paralysis disappeared. The patient was able to speak quite a number of words that could be understood; however, each word had to be formed slowly and always corrected again. The patient knew exactly what he wanted to say and had no difficulty in writing down his thoughts. If he attempted to speak slightly faster, however, the speech became gibberish. This pattern remained unchanged until the patient died from heart disease approximately 6 months after the onset of aphasia.

Gross postmortem examination of the brain revealed a small, embolic infarct measuring approximately 0.5 cm in diameter at the base of the left third frontal convolution. The lesion represented a coagulative necrosis (Prof. Krücke, Max-Planck Institute for Brain Research, Frankfurt/Main). The essential slices of the brain were studies on serial sections at the Research Laboratory for Brain Pathology and Psychopathology (Prof. Kleist). Dr. Sanides found on cytoarchitectonic grounds that the lesion had not destroyed the actual Broca's cortex but was located somewhat posteriorly in the lower third of the precentral convolution and extended through white matter slightly into the postcentral convolution (see Fig. 8.**24**).

Prefrontal Cortex (Frontal Association Areas)

Traditionally, the prefrontal cortex encompasses the areas 9, 10, 12, and 46 at the convexity and medial aspect of the frontal lobe, and also the areas 11 and 47 at its base, subsequently referred to as *orbital lobe*. Stimulation of all these areas elicits no motor response.

Phylogenetically, the prefrontal cortex expanded in primates and became particularly large in man. For this reason it has been considered for quite some time to be connected with higher psychic functions. Indeed, diseases damaging the frontal lobe cortex lead to psychic disorders. This is known from conditions such as frontal lobe injuries, frontal lobe tumors, tumors of the orbital lobes, general paresis, and Pick's disease of the frontal and orbital types. Frontal cortical areas have two-way connections with the medial thalamic nucleus. In addition, they receive impulses from hypothalamus and via fiber connections from most other cortical territories (see Figs. 5.**6** and 8.**14**).

Psychosurgery performed for the treatment of certain psychoses (such as frontal lobotomy, prefrontal leucotomy, and cingulotomy) revealed some of the importance of the prefrontal cortex for psychic functions (Moniz and Lima, 1936; Freeman and Watts, 1942; and others). These psychosurgical procedures have been almost totally discontinued because they proved to be more damaging than therapeutic in their results. Follow-up studies of various numbers of patients who had undergone psychosurgery revealed that they had developed characteristic psychic alterations if the damage was bilateral (Ström-Olsen and Tow, 1949; Tow, 1955). The alterations were personality changes characterized by a lack of mental and motor initiative or by breakdown of behavioral inhibitions associated with a decrease in judgement and ethical attitudes.

If one correlates the result of these and similar studies with observations on patients with frontal lobe disease, one finds that many patients show one or the other of two syndromes that appear to be related to the specific location of the focal alterations. Lesion involving the *prefrontal cortex at the convexity*, in other words, the anterior two-thirds of the frontal convolutions or their white matter, produce a loss of *initiative in motor activity as well as in active thinking* (Kleist, 1934). If the process destroys the cortex and white matter of the orbital lobes, the main characteristic of the personality change is a *lack of inhibition in social behavior*.

Syndrome of anterior frontal lobe damage

The term *anterior frontal lobe* refers to the anterior two-thirds of the three frontal convolutions at the convexity. If these convolutions become bilaterally damaged (atrophy as in frontal lobe Pick's disease; trauma; compression or infiltration by tumors), the patient loses spontaneity in motor as well as mental activities. He does not appear to realize that he is neglecting himself and his duties in the office or at home. Some patients can sit and look at a newspaper for hours without reading or stare out of a window without noticing what is before them.

A patient of this type may seem to suffer from an akinetic depression but is not depressed. The eyes are clear and not moist. The condition may be mistaken for catatonia, as it was in the case of a formerly efficient executive. The patient died four weeks later.

The cause of the akinetic condition was a glioblastoma of the knee of the corpus callosum which extended bilaterally into the white matter of first and second frontal convolutions. A similar tumor was found in a middle-aged woman who had become too slow to take care of her household and herself. On one occasion, after she opened the office door, she had to be asked over and over again to come in and sit down. When she was halfway inside, she lost control of her bladder and urinated on the floor. She slowly expressed embarrassment because she knew that the restroom was next to the office. She did not have the initiative to avoid the accident. At first she appeared to be demented but when questions were repeated several times, her answers were astonishingly knowledgeable and correct. The incontinence described also in other patients may be related to the lack of spontaneity. In the present patient and in other patients with frontal lobe tumors, it may be caused in part by oligemia in the paracentral lobule, stemming from pressure on the anterior cerebral arteries. (Both patients from Lindenberg's collection.)

Syndrome of orbital lobe damage

The clinical signs of bilateral damage to the orbital convolutions are quite different from those of prefrontal area involvement at the convexity. They consist of changes in character traits and in loss of inhibitions in social behavior. This was first observed by Welt (1888) in a patient who had old contusions in both orbital lobes discovered postmortem. The personality changes are particularly notable if the patient was formerly a serious, honest, and respectable person, because he is now hypomanic, flippant, garrulous, prankish and pugilistic and uses obscene and insulting language. He is negligent of his duties and responsibilities and exhibits no self-concern. He has no intellectual deficit but explains facts to his own liking. He cannot be serious and concentrate his thinking. He has no insight into his condition and volunteers no complaints of symptoms, such as headaches.

One of Lindenberg's patients had an old destruction of both orbital lobes from contrecoup contusions. He easily got into fights. This time, he was hit with the sharp side of a hatchet over the right convexity. He was taken to an emergency room, bleeding from the head and limping from left-sided weakness. He strongly resisted admission and ridiculed the physician for being so concerned about a minor injury that he could easily attend to at home. He limped home. Two days later, he was found dead from meningitis and brain abscess. In another of Lindenberg's patients, destruction of orbital lobes by contrecoup produced personality changes almost instantaneously. The patient fell on his occiput. As soon as he recovered from the resulting concussion, he was able to communicate again. His wife found that her quiet, considerate husband was euphoric and unconcerned about himself and his family and made joking and unfitting remarks. After his release from the hospital, he was sexually uninhibited and was finally arrested for molesting minors (Fig. 8.25).

In these cases of traumatic orbital lobe damage, the olfactory bulbs and tracts are almost invariably injured. Most of these patients have unilateral or bilateral *anosmia*, which is often the sole neurologic sign.

If trauma can be excluded and personality changes as well as anosmia develop slowly, a meningioma of the olfactory region is the most probable cause (see Fig. 8.31). Such a case, reported by Olivecrona and Urban (1935), may serve as example.

Case report: A 57-year-old pastor had noticed a decrease in his sense of smell after a cold approximately four years prior to his hospitalization. One year prior to hospitalization, he noticed a decrease in vision. He gradually lost his desire to work and became negligent in handling the paperwork connected with his office. Letters from his superiors remained unanswered in spite of repeated admonitions. At the same time he attracted much attention when he gave a sermon full of jesting and unfitting remarks at the funeral of one of his friends. When he continued to neglect his work, he was retired from his position approximately six months prior to hospital admission. Finally, his vision deteriorated further and he appeared to have headaches at times. In addition, he developed optical hallucinations in the form of snakes and similar animals. When his superiors arranged for hospitalization, he insisted that he was not ill and that he was feeling absolutely healthy.

It was found that he had lost his judgement and his drive to pursue his work. He was very euphoric and tended to joke constantly. Some of the humor was quite inappropriate. When he was found to have a bilateral anosmia and central scotoma on the right associated with an upper temporal field defect, an olfactory groove meningioma was diagnosed and soon removed without complication.

His psychological status returned to normal with extreme rapidity. Just a few days after the operation, the patient recognized that he had been ill. He felt ashamed of his former, obviously unfitting behavior, although he could barely remember it. The talkative, distrustful patient, slovenly in personal appearance and attire, changed again

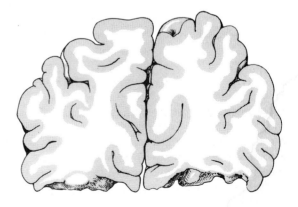

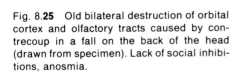

Fig. 8.25 Old bilateral destruction of orbital cortex and olfactory tracts caused by contrecoup in a fall on the back of the head (drawn from specimen). Lack of social inhibitions, anosmia.

into a quiet, friendly man, not without priestly dignity, in only a few days. Two months after discharge, he was back in his ministry and had not the slightest difficulty in administering it.

Psychological changes of this kind are rather common with tumors of the orbital lobes. In 1939 the present author personally reported more than 30 such cases in which tumors, predominantly meningiomas, were the cause of damage. The patients, inconspicuous before, became childish, superficial, silly, jocular, rude, ruthless, and unprincipled. They were often selfish, malicious, tactless, and impudent. They disregarded morality, were sometimes inflammatory, and got into conflicts with the law. At first they were usually euphoric and self-satisfied and proclaimed themselves to be in fine fettle. Later, when discomfort and pain developed, cheerfulness turned into discontent, dysphoria, and irritability. Uninhibited instinctive drives became stronger and led to increased sexual activity and masturbation and to excessive drinking and eating. At this time lapses of memory occurred.

In general, the early character changes are remarkably similar. Small differences regarding the preponderance of one or another character trait are probably related to the premorbid personality structure.

With gradual involvement of white matter and cortex of the frontal convolutions at the convexity, the clinical picture changes. The patients become quiet, neglect themselves, have no interest in their work, sit listlessly, and lose all spontaneity. Total loss of initiative overshadows the earlier personality changes. The mood becomes dull-euphoric. During the transitional period leading to the loss of spontaneity, some patients develop hallucinations. Finally, patients lose control of bladder and rectum because of lack of spontaneity or, as mentioned earlier, as a result of inadequate circulation in the paracentral lobules stemming from secondary involvement of the rostral stems of the anterior cerebral arteries by the tumors.

Because the patient has no insight into his condition, he sees no purpose in consulting a physician. Relatives usually do not realize the seriousness of the illness until severe headaches, vomiting, and visual disorders develop and convince them that medical attention is needed.

Epileptiform seizures occur fairly frequently. They are not bound to a particular phase of the disease but occur more often in its later course. Often they originate in the frontal adversive field. If the tumor is still growing, signs of brainstem involvement appear in the form of amnestic confabulations, delirious confusions, somnolence, and finally stupor. At this time frontal release phenomena, such as grasp reflex, 'gegenhalten' (counter-pressure reflex), motor perseveration, and tremor, are present.

Secondary Receptive Cortical Fields (Parietal, Occipital, Temporal Association Areas)

The *secondary* receptive fields or *association areas* of the parietal, occipital, and temporal cortex occupy by far the largest portions of these lobes (Fig. 8.**26**). Only secondary potentials can be recorded from these areas. When one or another sense organ is stimulated, the areas of response show definite overlapping. Thus, these areas cannot be attached to specific sense organs by electrophysiologic means. Only by coordinating clinical deficits with the location of focal lesions is it possible to draw conclusions as to the function of these fields.

Each primary sensory area has its adjacent secondary area. The somatosensory association region occupies much of the parietal lobe, commencing immediately caudal to the postcentral gyrus. It is represented by areas 5 and 7. Similarly, the primary visual area 17 is surrounded by areas 18 and 19, and the primary auditory area 41 is followed by areas 42 and 22. The olfactory area of association occupies area 28, which is located laterally from the primary olfactory cortex in area 34 in the medial half of the lower temporal lobe (see Fig. 8.**24**).

According to clinical experience, the information arriving at the primary sensory cortical areas is integrated in the secondary association areas and is compared there with formerly stored information or memories and thus becomes part of experience. This occurs particularly in the dominant hemisphere, to be discussed shortly.

Areas 39, 40, and probably 37 of the angular and supramarginal gyri occupy the transitional zone connecting the tactile or kinesthetic with the visual and auditory association territories. In the dominant hemisphere they are considered to be a *tertiary association region* of still higher order. In its structural features this region corresponds to association areas of frontal and temporal lobes. It has two-way connections with the pulvinar of the thalamus (page 186) and communicates with the ipsilateral occipital, temporal, and frontal lobes via short and long association fibers and with the corresponding contralateral areas via commissural fibers. In man, these convolutions cover by far a greater territory than they do in the lower primate brain and are believed to mature rather late (Luria, 1976). It is assumed that tactile, kinesthetic, vestibular, visual, and auditory information, already correlated in secondary association areas, is integrated in areas 39 and 40 at the highest level. It is suspected that this tertiary area represents the substrate for the most intricate forms of human perceptive and cognitive functioning.

Focal Signs Caused by Lesions in Association Territories

Somatosensory association area

A lesion limited to area 5 and 7 produces a *tactile agnosia*. The patient is still able to touch or feel an object; when the object is put into his hand while his eyes are closed, however, he is unable to recognize the object solely by touch. This inability is caused by the loss of formerly stored tactile experiences.

Tertiary parietal association area

If areas 39 and 40 of the dominant hemisphere are damaged, the patient has great difficulty in coordinating the information coming from the individual secondary association areas in such a manner that the essence of the total impression is recognized. Frequently, he cannot integrate the information

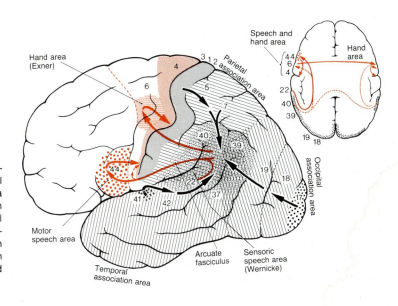

Fig. 8.**26** Secondary parietal, occipital, and temporal association areas adjoin in a tertiary association area in angular and supramarginal gyri (black arrows). It is connected, among others, with premotor areas for speech (Broca), face, and hand (red arrows).

so as to orient himself in a three-dimensional space. Although he knows his surroundings, he cannot find his way in his own neighborhood or even in his house or apartment. With a lesion in the angular gyrus. the patient loses feeling for the position of his own body in space and for the relationship of the individual parts of his body to one another. If the supramarginal gyrus is damaged by a lesion, particularly if it is the left gyrus, the patient loses feeling for his own body (*body-image agnosia* or *autotopagnosia* or *asomatognosia*). He also may not recognize the import of stimuli from the individual fingers (*finger agnosia*) and not be able to differentiate the right side of his body from the left (*right/left agnosia*).

Case Report: J. V., medical doctor, date of birth 26 July 1911, underwent glaucoma operations in 1974 and 1975. In 1978, a circumscribed gastric carcinoma, with healthy margins, was excised.

On 13 April 1980, when starting to write a thank-you letter to some friends, he noticed that he was no longer able to write properly. He could no longer find the right words, nor was he able to correct mistakes. He was no longer able to write prescriptions for patients. He had no signs of paralysis, but at the beginning of April he had briefly had a disturbed sensation in his right arm for a few minutes. When he was playing the violin, the bow had fallen out of his hand on one occasion. Writing became very difficult, so that he had to dictate everything. Recently, he had even become unable to make telephone calls. Even though he had the number he wanted to dial next to the phone, he always misdialed. At the beginning of May, he then noticed that he could no longer recognize numbers, and was therefore no longer able to do even the simplest arithmetic. About three weeks previously, he found that he was unable to read. He had to spell many words out letter by letter like a primary school child, before he could grasp what they meant. He also kept making mistakes when dealing with everyday objects. He had to think about how to hold a knife and fork. He was still able to play the violin, but could no longer read music, as he could not recognize the notes on the page. Reading was now so difficult for him that he had to have everything read to him. He had no difficulties at all with speaking or dictating.

A computed tomogram on 25 May 1980 showed a focal lesion of 1 cm in diameter in the left occipital region. An angiogram carried out at the Neurosurgical Clinic in Giessen confirmed this finding and also showed considerable arteriosclerotic vascular changes in the region of the internal carotid artery.

Mr. V., who was in excellent physical condition, decided to undergo conservative treatment with infusions. In the neurological examination, the PSR and ASR were found to be markedly reduced, but there was no other pathological neurological finding, apart from the focal symptoms described above. These improved slightly after infusion therapy with Rheomacrodex (dextran 40) and other electrolyte infusions, so that he gradually became able to formulate his thoughts in writing again, although still with numerous mistakes. He also regained the ability to carry out simple calculations and could read out short articles from the newspaper. But these activities quickly tired him, and he needed up to two hours to write a short letter. When writing, he often had to ask which letter he had written. *He could see everything, but it was very difficult for him to recognize what things were.* He could repeat anything that was said to him without any difficulty. Since it was difficult for him to recognize numbers, he was no longer able to count and failed completely even with the simplest written arithmetic exercises. He could recognize objects, but needed to concentrate intensely at breakfast to make sure that he did not pour the coffee into the sugar bowl. He was no longer able to measure blood pressure, since although he could see the numbers on the manometer, he could not recognize whether the blood pressure was normal or not. Nor could he carry out an ECG any more, since he could not remember how the electrodes were supposed to be attached. Writing became almost impossible for him, and even if he managed with a lot of patience to write something down, he was no longer able to read it later on. He was completely unable to write out a check.

Since he had the feeling that his condition was worsening again, he decided to undergo a further session of inpatient infusion therapy. At the end of this treatment, on 3 July 1980, he felt slightly better but still tripped up over certain words. In the following months and years, his condition improved sufficiently for him to be able to see patients again and examine them. He had had to abandon his practice immediately after the appearance of the acute focal symptoms. The focal symptoms remained, but they were weaker, so that he was able to resume a small amount of medical practice with the help of a receptionist.

To get an overall impression of the extent of the brain damage involved, I requested a magnetic resonance tomogram of the brain, which was carried out on an outpatient basis on 16 March 1990. The examination showed a substantial worsening of the findings.

Diagnostic summary: There was a substantial worsening of findings in comparison with the previous examination. Malacic demarcation in the area of a border zone insult in the left parieto-occipital region was found, with secondary leukodystrophic signal enhancement in the neighboring cerebral medulla. There was evidence of another apparently intercurrent partial insult (superior temporal artery) in the left temporal region (Fig. 8.26 A).

Multifocal, probably also vascular lesions were scattered through the cerebral medulla in both hemispheres, with more in the frontal area, and including the basal ganglia and thalamus. There was bilateral areolar signal enhancement in the peritrigonal area, probably also due to vascular leukoencephalopathy. No evidence of a space-occupying lesion was found.

On 6 July 1993, V. telephoned me and reported that he had been suffering from severe vertigo since that morning. He could not get out of bed, since when he tried to get up, the dizziness became so bad that he had to lie down again. I asked him to come to my clinic, but this was almost impossible for him. Finally, he arrived in a taxi and had to be carried into the room by the taxi driver and myself, as he could neither walk nor stand. He had no other complaints, apart from nausea, and no headache.

As V. could neither walk nor stand, I immediately had him admitted to hospital. The examination at admission showed that there had been an acute ischemic infarction in the medulla oblongata on the right, with a typical Wallenberg syndrome (Fig. 3.56, p. 150).

The neurological examination at admission showed slight miosis and ptosis on the right, corresponding to Horner's syndrome, considerable gaze nystagmus to the right, hypalgesia and thermohypesthesia on the left side of the face, absent innervation of the soft palate, marked difficulties in swallowing, and dysarthria. Muscle extension reflexes could not be stimulated in the arms, Babinski reflex negative. There were considerable ataxic disturbances on the

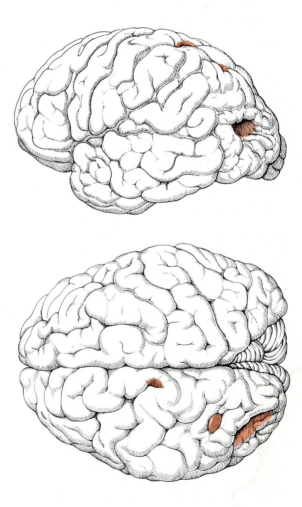

Fig. 8.26 A Malacic demarcation in the area of a border zone insult in the left parieto-occipital region, with secondary leukodystrophic signal enhancement in the neighboring cerebral medulla. Evidence of another apparently intercurrent partial insult (superior temporal artery) in the left temporal region.

right. Walking was only possible with support, with a tendency to fall to the right. There was hemihypalgesia and hemithermohypesthesia on the left side of the body.

On the day of admission, an emergency cranial CT was carried out, showing the old infarct in the left parieto-occipital region, with substantial regressive changes.

A cranial MRI carried out on 13 July 1993 showed findings of Wallenberg's syndrome. There was a small focal ischemic lesion on the dorsolateral right circumference of the medulla oblongata, as well as evidence of the previously known older insult area in the left parieto-occipital region.

The angiogram showed hypoplasia of the right vertebral artery.

During the further course of hospital treatment, the patient suffered several episodes of extreme confusion, and blood pressure values were markedly raised (195/140 mmHg). In spite of slight stabilization initially, the brainstem infarct further worsened his condition, and V. died on the evening of 16 July 1993.

If the body-image agnosia is unilateral, it may be associated with disregard for the left half of the body, particularly if the lesion involves the right parietal area. The patient does not recognize, for example, the paralysis of his left extremities or his unilateral loss of vision. This is referred to as *anosognosia* or *Anton's syndrome*. In such cases there is usually also visual *neglect* of the paralyzed half of the body. The patient has great difficulty putting on his clothes (*dressing apraxia*). Even if there is no paralysis present – for example in the parieto-occipital form of Alzheimer's disease – the patient with agnosia may still be confronted with great difficulties. For example, he will not be able to handle a fork properly with the left hand when eating. Equally, he will have problems walking and, above all, climbing stairs, as he is not able to perceive and supervise the movements of his left leg. If these signs are very marked, the lesion is almost always so large that it extends into the adjacent frontal, occipital, and temporal association territories. The disorder of spatial perception is most easily recognized by an impairment of constructive motor actions. The patient is unable to build a model house with building blocks; he is unable to assemble these blocks in the proper spatial order. This condition was referred to by Kleist as a *constructive apraxia*. The patient has difficulties as well with writing and drawing. When writing, he cannot maintain a straight line and has difficulty forming the various letters (*agraphia*). When drawing, he assembles various portions of the intended sketch in the wrong order. When calculating, he cannot register columns and rows of numbers; therefore, he cannot solve the problem (*acalculia*). The individual disabilities, such as right/left disorientation, finger agnosia, agraphia, and acalculia, are summarily referred to in the literature as *Gerstmann's syndrome*. It is believed that they are produced by a single lesion in the area of the angular gyrus of the dominant hemisphere. There is no full agreement on this syndrome; the individual signs also occur in different combinations.

These parietal defects are usually associated with functional losses of the adjacent occipital and temporal regions, for example, visual field defects, aphasic disorders, and abnormal difficulty in finding words and names.

For one to perform complicated and voluntary movements with dexterity, it is necessary that the feeling for body image and the storage of kinesthetic movement patterns be intact. A lesion in the supramarginal gyrus of the left lower parietal lobe may interfere with such skilled voluntary movements of the limbs even though there is no motor paralysis. According to Liepmann (1900), this kind of disorder is called *apraxia* or *dyspraxia*. It represents a disorder in planning a pattern of movements and in controlling voluntarily the sequence of actions. The patient is unable to move his limbs on command in the correct purposeful sequence. For example, instead of throwing a kiss or making a threatening gesture, the patient exhibits movements that are disconnected, searching, and without purpose.

Except for instinctive movements, all movements of head, trunk and extremities have been learned during life. By continual practice, patterns of movements have been acquired, and these engrams can be activated at any time. Each purposeful movement requires, however, that a certain stimulus first trigger an idea or plan of the action. The idea may come spontaneously or may be the response to a request or to a visual or acoustic stimulus. It is believed that the train of action activates motor movement patterns stored in the premotor area 6 by using long association fibers such as the arcuate and superior longitudinal fascicles. The ipsilateral premotor region is connected with the contralateral area by commissural fibers passing through the knee of the corpus callosum. From the premotor regions of both hemispheres, the planned impulses are transmitted in the proper order to the primary motor area 4. Motor pathways descending from this area finally activate muscle group of both sides for the performance of the desired movement. In short, each voluntary movement requires that a rather complex functional system be intact in all its subdivisions.

It is first necessary that all kinesthetic, visual, and vestibular impulses arriving from the periphery in the left parietooccipital region be integrated with one another by way of primary, secondary, and tertiary association areas for the individual to be fully oriented about the position of body and extremities in space, the state of joints, muscle tone, and other factors. Only then is it possible to plan movements in response to an existing situation and to perform them by way of the motor system. R. Jung believes that planning and early control of the sequence of actions are probably the result of cooperation between cerebral cortex, corpus callosum, brainstem, and cerebellum.

Apraxia: Earlier in the text, Liepmann's apraxia and Kleist's constructive apraxia were described. The literature mentions additional forms of apraxia; therefore, further comments are appropriate.

An apraxia caused by a lesion in the parietal lobe of the dominant hemisphere is known as *ideomotor apraxia*. It involves the left and right extremities and is often accompanied by sensory aphasic disorders and visual field defects because of the location of the auditory and visual association areas.

If the association fibers connecting the left parietal region and left premotor cortex are interrupted, there will also be bilateral apraxia. Should the facial movements be involved, the condition is called *facial apraxia*. In that case the patient cannot stretch out his tongue when asked to do so or blow out a burning match. These sequelae of interruption of interconnecting pathways are referred to as *disconnection syndrome* (Geschwind, 1965).

Lesions interrupting the commissural connections of both premotor areas in the region of the corpus callosum produce a *left-sided dyspraxia*.

An interruption of the commissural fibers near the ipsilateral left premotor cortex produces a right-sided hemiparalysis and motor aphasia together with a dyspraxia of the left, nonparalyzed arm. This is referred to as a *sympathetic apraxia* of the left arm.

A small lesion near the right or left premotor cortex that interrupts the short association fibers going to area 4 produces an *innervation* or *limb-kinetic apraxia*. Although no paralysis is present, the patient is unable to innervate various muscle groups in the proper sequence and strength and therefore cannot perform a fast, purposeful movement. The movement appears as awkward as if it were being performed for the first time. Presumably, the movement patterns required for fast and precise movements, such as typing or playing the piano, are no longer available in such cases.

There is also an *ideational* or *sensory apraxia*, usually seen if brain damage is more diffuse. This apraxia is a clear disorder of action sequence. For example, a patient given a pipe, tobacco, and matches no longer knows in which order these objects have to be used. He may, for example, rub the matchbox on the pipe.

Visual association area

If areas 18 and 19 are damaged, there is no blindness. On the contrary, the patient has good vision and avoids obstacles when walking. He has, however, lost the ability to recognize what he is seeing, particularly if the damage is bilateral. He has lost the stored optical engrams and cannot compare what he sees with visual memories; therefore, objects look strange to him. A patient with such *visual agnosia* tries to take the object he sees into his hand, hoping to recognize them by touch.

There are several types of visual agnosia. Agnosia for things is called *visual object agnosia*; for written or printed words, *alexia*; for colors, *coloragnosia*; and for faces, *prospagnosia*.

In 1921 Lenz published reports on two patients with bilateral central colorhemianopsia. The brains were carefully studied in serial section. In the first patient, an almost symmetrical softening involved the white matter at the base of both occipital lobes in the areas of the fusiform and lingual gyri. In the second patient, multiple smaller lesions were found; many of them occupied the same territory.

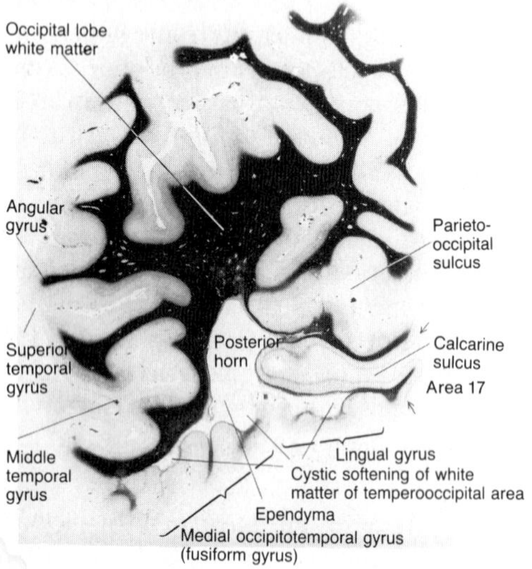

In 1930 Beringer and Stein reported a case of pure alexia. The brain was studied by Hassler (1954), who found one isolated infarct in the subcortical white matter of the lower portion of the left occipital lobe (Fig. 8.27).

If the right occipitoparietal region is damaged by a lesion, it is not unusual for the patient to show visual disorientation in space. Such a patient cannot walk through a dark room without difficulty. In order to perform this action successfully it is necessary to possess an optic image of the spatial arrangement of the room with all its furniture and to have intact tactile memories. By touching a chair or other piece of furniture, one knows one's position in the room immediately and is able to correct the direction of one's movements.

An occipital lesion producing optical agnosia often also involves the optic radiation and causes, in addition, a field defect.

Auditory association area

If areas 42 and 22 of the dominant hemisphere are destroyed, common noises, tones, and the like can be perceived, but their nature cannot be recognized. Thus, a rattling noise cannot be attributed to keys because the specific features of such noise, known from former experience, are lost. This condition is called *acoustic* or *auditory agnosia*. A lesion located more anteriorly in the temporal lobe may destroy the understanding of music, particularly if it involves the right temporal lobe. By the same token, destruction of the olfactory association areas 34 and 28 produces an *olfactory agnosia*.

Destruction of the posterior third of the first temporal convolution of the dominant hemisphere causes *Wernicke's sensory*

Fig. 8.27 Cross-section through the left occipital lobe of a patient with pure alexia shows cystic softening of the white matter of the basal occipitotemporal area. The softening is separated from the posterior horn by ependyma. Cortex of area 17 and subcortical U-fibers are preserved (indicated by arrows). (Finding by R. Hassler.)

aphasia. The patient can hear and can repeat words spoken to him, but has completely lost the ability to understand the words. He has lost the formerly stored sound symbols of words and cannot compare what he hears with former engrams and with words that have meaning. Because he does not understand the spoken word, he also cannot control his own speech. It becomes unintelligible because of *literal* and *verbal paraphasias*. In short, he has a *sensory aphasia*. Several additional types of sensory aphasia determined by the location and extent of damage, will be discussed later.

Penfield and Rasmussen (1950) stimulated the temporal lobe and angular gyrus of dominant and nondominant hemispheres electrically during operative procedures for temporal lobe epilepsy performed under local anesthesia. These patients reported seeing entire scenes and listening to conversations and to songs and melodies. Former experiences, some of them going back many years, were recreated. It is well known that temporal lobe epilepsy may be accompanied by acoustic, optic, and olfactory hallucinations, referred to as *uncinate fits*. Therapeutic temporal lobe resections usually include anterior portions of the hippocampus. As mentioned earlier in the text (page 205), removal of both Ammon's horns produces a loss of the ability to store recent memory, while formerly deposited memories remain intact. It was also mentioned that interruption of Meyer's loop of the optic radiation produces a contralateral upper quadrant hemianopsia.

It is not known how the cerebral cortex stores the unlimited number of sensory perceptions and marks them as memories that can be recalled from storage at almost any time. There are several theories that try to resolve the question of how single nerve cells are able to store memories or whether this can be done only by a large community of neurons arranged in reverberating circuits, and the issue of whether physical or chemical alterations takes place at synapses. Recently, the role of ribonucleic acid (RNA) and of deoxyribonucleic acid (DNA) has been discussed. Whatever the final answer is, it is agreed for the moment that the large association areas of the cerebral cortex are the warehouses of stored memories.

In contrast to other areas of the cerebral cortex, most of the temporal lobe has no specific thalamic projections (see Fig. 8.**22**). It is intimately connected with various association areas by association and commissural fiber systems, however (see Fig. 8.**15**). It has been suspected that a neuronal mechanism may exist in the temporal lobe that is concerned with the coding of long-term memories.

This supposition, voiced in the first (German) edition of this book in 1976, has been confirmed by recent investigations as discussed in the section about the entorhinal area (page 203 ff.). The anterior part of the parahippocampal gyrus in the temporal lobe is taken up by the entorhinal area (area 28). The allocortex consists of several layers and has two-way connections to all associative areas of the neocortex (isocortex). All incoming information is transmitted via the perforating tract to the hippocampal formation (Fig. 8.**28a**) where it is synthesized, processed, and transmitted back to the cerebral cortex. Only when both paths of this feedback circuit have been completed will the events be committed to memory. According to H. and E. Braak, it is precisely the entorhinal area with the origins of the neurons of the perforating tract that is prematurely destroyed in the limbic form of Alzheimer's disease (Fig. 5.**19b**). The consequence is a severe progressive impairment of the memory function.

In discussing the secondary sensory fields, it was mentioned that agnosias occur almost exclusively when the damage involves the *dominant hemisphere*. In 80 to 90 percent of patients, this is the left hemisphere, and its dominance is usually evidenced by right-handedness. In 10 to 20 percent of the patients, the right hemisphere is dominant or the two hemispheres are of equal value. In that case, some functions are carried out by

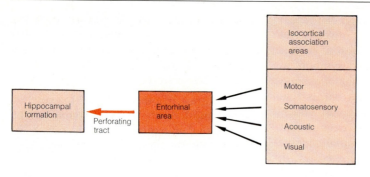

Fig. 8.28a Flow diagram showing transmission of information from isocortical association areas to the hippocampal formation (with kind permission of H. and E. Braak).

the right and other functions by the left hemispheres.

Hemisphere dominance is probably genetically determined. The left planum temporale, in the region of Wernicke's area, is supposed to be larger than the corresponding contralateral region in 65 percent of individuals, (Geschwind and Levitsky, 1968). It became known from hemispherectomies, however, that either hemisphere may become dominant until the age of 6 years. If a child suffers a severe injury to his dominant left hemisphere before he is 6 years old, it is usually not very difficult to make the right hemisphere dominant by training and exercises. The hemisphere is indeed able to take over all the functions of a dominant hemisphere. This is no longer possible in adolescents and adults.

Although one hemisphere may be dominant, sensory impressions and practical and emotional experiences are evenly stored in both hemispheres. In this process the corpus callosum and the anterior commissure play a large role. Because of the commissural fibers, there is a point-to-point connection between the two hemispheres except for the visual area 17, the primary auditory area 41, and the somatosensory areas for hands and feet. The importance of the corpus callosum for the storage of visual information has been demonstrated in animal experiments (Myers, 1956; Sperry, 1964; and others). For example, the corpus callosum, the anterior commissure, and the optic chiasm were split longitudinally in monkeys. With the left eye covered, each animal was taught to differentiate various objects with its right eye. When the right eye was covered, it was unable to differentiate the objects with its left eye. If the optic chiasm was transected but not the corpus callosum and anterior commissure, the animal had no difficulties in identifying with the left eye what it had learned to identify with the right.

These findings show that it is one of the functions of the corpus callosum to convey sensory impressions received and stored in one hemisphere simultaneously to the other hemisphere. Thereafter, the stored memories of both hemispheres can be recalled by the dominant hemisphere and integrated with one another. The role of the corpus callosum in transferring visual information from one side to the other applies also to other sensations, for example, touch sensation (*tactuokinesthetic learning*), studied in chimpanzees by Myers and Henson (1960).

The corpus callosum and anterior commissure have also been transected in human patients suffering from severe, otherwise intractable epilepsy. Detailed examination of such patients revealed that the transection did not influence their behavior, intellect, or affect. Bimanual skills learned prior to operation remained undisturbed. Skills learned by one hand after the operation, however, were no longer transferred to the other hand.

New information has become available, particularly in the field of speech. Gazzaniga and Sperry (1967) found that patients so operated could report on sensory information reaching the dominant left hemisphere verbally as well as in writing. If the sensory information was given to the nondominant right hemisphere, however, patients could report on it neither verbally nor in writing. Consequently, both speech and calculation seem to be tied to the dominant hemisphere. Probably both hemispheres do understand speech, but only the dominant hemisphere is able to communicate via the spoken word; the nondominant hemisphere remains silent and can express itself only by nonverbal reactions (Fig. 8.28b).

Based on studies of so-called split-brain patients, Levy-Agresti and Sperry (1968) came forward with the hypothesis that the hemispheres have complementary functions.

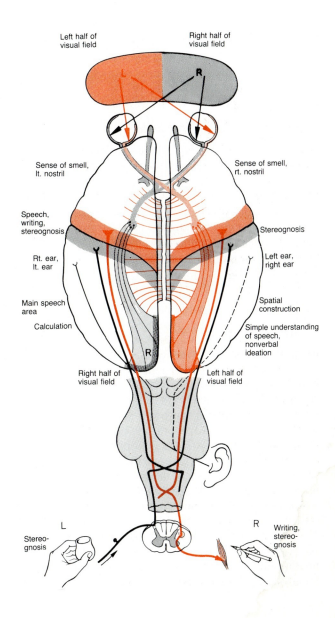

Fig. 8.28b Some of the functions of the dominant and nondominant cerebral hemispheres after commissurotomy.

Table 8.1 Complementary Functions of Both Cerebral Hemispheres.

Dominant Hemisphere	Nondominant Hemisphere
Connected with consciousness	No connection with consciousness
Verbal	Almost nonverbal; musical
Ideational	Feeling for forms and patterns
Analytical	Synthesizing
Segmental	Holistic
Arithmetic and computerlike	Geometrical and spatial

Eccles (1975) listed these complementary functions, as presented in Table 8.1 (from Eccles, J. C.: Das Gehirn des Menschen, Piper & Co, München, Zürich, 1975).

Sensory or Wernicke's Aphasia

According to the literature, there are several forms of sensory aphasia. Attempts have been made to correlate them with distinct areas of the cortex; there is, for example, a cortical sensory aphasia, a subcortical sensory aphasia, a conduction aphasia, a transcortical aphasia, an amnestic aphasia, and a jargon aphasia, to name only a few.

Sensory or *receptive aphasia* can best be understood if one remembers how speech develops during infancy. Between the first and second year of life, the infant becomes eager to speak. The mother is more than glad to help with words. One of the words is "mama", which the mother repeats over and over again until the child is able to say it. Because the mother is always being indicated when the word "mama" is spoken, the infant finally connects the word with the person of the mother. In other words, a symbolic sound becomes tied to the optic picture of the mother. Regardless of how many people are present, the child immediately recognizes his mother and calls for "mama". He also becomes familiar with her voice. He is able to identify it and says "mama" even if his mother is not visible but can be heard speaking in an adjacent room. The word symbol "mama" is now connected with a visual and acoustic engram, and the mother gradually becomes an idea. Similarly, the infant learns more and more words, which become meaningful by continual questioning and answering. For example, he immediately recognizes a small bell by the way it rings; he notices at the same time what such a bell looks like and can hear the word "bell." Having once had the bell in his hand, the child knows how the bell feels and how it can be rung. Thus, a tactile engram is added. Regardless of whether it is the name, the sound, the appearance, or the feeling of the bell that is the cause, the child identifies the object always as "bell." All these impressions appear as one unit as soon as the word "bell" is heard. For this process to occur, it is necessary that the primary, secondary, and tertiary cortical fields of the temporal, occipital, parietal, and frontal lobes and all their connections be mature and functional.

In order to say a word like "mama," the infant has to learn to innervate the musculature controlling respiration, larynx, and mouth simultaneously so that intelligible words and sentences can be spoken and ultimately compounded into speech. Gradually, corresponding motor engrams are stored, making it possible to speak fluently. The primary and secondary motor cortex, particularly the cortex of Broca's region and the face territory in the precentral gyrus are absolutely necessary for speech. Thus, the cooperation of additional extensive brain areas is needed for us to have an enjoyable chat with the neighbors.

Speaking is also connected with emotions. Therefore, subcortical structures, particularly the hypothalamus, thalamus, and limbic system, are important for speech. For example, the word "bell" may rekindle a whole chain of memories. Perhaps it reminds one of a Christmas Day in childhood, when one was permitted to enter the living room upon the ringing of a small bell and then saw the lights on the Christmas tree and all the presents beneath it. Such a memory may make one person melancholy and another, merry.

When a child is, on the average, 6 years old, the secondary and tertiary association areas are sufficiently mature for the child to go to school to learn to read and write. Now pictures of the written word – in other words, meaningful symbols – becomes stored. When learning to read, the child usually moves his lips at the beginning. The word to be written is spoken in a low voice; thus, reading and writing are usually learned via the spoken word.

If a lesion in Wernicke's cortical area damages the understanding of words, reading and writing are also damaged. In addition to sensory aphasia, there will be alexia and agraphia. Alexia, however, can also be the result of a circumscribed lesion in the visual association area; agraphia may be caused by one in the parietal association area.

Practically the entire brain participates in conversations, and it must be intact in order for us to understand others without effort and to be able to translate our own thinking into words. Although certain areas of the dominant hemisphere are the most important for understanding speech and others for speaking itself, it appears that an isolated speech center does not exist. These important areas can fulfill their task only in cooperation with other brain territories, including cortico-extrapyramidal-cerebellar feedback circuits, explaining why no two truly identical sensory aphasias exist. Although all of them have much in common, each always differs in some detail.

The *sensory aphasias* all involve *a deficit in the understanding of sounds, words, names, and sentences* and a *breakdown of speech control*. Words are heard, but their meaning is lost because they can no longer be compared with earlier. meaningful words. Depending on the extent and localization of the lesion in the sensory speech area, the loss of word comprehension may be minor or so severe that the patient's own language becomes a foreign language to him. As though he were learning a new language, he may be able to repeat a spoken word but it has no meaning for him. If the sensory aphasia is minor, verbal comprehension is only partial and requires much effort. With severe sensory aphasia, the speech of the patient becomes unintelligible, because he does not understand his own words and is, therefore, unable to correct them. Wrong words are used (*verbal paraphasia*), or syllables of words are exchanged or garbled (*literal paraphasia*).

The situation is such that a verbal communication is impossible. It is as if two people spoke to each other in different languages and neither understood the language of the other. If the speech defect is not too severe, an aphasic person usually gropes for the names of objects. He knows the objects but cannot name them, even if they are rather common. Thus, he replaces them with numerous expletives. This leads to bungled sentence construction. There may be *paragrammatism* and, not infrequently, *logorrhea*. There is a strong tendency to cling to one word (*perseveration*). If difficulties in finding names predominate, the condition is called *amnestic aphasia*. Inability to repeat multisyllabic spoken words is called *conduction aphasia*. The patient has no difficulty in speaking spontaneously but is not able to transfer multisyllabic words immediately into motor speech (possible interruption of arcuate or superior longitudinal fascicles).

As mentioned earlier, a severe inability to understand words is associated with difficulties in reading and writing. It is painful for the patient to read. He emphasizes the wrong words and syllables and has no comprehension of the words. If his sensory aphasia is moderate, he may be able to write at least familiar words, such as his name and address.

The temporoparietal speech area has two-way connections with the pulvinar of the thalamus, suggesting a functional relationship between the two (see Fig. 8.**22**). Penfield and Roberts (1959) described a patient in whom a small hematoma in the pulvinar of the dominant hemisphere had produced a severe aphasia. The pulvinar may have the task of integrating the impulses coming from the important parietal, occipital, and temporal areas.

There is still no general agreement on nomenclature, nature, or location of all individual forms of sensory aphasia. In addition to the classic *Wernicke's or total sensory asphasia*, however, the subforms in the following list have met with approval.

1. **Global or total aphasia:** This term stands for a severe, mixed, motor-sensory aphasia caused by a lesion involving the motor as well as the sensory areas for speech. The lesion is usually an infarct caused by an obstruction of the middle cerebral artery. Affected patients can utter only a few sounds or mangled remainders of speech and understand only a few sounds or words, which are immediately forgotten. They cannot repeat spoken words and are unable to read or write. This global aphasia is accompanied by hemiplegia, hemianesthesia, and hemianopsia.

2. **Jargon aphasia:** This term is applied if speech is unintelligible because of verbal and literal paraphasias, formation of new words (neologisms) and paragrammatism.

The following types of sensory aphasia have also been called *dissociative aphasias*, because they are supposedly caused by interruption of association fibers going to or coming from the individual areas of speech.

3. **Pure sensory aphasia:** This is a pure word deafness or auditory verbal agnosia that may exist while the patient is still able to differentiate between noises and tones. The deafness concerns only speech. Patients are unable to repeat spoken words and sentences or to write what is dictated. Spontaneous speech, writing, and reading are undisturbed. Postmortem examination reveals lesions in the middle third of the superior temporal gyrus. It is assumed that the clinical deficit is caused by an interruption of association fibers connecting Heschl's transverse convolutions with the secondary association territory of area 22 in the posterior and dorsal portion of the superior temporal gyrus.

4. **Conduction aphasia:** This condition is similar to Wernicke's aphasia. It differs from it in the good preservation of verbal comprehension, which is in contrast to the great difficulty affected patients experience in repeating spoken words. The patient simply cannot repeat multisyllabic words. The supramarginal gyrus of the dominant hemisphere – in other words, the transitional area between the posterior temporal lobe and the parietal lobe – has been found postmortem to be the site of a lesion. The difficulty in immediately repeating motorically a word just heard is believed to be caused by the interruption of the arcuate fascicle connecting the sensory and motor speech areas. In many instances the word that cannot be repeated can be said and pronounced without difficulty if it is presented to the patient in writing.

5. **Amnestic aphasia:** This condition is also called *amnesic, nominal,* or *anomic aphasia*. If not very severe, it is characterized by a continual groping for names of objects and ideas and by attempts to compensate for this difficulty by replacing these words with others. Patients recognize objects without difficulty but cannot remember their names. Postmortem findings suggest that this type of aphasia is

caused by lesions that interrupt the association fibers connecting the sensory speech area with the hippocampal region. The lesion is usually a tumor and occasionally an otogenous abscess in the deeper white matter of posterior and basal portions of the temporal lobe (possibly area 37) or an atrophic process, such as the temporal lobe version of Pick's disease.

6. **Transcortical aphasia** (Lichtheim): This is a severe aphasia that is associated with lack of auditory and visual comprehension of words and an inability to write or read with comprehension. Spoken words can be repeated, but their meaning cannot be understood. It is believed that this aphasia is caused by separation of the sensory speech area from the remaining cortex because of circulatory disorders in cortex and white matter along the arterial border zones between anterior, middle, and posterior cerebral arteries. This belief stems from the occurrence of the condition in cases of transient cardiac arrest regardless of its cause.

Additional Remarks

As mentioned earlier, visual as well as acoustic association areas are integrated by certain reflex arcs. A sudden light stimulus, such as lightning, produces an immediate averting of eyes and head because areas 18 and 19 have connections with the tegmentum of the midbrain, other parts of the brainstem and the cervical cord. The *pursuit reflex* and the *fixation reflex* of the eyes are related to efferent impulses coming from areas 18 and 19. They allow a moving object of interest to be held continuously in the fovea of the retina.

Similarly, a sudden noise, caused, for example, by an explosion, produces an immediate reflex averting of the head as part of a protection reflex. An interesting noise, voice, or melody, however, may cause a reflex turning of the head in the direction of the acoustic stimulus.

Summary. What has been discussed in this section may be condensed as follows: There are signs and syndromes caused by *focal* alterations involving various segments of the cerebral cortex and attached white matter. Analogously to the anterior horns of the spinal cord, the cortex in front of the central fissure subserves motor functions. Damage to the primary motor and the premotor areas produces signs of irritation or paralysis of muscles. Damage to the prefrontal area of the convexity impairs active thinking, leading to severe or total *loss of spontaneity* and *initiative*. Analogously to the posterior horns of the spinal cord, the cortex posterior to the central fissure is the primary cortex for somatic sensory inputs. In addition, visual inputs have their primary cortex in the calcarine area 17, and acoustic inputs their primary cortex in Heschl's transverse convolutions. Tactile, optic, and acoustic agnosias, the focal signs of motor and sensory aphasias, apraxia, alexia, and agraphia were discussed, as were focal disorders of taste and olfaction. Anosmia was mentioned as a potential neurologic sign accompanying pathologic states of the orbital cortex that lead to changes in character and personality, generally characterized by a loss of social inhibition. Most of these and other signs have become known through coordination of clinical observations with selected topical alterations found postmortem.

General Signs and Symptoms Accompanying Diseases of the Cerebrum

In diagnosing diseases of the Cerebrum, one must always remember that focal signs may be associated with or overshadowed by signs of general or distant involvement of the brain. This is particularly true if the disease is space-occupying, representing a tumor, a massive hematoma, or an early infarct. Under such circumstances, blockage of cerebrospinal fluid (CSF) circulation at one point or another may produce signs of in-

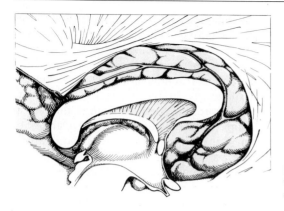

Fig. 8.29 Herniation of cingulate gyrus beneath falx, causing compression of branches of anterior cerebral artery (drawn from specimen).

creased intracranial pressure from hypertensive hydrocephalus. Other signs may be the result of pressure on blood vessels from either the tumor itself or midline displacement of one hemisphere beneath the margin of the falx (Fig. 8.29). This hemispheric shift may be associated with or followed by distortion of the hypothalamus and tentorial herniation of one parahippocampal gyrus, with displacement and compression of the midbrain (see Fig. 3.69). All these changes may produce additional signs and symptoms. Under such circumstances it is very important to ask for a detailed clinical history in order to establish the very first signs and symptoms and the subsequent symptomatology in chronological order. Establishing the symptomatology is particularly important if increased intracranial pressure has produced general symptoms and signs from distant areas.

When a space-occupying lesion, such as a tumor, enlarges, the crests of the convolutions become flat and the sulci compressed. The neighboring tissues of the hemisphere are displaced. This condition leads to a shift of the hemisphere across the midline through the opening of the falx. As the cingulate gyrus bulges to the opposite side, it displaces the anterior cerebral arteries and presses the branches of the ipsilateral artery against the almost unyielding margin of the falx (see Fig. 8.29). The lateral and third ventricles become distorted (see Fig. 7.8). The third ventricle, particularly its posterior portion, may become severely narrowed. Perifocal edema may spread and become generalized as a result of retardation of circulation from pressure on both arteries and veins, decreasing the supply of nutrients and oxygen and at the same time impeding the removal of acid metabolites. Finally, CSF circulation may be totally blocked and the tentorial opening impacted, causing compression of the midbrain with all its consequences (Figs. 3.68 and 3.69).

The increase in intracranial pressure is evidenced by headaches, nausea, retching, vomiting, and increasing papilledema. These symptoms are followed by clouding of the sensorium, somnolence, stupor, and, finally, coma.

This course may be the result of a gradually developing subdural hematoma following a minor head injury, a gradual bleeding into an old subdural hematoma (chronic subdural hematoma), or an extracerebral tumor. In most instances it is caused by an intracerebral glioma, particularly a glioblastoma multiforme, or by metastases or other fast-growing tumors that destroy the tissue they infiltrate. Slower-growing gliomas, such as astrocytomas, oligodendrogliomas, and spongioblastomas, are often clinically silent for some time, because the tumor cells grow along the nerve fibers without interfering with their function. An epileptiforme seizure may be the first dysfunction caused by such tumor and force a person to see a neurologist. He may find not more than a slight difference in the intensity of some reflexes and no signs of increased intracranial pressure. Nevertheless, if the patient is middle-aged or elderly, it always raises the level of suspicion sufficiently high to initiate diagnostic imaging in the hunt for a tumor without delay.

The cause of such a seizure may be a meningioma, which usually grows as slowly as an acoustic neurinoma (see Figs. 4.**14** and 8.**32**). It gives the brain ample time to adjust to displacement. Therefore, the tumor may be present for years without producing focal signs or signs of increased intracranial pressure. When finally diagnosed and operated upon, the tumor is usually much larger than was clinically expected. The postoperative prognosis is very good, provided the diagnosis is made before complications set in. The following remarks on the symptomatology of some meningiomas are intended to be helpful in this respect.

Meningiomas

These tumors represent approximately 20 percent of all intracranial neoplasms. They originate wherever pacchionian granulations of the arachnoid are present. Many develop along the superior longitudinal sinus as unilateral or bilateral parasagittal meningiomas. Next in frequency follow sphenoid ridge, olfactory groove, and suprasellar meningiomas.

Parasagittal meningioma

Located in front of the central fissure, a parasagittal meningioma is apt to trigger epileptic seizures sporadically over several years. Compression of the frontal convolutions may lessen spontaneity in movements and active thinking, as described earlier. Bitemporal hemianopic field defects are caused in such cases by the posterior gyri recti herniating into the anterior angle of the optic chiasm. If located posterior to the central fissure, the tumor may produce an occasional epileptic seizure but may also lead to hypesthesia or paresthesia in the perineal area (see Fig. 7.**8b**).

Olfactory groove meningioma

With this neoplasm a unilateral and, later, bilateral anosmia gradually develops of which the patient may be unaware. As the tumor involves cortex and white matter of the orbital convolutions (Fig. 8.**31**), the patient becomes uninhibited as described earlier. Finally, there may be papilledema, optic atrophy, or both (optic atrophy in the ipsilateral and papilledema in the contralateral eye is *Foster Kennedy syndrome*). With a posterior location in the olfactory groove, the tumor may approach the optic canals, as may be evidenced by visual field defects.

Tuberculum sellae meningioma

This condition has in common with a chromophobe pituitary adenoma that it presses from beneath against the optic chiasm and may produce a bitemporal hemianopsia. It does not alter the sella, however, and seldom causes hypothalamic signs. It has in common with the olfactory groove meningioma that it may grow into the optic canals and cause blindness in one and perhaps later the other eye. Olfaction, however, usually remains intact.

Sphenoid ridge meningioma

Complaints of poor vision and pain within or about one eye, protrusion of the painful eye, visual field defects, and, perhaps, bulging of the ipsilateral temple suggest this tumor, illustrated in Fig. 8.**30**. A regular roentgenogram may show a density in the area of the lesser sphenoid wing. A paralysis of ocular muscles (see Fig. 3.**17**) may be another sign and suggests that the tumor is located over the medial third of the sphenoid ridge. Compression and displacement of the anterior temporal lobe may produce so-called *uncinate fits*.

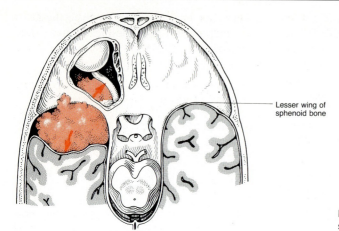

Fig. 8.**30** Meningioma of lesser sphenoid wing.

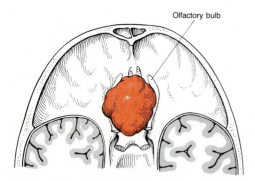

Fig. 8.**31** Meningioma of olfactory groove.

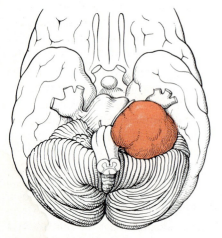

Fig. 8.**32** Neurinoma of VIII in pontocerebellar angle.

Protrusion of one eye may be caused by a variety of retrobulbar and even retroorbital processes, such as a malignant metastatic tumor, lipoma, epidermoid, angioma, arteriovenous fistula, Hand-Schüller-Christian disease (histiocytosis X), or even by a malformation, such as oxycephaly.

Occasionally, a meningioma is part of neurofibromatosis (von Recklinghausen's disease). In this disease it is not unusual to find multiple meningiomas; in fact, the inner surface of the dura may be covered with innumerable small tumor nodules. Also, neurinomas of spinal, not only cranial, nerves are seen in this condition. This tumor most often involves nerve VIII (Fig. 8.**32**). Bilateral involvement of the acoustic nerves is symptomatic of von Recklinghausen's disease. The clinical features of the tumor have been discussed earlier, on pages 177, 178.

Epileptic Seizures

Ictal conditions with the characteristics of epileptic seizures have repeatedly been mentioned (pages 36, 205 f, 279, 284, 298 f). These seizures are manifestations of repetitive functional disorders of the brain and are triggered by paroxysmal synchronized discharges of individual groups of neurons in cerebral gray matter. It is not fully understood how such focal epileptic discharges come about. There may be related to the hyperexcitability of neurons in or around an area of cortical atrophy from former selective loss of neurons, such as the Ammon's horn sclerosis, a traumatic corticomeningeal adhesion, a tumor, a malformation, or a focal inflammation. Epileptic discharges of more diffuse origin are often the result of a systemic metabolic disorder, such as uremia.

The great number of epileptic manifestations are listed in the "International Classification of Epileptic Seizures" (Gastaut, 1970). We can discuss here the large groups of *partial* and *generalized attacks*, only in general terms.

Focal motor seizures, such as Jacksonian attacks, belong to the first group. In general, these seizures are not accompanied by an impairment of consciousness and are not followed by lasting neurologic deficits. Electroencephalography often shows transient spikes. They may suggest the location of the irritating lesion. In this respect the specific nature of the clinical signs and symptoms is by far more indicative.

A cortical alteration in the visual area may cause the complaint of seeing flashes of light. Involvement of the somatosensory region produces symptoms such as dysesthesias, tingling, or numbness in the corresponding areas of the body. A focus in the motor cortex is responsible for a motor partial seizure that may consist, for example, of clonic twitching of the facial muscles of one side or the muscles of a hand or a foot. The seizure may terminate in seconds or minutes. It is possible, however, for the epileptic discharges to spread over other parts of the ipsilateral motor cortex, causing the convulsion to "march" (Jacksonian seizure), for example, from face to arm or from foot to leg, finally involving half of the body. A partial seizure may follow this pattern from the beginning and may be followed by a temporary paresis, referred to as *Todd's paralysis* or *hemiconvulsion hemiplegia syndrome*.

A focus in the premotor cortex tends to produce adversive attacks usually consisting of contralateral turning of eyes, head, and trunk (page 279).

A focal alteration in the inferior temporal lobe may produce complex emotional experiences that may be associated with complex motor manifestations, as mentioned in the section on psychomotor attacks (page 205). On cause is gliosis following pressure of the uncus on the tentorium cerebelli when the head is squeezed during birth.

After careful analysis of focal clinical signs and electroencephalographic findings, partial seizures require immediate application of all diagnostic techniques available.

Generalized seizures often commence as partial attacks that rapidly turn into fits of grand mal type characterized by total loss of consciousness, generalized tonic-clonic convulsions, cyanosis, foaming at the mouth, tongue biting, and enuresis.

The group of generalized seizures includes periods of absence characterized by a lack of awareness for only seconds, and states of petit mal in which the lack of awareness is associated with some discrete motor phenomena such as myoclonic twitchings of face or other muscles, changes in postural tone, or automatisms. These types of attacks are seen predominantly in children and adolescents. Characteristically, the electroencephalogram shows rhythmic, 3 Hz (petit mal) or 2.5 Hz spike-and-wave patterns (variant petit mal).

Occasionally, a generalized seizure may repeat itself at such brief intervals that the patient fails to regain consciousness. This is called *status epilepticus*.

Circulatory System of the Cerebrum

Arterial Supply

The blood is supplied to the brain by two pairs of arteries: the internal carotid and the vertebral arteries. These four *feeders* are independent until they enter the cranium and become interconnected by the anastomotic safeguard system of supply, the *arterial circle of Willis and basilar artery*. Peripherally, this system is followed by the *cerebral arteries proper*.

Internal Carotid Arteries

These arteries ascend from the common carotid arteries, which derive on the right from the brachiocephalic trunk and on the left from the aortic arch. At the level of the thyroid cartilage the common carotids divide into external and internal carotid arteries. The external carotids supply the upper portion of the anterior neck and face and the frontotemporal regions of the cranium. The internal carotids ascend through the deep neck without giving off branches. On their way through the carotid canals of the petrous bones and cavernous sinuses, they deliver small branches to the floor of the middle ear, the dura of the clivus, the semilunar ganglion of the trigeminal nerve, and the pituitary gland. Beneath the cranial opening of the optic canals, the internal carotids enter the subarachnoid space and give off the *ophthalmic arteries*, which immediately turn rostrally and pass beneath the optic nerves through the optic canals and into the orbits. They supply all orbital structures; the mucosa of the sphenoid sinus, the ethmoidal cells, most of the nasal cavity, and the dura of the anterior cranial fossa. They terminate in branches supplying the skin of forehead, root of nose, and eyelids and anastomose with the facial and internal maxillary arteries, which are branches of the external carotid arteries.

Vertebral Arteries

These arteries are the first branches of the subclavian arteries. They ascend through the transverse foramina of the upper six cervical vertebrae and enter the skull between the atlas and the lateral margin of the foramen magnum.

Before entering the cranium, the vertebral as well as the internal carotid arteries form S-shaped *siphons* which probably serve the purpose of dampening the incoming pulse waves. The carotid arteries form their siphons within the cavernous sinuses. The vertebral arteries do so after emerging from the transverse foramina of the atlas. These arteries first run posteriorly alongside the lateral masses of the atlas, then turn upward and medially and enter the cranial cavity on either side of the medulla oblongata (Fig. 8.**33**).

In front of the pontomedullary junction, the vertebral arteries merge to form the basilar artery, which divides into posterior cerebral arteries at the pontomesencephalic border. The supply territories of vertebral and basilar arteries have been described earlier (see Figs. 3.**52**, 3.**53**, 3.**54**, 4.**7**, 4.**8**, and 4.**9**).

Arterial Circle of Willis

After entering the subarachnoid space, the internal carotid arteries proceed posteriorly beneath the optic nerves and then laterally from them to the level of the optic chiasm, where they make right-angled turns in order to enter the sylvian fissures. At these turns they give off the *posterior communicating arteries*, which join the proximal stems of the posterior cerebral arteries and form together with them and the rostral basilar artery the posterior arc of the circle of Willis.

The internal carotids also give rise to the anterior choroidal arteries before they terminate by dividing into anterior and middle cerebral arteries (Fig. 8.**35**). The stems of the anterior cerebral arteries immediately converge to the midline and become connected by the anterior communicating artery. Thus, the anterior arc of the circle of Willis is closed.

The "normal" circle of Willis seen in Figs. 8.**34** and 8.**35** exists in not more than half of all persons. The circle varies considerably in the others. This is particularly true of the posterior arc (Fig. 8.**40b**). In rare in-

Circulatory System of the Cerebrum 303

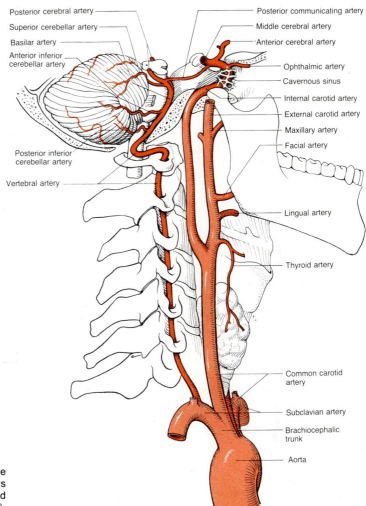

Fig. 8.33 Extracranial course of the large arterial feeders (common and internal carotid arteries and vertebral arteries).

stances one or even both posterior communicating arteries may be absent.

These anomalies are not significant under normal circulatory conditions, but become so if supply by the feeding arteries becomes reduced or interrupted. In such a situation the state of the circle largely determines whether the circle is still able to distribute the blood in sufficient amount or if ischemia cannot be prevented and thus produces a small or larger infarct. The rate at which the circulatory crisis develops is also important. With acute onset there is usually not enough time for an efficient redistribution of blood flow. With gradual development there is a chance that good collateral flow will become operative. A well-developed circle usually has no difficulty in handling such an emergency. If, for example, one of the internal carotids is compressed or ligated, blood is immediately shunted by anterior and posterior communicating arteries to the area for which the nonfunctioning artery was responsible. Successful endarterectomy of the internal carotid artery depends on this mechanism.

In addition to the circle of Willis, there are

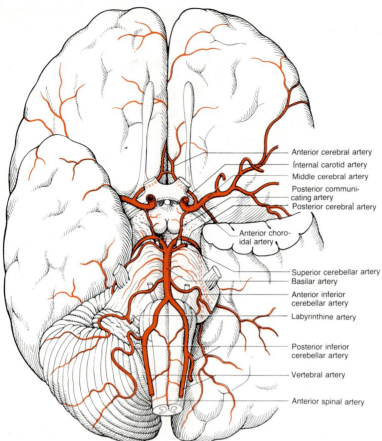

Fig. 8.**34** Arteries at base of brain.

a few other, less effective collaterals which may become active. It was mentioned earlier that the ophthalmic arteries anastomose with facial and internal maxillary branches of the external carotid arteries. Under certain conditions they may carry blood from these branches back into the intracranial internal carotids. Similar extracranial anastomoses exist between the occipital branches of the external carotids and the vertebral arteries. Anastomoses between cerebral arteries are mentioned later.

Cerebral Arteries Proper

Branches of the posterior communicating arteries

As illustrated in Fig. 8.**35**, the posterior communicating arteries give rise to a number of small branches that supply the tuber cinereum, mamillary bodies, anterior third of the thalamus, subthalamus, and part of the posterior limb of the internal capsule.

Anterior choroidal artery

This artery descends from the internal carotid lateral to the posterior communicating artery or from the stem of the middle cerebral artery (see Figs. 8.**34** and 8.**35**). It accompanies the

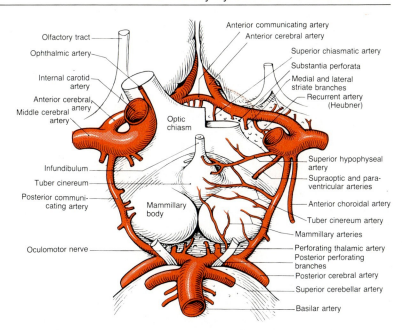

Fig. 8.35 Circle of Willis and its branches.

optic tract to supply the lateral geniculate body and choroid plexus of the inferior ventricular horn. In addition to the optic tract, it supplies the medial two-thirds of the pallidum and parts of the amygdaloid complex, the uncus, and the anterior hippocampal gyrus. It also serves the ventral two-thirds of the posterior limb of the internal capsule; the lateral portion of the lateral geniculate body, including the very rostral part of the optic radiation as it emerges from the lateral geniculate body; and the rostral portions of the midbrain, particularly the medial substantia nigra, part of the red nucleus, the medial third of the peduncle, and the lateral half of the subthalamic nucleus. It enters the choroid plexus of the inferior ventricular horn near its anterior tip and communicates with the posterior choroidal artery, a branch of the posterior cerebral artery. The efficiency of the anastomosis is believed to be the reason that ligation of the posterior choroidal artery produces no clinical deficits.

Anterior cerebral artery

Immediately after originating from the internal carotid artery, the anterior cerebral artery gives off a number of small branches that enter the anterior perforated substance and supply the ventromedial half of the anterior striate body, the ventral anterior limb of the internal capsule, the septal region, and the anterior commissure. The striatum artery is usually the strongest of these branches. It may originate near the anterior communicating artery and must proceed caudally in order to reach the anterior perforated substance. This is the reason why Heubner described it as a *recurrent artery*. Other small branches originating near the anterior communicating artery supply part of the optic chiasm and adjacent portions of the optic nerves (see Fig. 8.35).

The two anterior cerebral arteries run side by side through the length of the interhemispheric cistern, each giving off five major branches, the orbital, frontopolar, pericallosal, callosomarginal, and parietal branches (see Fig. 8.37). These branches can

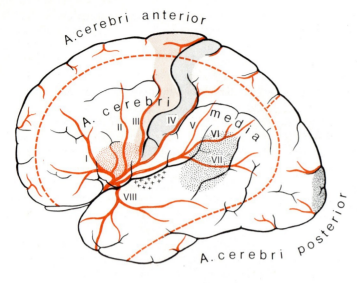

Fig. 8.36 Supply area and distribution of branches of the middle cerebral artery at the convexity of the brain. I, orbitofrontal artery; II, prerolandic artery; III, rolandic artery; IV, anterior parietal artery; V, posterior parietal artery; VI, angular artery; VII, posterior temporal artery; VIII, anterior temporal artery.

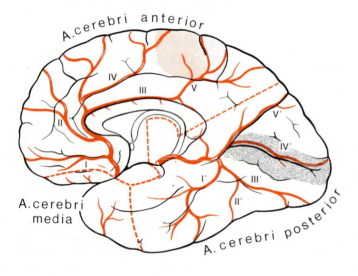

Fig. 8.37 Supply areas and distribution of branches of anterior, posterior, and middle cerebral arteries at the median and inferior aspects of the right hemisphere. I, orbital artery; II, frontopolar artery; III, pericallosal artery; IV, callosomarginal artery; V, parietal artery; I', anterior temporal artery; II', posterior temporal artery; III', posterior occipital artery; IV', calcarine artery; V', parietooccipital artery.

be identified readily on angiography. The pericallosal branch is the direct extension of the anterior cerebral artery and supplies the corpus callosum, with the exception of the splenium, which belongs to the territory supplied by the parietooccipital branch of the posterior cerebral artery.

All cortical branches cross the orbital, frontal, and parietal margins of the hemisphere and supply a strip of marginal cortex and white matter of the orbital lobes and of the frontal and parietal convexity, as indicated in Figs. 8.36 and 8.39.

Middle cerebral artery

After giving off the anterior cerebral artery, the internal carotid artery becomes the middle cerebral artery, the largest of all cerebral arteries. As its stem circles around the limen of the insula, it delivers its first branches, which enter the caudal portion of the anterior perforated substance as striatum branches. They supply almost all of the putamen and caudate nucleus, the lateral third of the pallidum, and the dorsal segment of the internal capsule, passing between putamen and caudate nucleus (see Fig. 8.39). The largest of the striatum branches is located most laterally and supplies the lateral putamen as well as the external capsule. Because it is most often the source of an apoplectic hypertensive hematoma, Charcot called it "l'artère de l'hémorrrhagie cérébrale."

Before the stem of the middle cerebral artery leaves the limen of the insula, it gives off a small branch that supplies the anterior insula, extreme capsule, and claustrum. Thereafter, the stem divides into three or four major branches, which subdivide within the fissure. Their subbranches emerge from the fissure and supply most of the cortex and white matter of the lateral aspect of the hemisphere. The subbranches, which can be seen with regularity and can usually be identified without difficulty on angiography, are the orbitofrontal, prerolandic, rolandic, anterior parietal, posterior parietal, angular, posterior temporal, and anterior temporal branches.

Figure 8.36 illustrates that the middle cerebral artery supplies most of the convexity of the hemisphere except for its dorsal margin (anterior cerebral artery) and the occipital pole (posterior cerebral artery). It is responsible for all those regions of frontal, temporal, and parietal lobes that, when damaged in the dominant hemisphere, produce important focal signs such as motor and sensory aphasia, alexia, agraphia, apraxia, acalculia, and disturbance of body image. The longest branch, the angular artery, almost reaches the occipital pole.

Posterior cerebral artery

These arteries are usually the terminal branches of the basilar artery. Occasionally, they are extensions of the internal carotid arteries. The nerve fibers accompanying them are part of the plexus of the carotid arteries.

Small branches of the basilar artery and of the proximal stems of the posterior cerebral arteries supply the midbrain (see Fig. 3.54a). Paramedial branches among the *peduncular arteries* descend into the tegmentum of the rostral half of the pons. The posterior cerebral arteries are also responsible for the thalami (see Fig. 8.39). Most of the lateral and ventral nuclei are supplied by the *thalamoperforating branches*, which ascend through the posterior perforated substance (see Fig. 8.35). The lateral and medial geniculate bodies and their vicinity are supplied by the *thalamogeniculate branches* (see Fig. 5.8). The medial posterior choroidal arteries, which leave the posterior cerebral arteries already in front of the midbrain (see Fig. 3.54a) and accompany the arteries on their way through the cisternae ambientes, swing around the pulvinars and, taking a rostral course, supply dorsal portions of the thalami until they terminate in the anterior thalamic nuclei. They also enter the choroid plexus of the third ventricle and that of the cella media of the lateral ventricles.

Within the cisternae ambientes one or, more often, two additional choroidal arteries, the *lateral posterior choroidal arteries*, branch off laterally and enter the choroid plexus of the inferior ventricular horns. They have strong anastomoses with the anterior choroidal arteries.

Three to five additional small arteries descend in each cisterna ambiens and proceed laterally into the hippocampal fissure, where they form anastomoses from which the Ammon's horn arteries derive, among them the long arteries of Uchimura, supplying Sommer's sector of the Ammon's horn. Because these arteries cross the margin of the tentorium at only a slight distance, they are vulnerable to compression during hippocampal herniation (Fig. 8.38). The Ammon's horn arteries connect rostrally with branches of the anterior choroidal arteries.

Five large peripheral branches supplying cortex and white matter originate within each cisterna ambiens. They are the anterior tem-

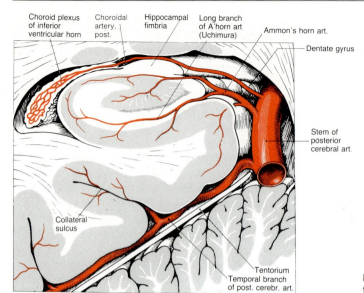

Fig. 8.**38** Arterial supply of the Ammon's horn.

poral, posterior temporal, posterior occipital, calcarine, and parietooccipital arteries or branches. Their supply territories are shown in Figs. 8.**37** and 8.**39**.

Peripheral Anastomoses of Cerebral Arteries

It is known from acute embolic infarcts that the supply territories of the major cerebral arteries are sharply delineated, as shown in Figs. 8.**36**, 8.**37**, and 8.**39**. Circulation ceases in such cases too rapidly for peripheral anastomoses to overcome the stagnation and to keep the blood flowing in at least a marginal area of the involved territory.

It was mentioned earlier that anastomoses exist between the anterior choroidal and posterior choroidal as well as the Ammon's horn arteries. They are present also among the various terminal branches of the anterior, middle, and posterior cerebral arteries and may measure up to 0.3 mm in diameter. These anastomoses represent persisting connections of the early embryonal network of blood vessels. They vary in number and location. They are strongest between the anterior and middle cerebral arteries in the precentral and central areas, between the middle and posterior cerebral arteries in the caudal interparietal fissure, and between the anterior and posterior cerebral arteries in the region of the precuneus (Vander Eecken and Adams, 1953).

These peripheral anastomoses may be regarded as a peripheral safeguarding system of supply that is effective if focal ischemia develops slowly or is transient. It is well known that anastomotic branches of the middle cerebral artery may save the calcarine cortex at the convexity of the occipital pole while the remainder of the cortex becomes necrotic from an obstruction of the calcarine artery. This phenomenon explains the finding of a hemianopsia with sparing of the macula. The pathology of the cerebrovascular diseases is richly illustrated in the atlas by McCormick and Schochet (1976).

Signs and Syndromes of Cerebral Circulatory Deficiencies

Inadequate cerebral circulation may be caused by a *vertebrobasilar insufficiency* or by a *stenosis or obstruction of one or both internal carotid arteries*.

Circulatory System of the Cerebrum 309

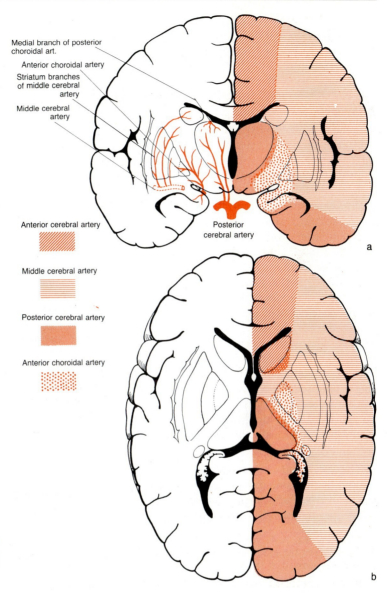

Fig. 8.39 Arterial supply of inner structures of brain. **a** Coronal section; **b** horizontal section.

Vertebrobasilar Insufficiency

Signs and symptoms of insufficiency are: dizziness, vertigo, disequilibrium, tinnitus or other head noises, visual disorders, dysarthria, dysphagia, dysphonia, headaches, and possibly disorder of consciousness, or so-called *drop attacks*, in which the patient suddenly loses postural tone, falls to the ground while conscious, regains postural control, and rises quickly. These signs may appear suddenly in any combination.

They may stem from a *subclavian steal* brought on by stenosis of a subclavian artery proximal to the origin of the vertebral artery. If such a stenosis involves, for example, the left subclavian artery, part of the blood carried by the right vertebral artery into the cranium is siphoned back into the left vertebral artery to fill the need of the left axillary artery. If the left arm is exercised or used more than usual, it needs more blood, and this blood is "stolen" from the vertebrobasilar supply territory.

Stenosis or severe hypoplasia of one vertebral artery may be asymptomatic until the intact artery becomes obstructed or compressed. Compression may occur if the head is held in a damaging position during the night. If the head is turned to one side and is bent backward at the same time, the contralateral artery will be under pressure at the cervicooccipital junction (Brown, 1963; Chroost & Corbier, 1962; Herrschaft, 1970) (Fig. 8.**40a**). If this artery is intact and this position is maintained for some time during sleep, oligemia will occur throughout the supply territory of the vertebral arteries. The patient, who went to bed without feeling ill, will awake in the morning with severe vertigo, disorders of equilibrium, and retching, and these symptoms may continue for several days. The vertigo is clearly positional and can be provoked by holding the head in a certain position. Occasionally it is associated with nystagmus.

The transient circulatory insufficiency caused by the same mechanism may produce a so-called *global transitory amnesia*. This is illustrated by the following two cases.

Case report 1: A 41-year-old woman drove all by herself into the mountains. After $5\frac{1}{2}$ hours of driving she arrived at the ski lift and went to the top of the run. First, she did some sunbathing lying flat on a cot and having her head dangling over its head end. She fell asleep. When she awoke, she felt ill. On the way down on her skis, she met several friends. Later, she could not remember having seen them. Back in the village, she bought a hat. Walking with a friend to the hotel, she wondered what she was carrying in a plastic bag. It was the hat, but she had no memory at all of having bought it. During the remainder of the day she forgot everything immediately and repeated over and over again the same questions. At first, her friends found it amusing and thought that she was jesting. Soon, it became obvious that she was utterly helpless because of the forgetfulness. The next morning, she was herself again and could take note of everything. The preceding day, however, was a blank in her memory. She had had similar, but shorter episodes of amnesia previously. They were usually associated with vertigo and headaches. Neurologically she showed a positive Babinski on the right. The EEG and CT-scan failed to reveal an abnormality. A catheter angiogram, however, showed that the left vertebral artery was hypoplastic to the degree of a thread.

Case report 2: The 57-year-old man enjoyed the Sunday morning and was looking forward to a tennis competition to be seen on TV at 3:00 p.m. This gave him time to take a nap after lunch. When he awoke, he felt ill, had vertigo and a loss of equilibrium. During the tennis game he fumbled thoughtlessly with a note block, walked aimlessly up and down the room, and showed no interest in the play. Continuously, he asked the same questions. He did not know anything about the game when the show was over. Next morning, he felt well again, but had no memory of the Sunday events and was quite upset about his "blackout". He reported that he had had similar, but less severe episodes three times in the past. A neurologic examination proved negative. An angiogram showed a thread-like hypoplastic vertebral artery on the right and a kinking of the left vertebral artery near its point of origin.

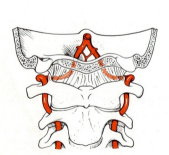
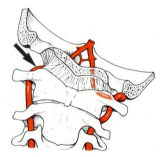

Fig. 8.**40a** Mechanical involvement of vertebral artery at atlanto-occipital joint upon tilting of the head.

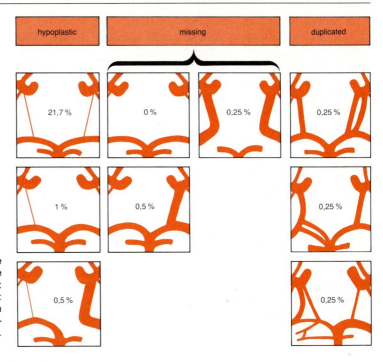

Fig. 8.**40b** Variations of the posterior segments of the Circle of Willis. (From: Krayenbühl, H. M. G. Yasargil: Die vaskulären Erkrankungen im Gebiet der Arteria vertebralis und Arteria basilaris. Thieme, Stuttgart 1957.)

Such global transient amnesia is usually not part of the spectrum of signs caused by vertebrobasilar insufficiency. The finding of one vertebral artery being hypoplastic is not unusual. A global transient amnesia, however, is quite rare. In the literature, this sign is attributed to bilateral insufficiency of circulation in the hippocampal areas due to arteriosclerosis or embolizations. Had this mechanism been operative in our cases, the amnesia should have lasted much longer.

The short duration of the amnesia in these two cases suggests that the insufficiency in circulation was functional. It could be explained by assuming that the hypoplasia of one of the two vertebral arteries in each case may have been associated with anomalies in the posterior parts of the circle of Willis. Indeed, cases have been described, in which one or both posterior communicating arteries were hypoplastic or even missing (Fig. 8.**40b**). Under such circumstance, the transient compression of the normal vertebral artery during the afflictive positioning of the head in the recumbent position may temporarily produce the critical reduction of blood flow in the small hippocampal branches of the posterior cerebral arteries.

Internal Carotid Artery Insufficiency

A stenosis or obstruction of an internal carotid artery at the site of its origin may be asymptomatic unless the circle of Willis is incompetent or the systemic blood pressure is low from cardiac or other disease. If this is the case, the symptomatology is usually like that of oligemia without focal signs. The same pattern may develop if, in the presence of an efficient circle of Willis and normal or elevated blood pressure, both internal carotids are obstructed in the neck and the two vertebral arteries have to supply the entire brain. In that case the oligemia will be generalized and also involve the brainstem, because much of the blood entering the basilar artery is diverted to the cerebrum. Therefore, the brainstem may show signs of an "*internal steal syndrome.*"

In general, signs and symptoms of internal carotid artery obstruction depend on the site of the obstruction, on whether the obstruction is acute or subacute, and on the quality of collateral circulation, primarily the quality of that provided by the circle of Willis. Consequently, the clinical manifestations may show one of three degrees of severity:

1. They may be mild and fleeting, indicating a short-lasting oligemia.
2. They may slowly progress to a stroke, indicating that oligemia is probably worsening to ischemia. This may be caused by an advancing arterial thrombosis.
3. They may from the beginning consist of a complete stroke. This finding suggests that the obstruction involves not only the carotid but also the middle and perhaps the anterior cerebral arteries and produced an irreversible infarct.

What is called *transient ischemic attack* (TIA) is usually brought on by one or another factor becoming operative in addition to a stenosis of the internal carotid and its branching point from the common carotid. There may be a transient low in systemic blood pressure. One or both arteries may be abnormal and may have developed kinking and coiling over the years from loss of elasticity, making them vulnerable to transient narrowing of their lumen with certain positioning of the head. There may be additional stenosing arteriosclerosis at the branching points of the large arteries, its sites of predilection (Fig. 8.**40c**). It appears that in many instances the attacks are caused by soft, fast-dissolving emboli originating at so-called ulcerating arteriosclerotic plaques at the site at which the internal branches from the common carotid artery.

Signs of a circulatory insufficiency in the supply territory of an internal carotid artery are: transient hemiparalysis or paresis, especially of face and arm, associated with mild dysesthesias (tingling, numbness) in the contralateral extremity and a transient disorder of speech if the dominant hemisphere is involved. The arterial pressure in the ipsilateral eye may be low. There may be episodes of *amaurosis fugax*. The blindness may not be associated with darkening of the visual field; instead, the eye may be blinded by what appears to be bright white steam. Ipsilateral headaches in the frontal areas are quite frequent.

A thrombosis may occur in the distal portion of the internal carotid artery as it passes through the cavernous sinus and may extend beyond the point of origin of the ophthalmic artery. In such a case there is a contralateral hemiparesis or paralysis associated with cortical sensory disorders and an ipsilateral blindness because of thrombosis of the ophthalmic artery supplying the central retinal artery. Should the carotid obstruction extend

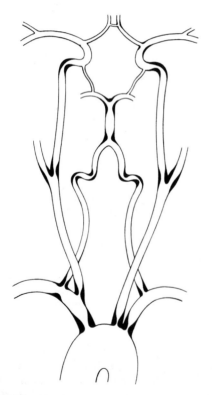

Fig. 8.**40c** Most frequent location of arteriosclerotic stenoses in the large supplying arteries and arteries at the base of the brain.

into the posterior communicating and the adjacent anterior choroidal arteries, involvement of optic tract and lateral geniculate body may produce a contralateral hemianopsia. Propagation of the thrombus into the stems of anterior and middle cerebral arteries transforms the supply territory of both arteries into a huge infarct, leaving only that of the posterior cerebral artery intact. There may be many additional focal signs; they are listed later in the text as results of obstruction of the stem of a middle cerebral artery. It is, however, more likely for them to be abolished when the patient slips into coma.

Infarcted tissue begins to swell very soon and turns the lesion into a space-occupying alteration, causing displacement of the remaining hemispheric tissue across the midline (Fig. 8.**41a**) and into the tentorial opening. Compression of the midbrain, rather than tissue loss, is the cause of coma and usually also of death by respiratory failure. It should be mentioned that a faint pulse in the internal carotid artery in the neck and a bruit over its area are indicative of arterial stenosis.

Obstruction of the stem of the middle cerebral artery is rare and is usually the result of embolization and not of arteriosclerotic thrombosis. The embolus may be part or all of a mural thrombus of the left heart caused by an endocardial irritation usually in response to ischemia of the heart muscle. It may also have originated from an ulcerating atherosclerotic plaque in the internal carotid artery at the branching point of the common carotid artery.

The clinical sequelae of such a large infarct in the dominant hemisphere include contralateral hemiparalysis, particularly of face and arm; contralateral cortical hemianesthesia; 'total aphasia; agraphia; alexia; apraxia; and contralateral homonymous hemianopsia. At the beginning there may be head turning and conjugate deviation of the eyes to the opposite side. If the infarct involves the nondominant hemisphere, there will be contralateral hemiplegia and hemianesthesia as well as hemianopsia, apraxia, and possibly anosognosia.

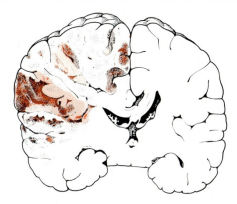

Fig. 8.**41a** Recent softening in the supply areas of anterior and middle cerebral arteries after thrombosis of internal carotid artery. Because of space-occupying swelling of infarct, there is herniation of cingulate gyrus under falx (drawn from specimen).

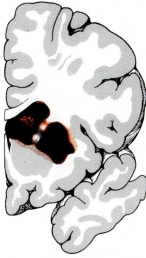

Fig. 8.**41b** Recent hemorrhagic infarction of rostal portion of caudate nucleus and putamen (striatum) caused by embolic obstruction of striate body branches of right middle cerebral artery. The preserved ventromedial part of the striatum represents the supply territory of Heubner's recurrent branch of the anterior cerebral artery (drawn from specimen).

Obstruction of the striatum arteries causes infarction of the caudate nucleus and putamen as well as of the dorsal portion of the internal capsule lying between the two. Consequently, there will be a contralateral hemiplegia without aphasia (Fig. 8.**41b**).

Obstruction of the prerolandic branch of the middle cerebral artery produces a contralateral facial and hypoglossal paralysis. If the lesion involves the dominant hemisphere, there will also be a motor aphasia because of damage to Broca's region in the posterior third of the third frontal convolution (see Fig. 8.**36**).

Obstruction of the rolandic branch, which mainly supplies the lower two-thirds of the precentral gyrus, produces a contralateral, predominantly brachiofacial hemiparalysis. The lower extremity is involved less or not at all, because the area for its cortical innervation is supplied by the anterior cerebral artery.

Obstruction of subsequent branches supplying parietal, occipital, and temporal areas of the dominant hemisphere produces cortical sensory deficits and contralateral quadrantanopsia or hemianopsia from involvement of the optic radiation, sensory aphasia, and possibly alexia, agraphia, acalculia, ideokinetic apraxia, left/right disorders, finger agnosia, and other disturbances.

Obstruction of the anterior cerebral artery (see Fig. 8.**37**) is rare. Obstruction of Heubners recurrent artery produces a contralateral weakness of face and tongue and perhaps of arm. Obstruction of the anterior cerebral artery above the corpus callosum and proximal to the paracentral lobule causes a spastic paralysis and a cortical sensory disorder in the contralateral leg. In addition there may be a weakness of the sphincter of the urinary bladder. A large and space-occupying lesion may cause additional transient paralysis of the contralateral arm.

If a unilateral space-occupying process displaces corpus callosum and cingulate gyrus over the midline, the margin of the falx may compress branches of the herniating anterior cerebral artery (see Fig. 8.**29**), and this may produce clinical signs of insufficient blood supply, particularly from the paracentral lobule.

Should thrombosis or embolization of the anterior cerebral artery result in infarct of the rostral corpus callosum, there may be a dyspraxia of the left arm. Such an infarct interrupts fibers that cross from the left parietal lobe via the corpus callosum to the motor region of the right hemisphere. Obstruction of both anterior cerebral arteries causes spastic paralysis of the legs, urinary incontinence, and particularly a loss of spontaneity. In addition, there may be snapping and grasping reflexes, apraxia, and a conjugate deviation of the eyes.

Obstruction of the anterior choroidal artery causes ischemia in the lower portion of the posterior limb of the internal capsule, part of the optic radiation, the medial two-thirds of the pallidum, and halves of the lateral geniculate body and subthalamic nucleus. The clinical sequelae are contralateral hemiparalysis and hemihypesthesia as well as hemianopsia. Involvement of the optic tract produces an ipsilateral dilatation of the pupil with slow reaction to light. Because of the good anastomoses of the artery, motor and sensory disorders may soon improve. The hemianopsia usually persists. An infarct involving the medial two-thirds of the pallidum interrupts pathways that extend from cortex and striate body through pallidum to thalamus and structures in subthalamus and brainstem. Extrapyramidal motor signs with lack of spontaneous movements and lack of mimetic facial expressions may result.

Obstruction of the posterior cerebral artery usually causes ischemia in the calcarine cortex. This is one reason for homonymous contralateral field defects. The hemianopsia is total if all of the visual cortex is destroyed by the infarct. Anastomoses between posterior and middle cerebral arteries over the occipital pole may save the cortex representing the macula and be responsible for the sparing of central vision in the hemianopic fields. The infarct may destroy only white matter of the inferior temporal convolutions and leave the calcarine cortex intact, as illustrated in Fig. 8.**27**. Such a lesion destroys the ventral half of the optic radiation, which passes around the floor of the posterior ventricular horn on its way to the ventral lip of the calcarine cortex. The result is a contralateral homonymous upper quadrantanopsia. Occasionally, the calcarine cortex is damaged only in spots. This may produce elusive scotomas in the contralateral fields. If a more substantial infarction involves the dominant hemisphere, the hemianopsia may be associated with optic agnosia, alexia, or agraphia (see Fig. 8.27).

An embolus riding the bifurcation of the basilar artery may cause obstruction of both posterior cerebral arteries with involvement of both calcarine areas (Fig. 8.42). This may result in blindness from bilateral hemianopsia. The blindness may be total, and the patient may act accordingly. It is also possible for the patient to deny the total blindness. This indicates that he has, in addition, an anosognosia, or an inability to recognize that he has a physical disability. This is called *Anton's syndrome*. It may be associated with a Korsakoff-like confabulation about the disability.

In a case of bilateral hemianopsia, the preserved central fields may be so small that the patient acts as if he is blind and even complains of blindness. His condition should not be mistaken for functional blindness. When his vision is tested, no large letters should be used, because they exceed his visual fields and he may not be able to read them. When he is shown letters that fit into the smallness of his fields, he will recognize them without hesitation.

Blindness from bilateral hemianopsia may be the result of bilateral compression of posterior cerebral or, more specifically, calcarine arteries by the tentorial margin if a space-occupying supratentorial lesion such as a subdural hematoma, an intracerebral hematoma, or a tumor led to tentorial impaction. The same result may occur in the absence of a space-occupying lesion if swelling of the brain develops during acute shock. Cortical blindness is also known to be a sequela of transient cardiac arrest. The vulnerability of the calcarine cortex in such a case is related to the fact that the cortex, together with the posterior parietooccipital region, is farthest from the heart. Therefore, it is there that stasis occurs first and circulation returns latest.

Obstruction of both thalamoperforating arteries produces butterfly-like softenings extending up into the thalami and involving particularly the centrum medianum (see Figs. 5.8 and 5.9). The most notable sign is severe somnolence for weeks and months after initial unconsciousness. The patient can be awakened, recognizes his surroundings, and takes nourishment but falls asleep again immediately thereafter.

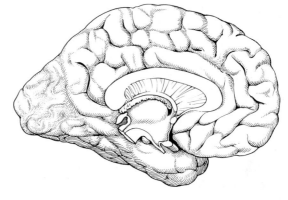

Fig. 8.42 Necrosis of both occipital lobes (right not shown) after thrombosis of posterior cerebral arteries (riding embolus) (drawn from specimen).

Arterial Aneurysms

By far the greatest number of aneurysms are congenital and are found at the base of the brain, involving most often the rostral half of the circle of Willis (Fig. 8.**43a**). They are usually asymptomatic until they become large enough to involve adjacent structures, such as the optic and oculomotor nerves. In other cases the only sign suggesting the presence of an aneurysm is sudden headaches associated with subarachnoid hemorrhage, usually from oozing of blood. With true rupture of an aneurysm, the subarachnoid hemorrhage is fulminant and often fatal.

Occasionally, an aneurysm is arteriosclerotic; in those cases it usually involves a carotid, vertebral, or basilar artery. Traumatic (Krauland, 1982) and mycotic aneurysms do occur and may be found in areas other than the base of the brain.

A *microaneurysm* is a pouching of the arterial wall so small that it is difficult to identify it on arteriograms or computed tomographic scans. Most aneurysms are *sacculated* or *berry aneurysms* of various sizes, usually with narrow entrances or necks. *Fusiform aneurysms* are spindle-shaped, local widenings of an entire segment of an artery. Fusiform aneurysms usually involve one of the large feeding arteries or the basilar artery. Those of the internal carotid artery prefer the segment passing through the cavernous sinus, as was demonstrated earlier (see Fig. 3.**17**). They may be the cause of severe neuralgia, particularly in the distribution areas of ophthalmic and maxillary branches of the ipsilateral trigeminal nerve, and may be associated with palsies of oculomotor, trochlear, and abducens nerves.

Such aneurysms may rupture spontaneously or from trauma. The *carotid-cavernous fistula* produces ipsilateral exophthalmus, paralysis of eye muscles, headaches, a bruit synchronous with the pulse, and edematous swelling of the eyelid. A subarachnoid hemorrhage does not occur because the aneurysm is located outside the dura or, more precisely, between the dural leaves forming the sinus. A traumatic carotid-cavernous fistula may occur in the absence of an aneurysm.

Aneurysms of the intracranial carotid may press on optic nerve, chiasm, or optic tract and produce visual field defects and optic atrophy. Waxing and waning of the visual disorder is highly suggestive of an aneurysm.

A unilateral optic atrophy is, in rare instances, the result of an aneurysm of the ophthalmic artery in the area of the optic canal. A larger aneurysm of the anterior communicating artery may bear down on the optic chiasm and be the cause of a bitemporal hemianopsia (Fig. 8.**43b**). An aneurysm of the posterior communicating artery may produce an isolated oculomotor palsy, not unlike a diabetic palsy. An aneurysm of the rostral basilar artery may damage both oculomotor nerves, peduncles, and mamillary bodies.

Blood from a leaking aneurysm collects in the subarachnoid space (Fig. 8.**45**). Signs are those of a rapidly increasing intracranial pressure, characterized by headaches, nausea, retching, vomiting, stiffness of the neck, and clouding of consciousness deteriorating to unconsciousness. A smaller bleeding may produce only local signs, their nature depending on the site and intensity of bleeding.

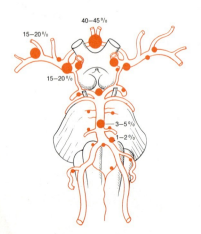

Fig. 8.**43a** Frequency of location of congenital cerebral aneurysms.

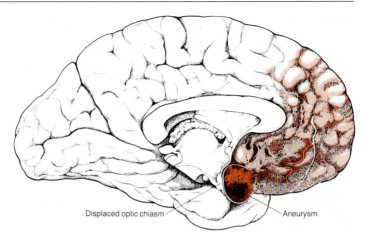

Fig. 8.**43b** Sagittal section through large aneurysm of anterior communicating artery displacing the optic chiasm in caudal direction and causing subarachnoid hemorrhage from leakage (drawn from specimen).

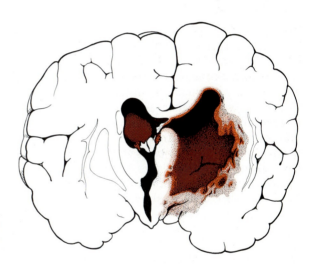

Fig. 8.**44** Apoplectic hematoma in basal ganglia and internal capsule with rupture into ventricles (drawn from specimen).

Occasionally, the blood penetrates into the brain tissue. If such bleeding derives from a middle cerebral artery in the sylvian fissure, it may produce an intracerebral hematoma of the same location and extent as a hypertensive apoplectic hematoma, shown in Fig. 8.**44**. It is also possible for the bleeding spot to face the arachnoid and for the blood to perforate the arachnoid and accumulate in the subdural space in a space-occupying amount simulating a traumatic subdural hematoma.

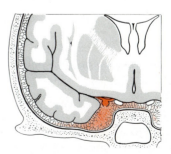

Fig. 8.**45** Subarachnoid hemorrhage from ruptured aneurysm.

If bleeding from an aneurysm is not fatal within the first few hours, it may be survived with proper treatment (Pia et al., 1979). The blood in the subarachnoid space may impede CSF circulation, producing a further increase in intracranial pressure and often a papilledema. Retardation of venous outflow associated with a decrease in arterial pressure may lead to brain edema. Later, subarachnoid adhesions may be the cause of communicating internal hydrocephalus. Recurrence of subarachnoid hemorrhage from aneurysms is rather frequent. The signs and symptoms of subarachnoid hemorrhage may be brought on by an arteriovenous fistula or angioma at or near the surface of the brain.

Arterial dolichoectasia

The term *dolichoectasia* represents a disease entity of larger arteries (including intracranial arteries) characterized by gradually progressing elongation and distention of the arteries caused by changes in their elastic tissue (Sacks and Lindenberg, 1969). This condition has been variously termed *cerebral artery ectasia, fusiform aneurysm,* and *fusiform enlargement*. The large arteries at the base of the brain become very tortuous and giant in caliber. Consequently, they may distort, compress, or erode cranial nerves and brain structures, such as the floor of the third ventricle, the base of the pons, and the ventral medulla oblongata, including the pyramids. Thus the disease may produce one or multiple focal signs, usually simulating involvement by a space-occupying lesion or a disease such as multiple sclerosis.

Hypertensive Arterial Disease and Intracerebral Bleeding

Chronic arterial hypertension is the most frequent cause of necrosis and hyalinosis of arteries. With or without arteriosclerosis of the main arterial stems and branches, these peripheral vascular changes may lead to bleeding into the cerebral tissue.

If the disease is limited to the arterioles, small ball hemorrhages measuring up to 1 to 2 mm in diameter will be found in the gray matter, particularly in the cerebral cortex. They produce no particular focal signs. The small hemorrhages may be associated with slightly larger hematomas extending into the subcortical white matter and spreading along arcuate fibers or into the subarachnoid space.

Focal necrosis and hyalinosis of the media of larger intracerebral arteries is the cause of massive hypertensive hematomas. They occur most often in the striatum (42 percent of 393 fatal cases analyzed by E. Freytag, 1968). The lateral, rather large striatum artery of Charcot is the most frequent source. Next in frequency follow hematomas in pons (16 percent), thalamus (15 percent), cerebellum (12 percent), and various areas of the cerebral white matter (10 percent). Rupture into the ventricles is usually fatal (see Fig. 8.**44**).

In contrast to infarcts, the tissue destruction from bleeding does not respect borders of arterial supply. The hematoma tends to follow the course of least resistance, splitting the tissue rather than crushing it. Perifocal edema may develop rapidly and contribute to a considerable increase in intracranial pressure. With supratentorial hematomas there is the imminent danger of midbrain compression. With cerebellar hematomas the medulla oblongata is likely to be compressed by herniated cerebellar tonsils.

The typical apoplectic hematoma in the striatum (see Fig. 8.**44**) is of sudden onset. The patient collapses as if felled by a stroke and is almost immediately unconscious. Interruption of the internal capsule produces contralateral hemiplegia which is flaccid at first. Because of increasing intracranial pressure, breathing becomes deep and changes to Cheyne-Stokes respiration. The face is flushed. The paralyzed cheek blows with each expiration. The skin is red and moist. Corneal and conjunctival reflexes are absent, as are tendon reflexes. The muscles are flaccid. The paralyzed leg, when dropped, falls down heavily because of its flaccidity. The pupils are wide and react poorly to light because of oculomotor nerve involvement by pressure. Among autonomic signs, bradycardia and hyperthermia are present. The sphincters of rectum and bladder are paralyzed. There is usually a conjugate deviation of the eyes and turning of the head to the side of the lesion. The pressure on the midbrain from tentorial impaction is responsible for coma and death from central respiratory failure. If the patient survives the crisis, the focal signs caused by the lesion will gradually become apparent when consciousness returns.

Not all intracerebral hematomas produce such a dramatic picture. Smaller hematomas (Fig. 8.46) produce at first headaches, dizziness, contralateral weakness, and some clouding of the sensorium. The weakness progresses to hemiplegia as the patient becomes unconscious. Whatever the size of a hematoma may be its breakthrough into the ventricles is always ominous. Deep coma is associated with severe autonomic disorders, such as hyperthermia. The event is rarely survived.

With survival, blood and necrotic brain tissue are gradually resorbed by macrophages. The resulting cyst usually contains scar tissue consisting of connective tissue, proliferated astrocytes, new blood vessels, and many hemosiderin-containing macrophages, giving the scar a yellow tint. The clinical symptomatology may improve, but, as a rule, some degree of spastic hemiplegia, some hypesthesia, and, if the dominant hemisphere was damaged, aphasia and other focal deficits persist.

Epidural hematoma

This lesion is always traumatic and is almost always associated with a skull fracture. A separation of dura and bone during deformation and fracturing of the skull is a prerequisite for the extradural collection of blood from injured dural (meningeal) arteries running in the outer, periosteal layer of the dura (page 239). Once this initial space is filled, continuing bleeding will force the dura to separate further, causing the hematoma to become a considerable, space-occupying mass (Fig. 8.47). Most hematomas are situated over the lateral convexity of a hemisphere, forcing it to shift over the midline and toward the tentorial opening. Pressure of the herniated ipsilateral uncus on the oculomotor nerve where it crosses the sphenoparietal ligament produces a most valuable lateralizing sign: an ipsilateral dilated pupil nonreactive to light and convergence – if the latter can still be tested. Once the diagnosis is made, immediate surgical intervention is a necessity, because fatal respiratory failure from midbrain compression may occur at any time. The finding of bilateral wide pupils, nonreactive to light, indicates that death is imminent. With an extradural hematoma in the posterior

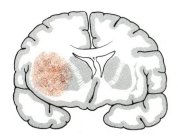

Fig. 8.46 Beginning "claustrum apoplexy" in arterial hypertension.

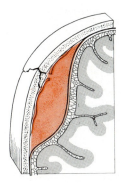

Fig. 8.47 Epidural hematoma (arterial) after skull fracture and injury of middle meningeal artery.

fossa, the medulla oblongata and not the midbrain is in danger of being compressed. In such a case the patient, who may have been conscious for some time, may suddenly and unexpectedly stop breathing and die.

Subdural hematoma

The *acute subdural hematoma* is always traumatic (Fig. 8.**48**). It is most often caused by tears in regular or ectopic bridging veins, those segments of the cerebral veins that cross the subdural space on their way to the dural sinuses. Some hematomas are the result of small contusional holes in branches of cerebral arteries, particularly those of the middle cerebral artery, and in the attached arachnoid at crests of convolutions (Krauland, 1982). There is usually little or no bleeding into the subarachnoid space. The arterial blood may spurt into the subdural space as if coming from a miniature fountain. In cases of more severe head injury, subdural hematoma may result from cortical contusion hematomas bleeding through rents in the arachnoid into the subdural space. The acute subdural may develop as quickly as the epidural hematoma. If the midbrain is damaged by secondary hemorrhages and necroses before the hematoma can be drained, the patient may never regain consciousness during a survival period that may last months or even years.

Subdural blood is organized by cells sprouting from the inner surface of the dura into the blood and by their growth over the free surface of the clot, encapsulating it. During the process of organization, numerous thin-walled blood vessels are formed. These sinusoids may bleed again into the enclosed and often liquefied remainder of the original mass of blood.

The *chronic subdural hematoma* represents such bleeding into membranes or sack of an older subdural hemorrhage that may have been too small to produce symptoms. The new extravasation is often recurrent. It may have no obvious cause or may have been initiated by another, usually trivial head injury (Lindenberg, 1976).

The patient complains of headaches, becomes detached, loses initiative, and shows forgetfulness and perhaps confusion. Neurologic examination is usually normal except for a mild difference in reflexes. A brain tumor may be suspected or, in an elderly person, a beginning senile dementia, a multifocal encephalopathy or a confusional syndrome caused by cardiac insufficiency. Angiography or computed tomography will reveal the true lesion. As much as the patient may have denied a head injury, he probably will remember it when his sensorium clears after removal of the hematoma.

The blood in the encapsulated hematoma may totally dissolve and be replaced with a watery liquid, which acts as space-consuming lesion. This occurs most often in young infants and is referred to as *hygroma*. The enclosing membrane is usually paper-thin.

Veins and Dural Sinuses

External Veins

The capillary blood entering the veins leaves the brain through external and internal veins draining into the large dural sinuses (Figs. 8.**49** to 8.**53**). From the sinuses the blood returns to the heart via internal jugular veins, brachiocephalic veins (venae anonymae), and superior vena cava. A very small

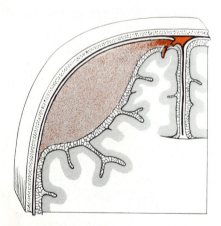

Fig. 8.**48** Subdural hematoma (venous) after injury to bridging veins.

portion of the blood leaves the cerebrum through the venous plexus of the spinal canal and by emissary veins that connect the sinuses with diploic veins and veins of the scalp. The course of many cerebral veins is independent of that of the arteries that supply their territories. These veins drain into the superior longitudinal and transverse sinuses. Other veins run almost parallel to arteries of like names and connect with sinuses at the base of the skull.

The former group consists of the superior cerebral veins, subdivided into dorsal, and medial veins, and of the inferior cerebral veins. The latter group of veins includes the anterior, middle, and posterior cerebral veins (see Figs 8.49 and 8.50).

The *dorsal superior veins* drain the dorsal convexity of the cerebral hemispheres and cross the subdural space as bridging veins before they enter the superior longitudinal sinus. The *medial superior veins* drain most of the medial aspects of the hemispheres and connect more directly with the same sinus. The drainage territories of the superior veins

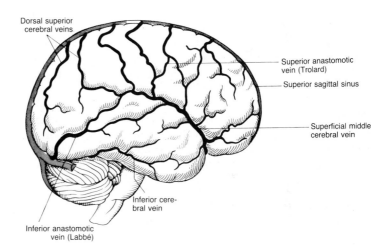

Fig. 8.49 Cerebral veins (lateral view).

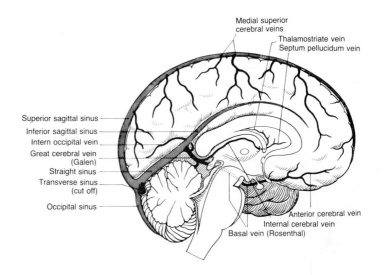

Fig. 8.50 Cerebral veins (medial view).

are bordered by those of the anterior, middle, and posterior veins.

The *inferior cerebral veins* carry the blood of the lower convexity and lateral basal portion of the temporal and occipital lobes and connect with the transverse sinuses after bridging the subdural space.

The *anterior cerebral veins* drain orbital and medial frontal convolutions as well as the rostral corpus callosum. Their blood reaches the straight sinus via the basal veins of Rosenthal.

The *middle cerebral veins* are rather large and form one deep and one superficial channel. The *deep veins* drain the blood from convolutions within the sylvian fissures; the *superficial veins*, that from convolutions surrounding the sylvian fissures and those of the lateral frontal convexities and the lateral orbital lobes. The superficial middle cerebral veins empty into the cavernous sinuses and the deep veins into the basal veins of Rosenthal. The deep and superficial veins anastomose with each other. The superficial veins running over the external sylvian fissures communicate with those dorsal superior veins responsible for the central regions via the *superior anastomotic veins of Trolard*. They are also connected with the inferior cerebral veins at the convexity of the temporal lobes via the *inferior anastomotic vein of Labbé* (see Fig. 8.**49**).

The *basal veins of Rosenthal* and their tributaries are illustrated in Fig. 8.**52**. They run through the basal cisterns and cisternae ambiens to the transverse cistern behind the pineal gland and beneath the splenium of the corpus callosum. There they meet the *internal cerebral veins* and also the *posterior cerebral veins*, which drain the calcarine regions in an occipitofrontal direction (see Fig. 8.**50**). Together, these veins form the *great vein of Galen* which is the largest bridging vein and drains into the straight sinus.

Internal Veins

Whereas the external cerebral veins remove the blood from the cortex and subcortical white matter and also from the lower halves of pallida, striate bodies, and thalami, the internal veins drain the main bulk of the white matter and the dorsal halves of pallida, striata, and thalami. They radiate through the deep white matter toward the lateral ventricles, where they run in the ventricle wall to the lateral angles of the ventricles. There they form longitudinal anastomoses which at various intervals connect with the *thalamostriate veins (terminal veins)* lying on either side in the groove of the ventricle wall flanked by caudate nucleus and thalamus. Only the veins of the medial frontal white matter proceed straight caudally and join the veins of the septum pellucidum.

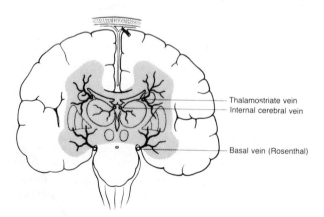

Fig. 8.**51** Internal cerebral veins and drainage areas on coronal section.

Circulatory System of the Cerebrum 323

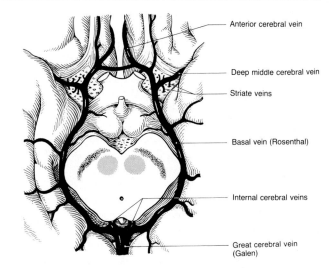

Fig. 8.52 Veins at base of brain.

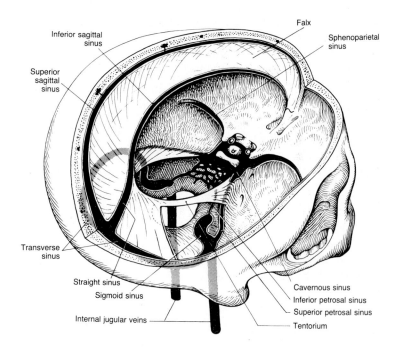

Fig. 8.53 Sinuses of dura mater.

The thalamostriate veins run rostrally toward the foramina of Monro. There they meet the veins of the septum pellucidum and veins of the choroid plexus and form the *internal cerebral veins*. These veins follow the stroma of the choroid plexus in a caudal direction and finally join the basal veins of Rosenthal and the posterior cerebral veins on their way to the great vein of Galen (see Figs. 8.50, 8.51, and 8.52). Also the dorsomedial cerebellar veins drain into this large receiver.

Symptomatology of Venous and Sinus Thromboses

From what has been stated, it is evident that the cerebral veins substantially have their own drainage territories. If venous outflow is obstructed by venous or sinus thrombosis, capillaries and venules in the involved drainage area become engorged, and smaller or larger congestive hemorrhages develop in gray and white matter, leading to necrosis and edema of the tissues in between. Confluence of the individual bleeding spots creates a lesion that may grossly simulate an apoplectic hematoma. The fact that these infarcts are largely limited to the drainage territories of external or internal veins has clinical importance and permits us to speak of syndromes of venous drainage areas (Noetzel and Jerusalem, 1965; Krücke, 1971). For an infarct to occur it is necessary that the stems of the veins at their site of entrance into a sinus be thrombosed. A thrombosis limited to a sinus may remain asymptomatic.

Venous and sinus thromboses are caused by, among other conditions, cardiac and circulatory disorders; toxic diseases; trauma; space-occupying processes; inflammatory diseases of brain, cranium, or cranial sinuses; and also by cachexia, complications during puerperium, epilepsy, leukemia, anemia, coagulopathies and, in newborns and infants, congenital heart defects, infections, and toxic conditions.

Thromboses of cerebral veins are often associated with venous obstruction in other portions of the body, such as pelvis, legs or lungs.

As cerebral veins become thrombosed, there is usually an acute increase in intracranial pressure, causing headaches, nausea, vomiting, depression of sensorium, stiffness of the neck, fever, focal or generalized seizures, papilledema, and, depending on the location of the hemorrhagic infarct, motor and sensory disorders as well as focal signs such as aphasia, visual field defects, ataxia, paralysis of cranial nerves, and extrapyramidal disorders. Leukocytosis and acceleration in the sedimentation rate are common. According to Noetzel and Jerusalem, only one-third of patients exhibit a subacute, chronic, or recurrent course. With supratentorial lesions the increase in cranial pressure usually leads to tentorial impaction, with all its consequences.

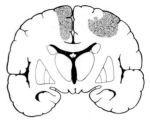

Fig. 8.54 Thrombotic hemorrhagic infarction in drainage area of medial superior cerebral veins (right) and dorsal superior cerebral veins (left).

A thrombosis of the dorsal superior cerebral veins causes a hemorrhagic lesion in the dorsal portion of the hemisphere, resulting in contralateral weakness or hemiplegia, sensory disorders, and perhaps focal signs such as aphasia if the lesion involves the dominant hemisphere (Fig. 8.54). An infarct from thrombosis of the medial superior veins leads to contralateral paralysis of the leg. If the infarct is bilateral, there will be paraparesis of the legs, associated with disorders of bladder control (see Fig. 8.54).

If the inferior cerebral veins are thrombosed, the lesion involves the lower margin of the temporal lobe and part of its convexity and may extend to the occipital lobe (Fig. 8.55). There may be contralateral homonymous hemianopsia from involvement of the optic radiation. If the dominant hemisphere is damaged, aphasia and other focal disorders also will be noted.

Thrombosis of the internal cerebral veins causes stupor that rapidly progresses to coma (Fig. 8.56). There may be signs pointing to bilateral interruption of the pyramidal tract, but the patient's severe state will obscure all other signs. Thrombosis of only a small branch of the thalamostriate vein may produce rigor, trismus, and salivation.

Circulatory System of the Cerebrum

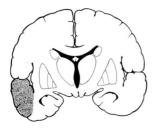

Fig. 8.55 Thrombotic hemorrhagic infarction in right temporal lobe in drainage area of inferior cerebral veins.

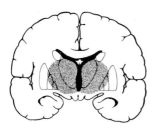

Fig. 8.56 Symmetrical hemorrhagic infarction of thalami and basal ganglia in drainage area of internal cerebral veins.

In the case of venous infarction of the deep cerebral ganglia illustrated in Fig. 8.56, it is notable that the hemispheric white matter shows no such alteration even though it is also primarily drained by the internal veins. This finding indicates that the numerous anastomoses existing between white matter veins and cortical and subcortical veins are able to function under these circumstances. The situation is different if the drainage problem is not limited to a focal area, however large it may be, but is systemic and caused, for example, by an insufficiency of the right heart.

Because of such insufficiency, all cerebral veins will be passively engorged, the white matter veins most severely because their pattern of drainage is not as simple as that of the peripheral veins. As long as the arterial pressure remains normal, the increased intravenous pressure has no detrimental effect on the capillary circulation. If the systemic arterial pressure drops, however, the capillary flow is reduced throughout the brain, and most prominently in the deep white matter where the intravenous pressure to be overcome is the greatest. Consequently, the white matter is under such circumstances more easily exposed to episodes of capillary stagnation than is any other structure of the brain. This is why it occasionally is the only area of the brain that is symmetrically swollen from edema with or without petechiae or shows symmetrical infarctions centered along its arterial border zones (illustrated in Fig. 8.39). Because of the swelling of the brain, the pathologic picture may be complicated by additional alterations related to vascular compression.

These alterations, when occurring during the perinatal period or in early infancy, may be survived and are one of the morphologic substrates of *infantile spastic diplegia.*

Terminal states of venous infarction are very rare in adults, although it may be assumed that smaller infarcts can undoubtedly be survived (Krücke). Larger infarcts, however, are extremely dangerous, and most patients die within the first few days.

Acute cerebral venous thrombosis

The history of one patient of the author is presented as an example of acute thrombosis of the right inferior cerebral veins, the transverse and sigmoid sinuses bilaterally, and the superior longitudinal sinus.

Case report: A 26-year-old woman was admitted four days prior to death on September 4, 1964. She had had occasional frontal headaches during the previous year. On August 26, 1964, frontal and occipital headaches became most severe. The patient became drowsy and somnolent and vomited repeatedly. She noted a tendency to fall to the right. When admitted on September 1, she was drowsy and somnolent but oriented as to time and place. Examination revealed the following: meningism and positive Brudzinski's sign; hematoma of the right eyelid; bilateral abducens palsy, more on the left; papilledema 2 diopters with fundus hemorrhages on the right; mild weakness of the right side of the mouth; increased right arm reflexes; ataxia during finger-nose test, more on the left; decreased abdominal reflexes; decreased strength in both legs, more on the left;

increased patellar and Achilles tendon reflexes on the right; and bilateral ataxia during knee-heel test. She had no sensory disorders and no spastic toe reflexes. Electroencephalography showed moderately severe, generalized changes in the parietooccipital areas, with slow waves left parietooccipital and signs of focal irritation. Left angiography revealed the branches of the anterior and middle cerebral arteries to be somewhat narrow and stretched. The position of the arch of the pericallosal artery appeared lower than normal. After a poorly focused capillary phase, the usual picture of cortical veins was missing bilaterally. The angulus venosus and a number of descending basal veins showed good filling. Arterial circulation was delayed. The poor representation of the marginal veins, the relative engorgement of the internal cerebral veins, and the stretching of the arteries strongly suggested a thrombosis of the longitudinal sinuses. Scintigram was normal. Blood sedimentation rate was: first hour, 21; second hour 49. Leukocyte count was 18,000.

The intracranial pressure increased acutely on the third day of hospitalization. The patient slipped into coma. The left pupil was dilated, the right was rather narrow, and neither reacted to light. Cardiac dysrhythmias were followed by central respiratory failure.

Postmortem examination (Dr. Hübner) revealed a not very fresh thrombosis obstructing the superior longitudinal sinus, the superior veins, and the transverse and sigmoid sinuses bilaterally. There was severe brain swelling with flattening of convolutions and pressure notches along hippocampal gyri and herniated cerebellar tonsils. All ventricles were narrow. The white matter of the entire right cerebral hemisphere was swollen. There was a massive recent confluent hematoma in the right temporal lobe extending from the level of the insula to the temporooccipital border. The cortex near the hematoma was interspersed with petechial hemorrhages. The left frontal lobe showed an older hematoma the size of a prune. Microscopic examination of the superior longitudinal sinus revealed a not very fresh thrombosis. Sections of the hematoma and its neighboring areas failed to reveal a hemangioma as cause of the hematoma. Findings thus indicated a not very fresh thrombosis of several dural sinuses causing fresh massive hematoma in the right temporal lobe.

What has been called "massive hematoma" in this report is probably a hemorrhagic venous infarct characterized by the confluence of numerous congestive bleedings. Bilateral neurologic signs resulted from swelling of the brain and the considerable increase in intracranial pressure. The presence of exaggerated reflexes ipsilateral to the right-sided temporal lobe lesion is explained by the notching of the left cerebral peduncle from being pressed against the tentorial margin as a result of midbrain displacement to the left (Kernohan's notch or crus syndrome).

Undoubtedly, such cases of extensive venous and sinus thrombosis are rare. One must assume that less dramatic obstructions of these drainage channels do occur but often fail to produce characteristic signs. In view of the extensive network of venous collaterals, it is not surprising that the obstructions remain asymptomatic. They do, however, produce brain swelling and increased intracranial pressure and therefore headaches, nausea, vomiting, clouding of the sensorium, and perhaps seizures or focal signs, depending on the location of the ischemic or at least oligemic drainage territory. Papilledema occurs and raises the danger that venous or sinus thrombosis will be mistaken for a brain tumor. A serial phlebogram should help in arriving at an accurate diagnosis. It is true that in time the thrombi become recanalized, but this does not remove the danger of recurrence of thrombosis. Perhaps this condition will be diagnosed more frequently if one remembers to consider it among differential diagnostic possibilities. It is much easier to diagnose phlebitic or septic venous or sinus thromboses, often caused by inflammatory processes involving adjacent cranial sinuses. The condition is sometimes suggested by general signs of an infection (fever, leukocytosis, and accelerated sedimentation rate).

It must be mentioned at this point that a tumor and not a thrombus may be obstructing a dural sinus and may be the cause of pseudotumor cerebri. A phlebogram may demonstrate the site of the obstruction. The tumor may be a meningioma that grew within the confines of the sinus. The diagnosis was missed in the patient described in the following report.

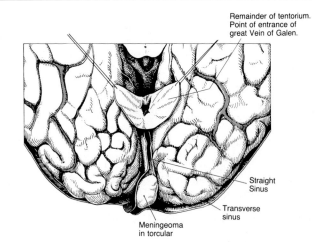

Fig. 8.57 Meningioma in confluence of sinuses (torcular) caused brain swelling from impeded venous drainage (drawn from specimen).

Case report: A 51-year-old man developed headaches, weakness in both legs, and blurring of vision. Blood pressure was elevated, and his condition was diagnosed as stroke. Electrocardiography and radiography of the skull showed no abnormalities. CSF was normal. Shortly after the spinal tap, the patient stopped breathing and fatal cardiac arrest followed. The brain was swollen and hyperemic postmortem. The midbrain was edematous from pressure. When the superior longitudinal sinus was opened, a meningioma was found within the torcular (Fig. 8.57), blocking the outflow from the superior longitudinal sinus and, partially, that from the straight sinus (Lindenberg, Walsh, and Sacks, 1973).

References

Adams, R. D., V. Maurice: Principles of Neurology. McGraw-Hill, New York 1977

Adrian, E. D.: Afferent discharges to the cerebral cortex from peripheral sense organs. J. Physiol. (Lond.) 100 (1941) 159–191

Adrian, E. D.: The Physical Background of Perception. Clarendon Press, Oxford 1947

Alling, C. A.: Facial Pain. Lea & Febiger, Philadelphia 1968

Aminoff, M. J.: Electrodiagnosis in Clinical Neurology. Churchhill-Livingstone, Edinburgh 1980

Anochin, P. K.: Beiträge zur allgemeinen Theorie des funktionellen Systems. VEB Fischer, Jena 1978

Asbury, K., P. C. Johnson: Pathology of Peripheral Nerve, Saunders. Philadelphia 1978

Bailey, P.: Die Hirngeschwülste, Enke, Stuttgart 1936; 2nd ed. 1951

Bailey, P., C. v. Bonin: The Isocortex of Man. University of Illinois Press, Urbana/III. 1951

Barr, M. L.: The Human Nervous System. Harper & Row, New York 1972

Bartholow, R.: Experimental investigations into the functions of the human brain. Amer. J. med. Sci 67 (1874) 305–313

Basset, D. L.: A Stereoscopic Atlas of Human Anatomy, Section I. Sawyers, Portland/Oregon 1952

Bay, E.: Der gegenwärtige Stand der Aphasieforschung. Nervenarzt 44 (1973) 57–64

Beck, E.: Zur Exaktheit der myeloarchitektonischen Felderung des Cortex cerebri. J. Psychol. Neurol. 31 (1925) 5

Beck, E.: Die Myeloarchitektonik der dorsalen Schäfenlappenrinde beim Menschen. J. Psychol. Neurol. 41 (1930) 129–262

Beevor, C. E., V. A. Horsley: An experimental investigation into the arrangement of the exitable fibres of the bonnet monkey. Phil. Trans. 181 B (1890) 49–68

Beringer, K., I. Stein: Analyse eines Falles von "reiner Alexie". Z. ges. Neurol. Psychiat. 123 (1930) 472–478

Biemond, A.: Brain Diseases. Elsevier, Amsterdam 1970

Bing, R.: Kompendium der topischen Gehirn und Rückenmarksdiagnostik, 9th ed. Urban & Schwarzenberg, Wien 1934; 14th ed. Schwabe, Basel 1953

Bing, R.: Lehrbuch der Nervenkrankheiten. Schwabe, Basel 1952

Bodechtel, G.: Differentialdiagnose neurologischer Krankheitsbilder, 3rd ed. Thieme, Stuttgart 1974; 4, Aufl. 1984

v. Bonin, G.: The Evolution of the Human Brain. University of Chicago Press, Chicago 1963

Bossy, J.: Atlas of Neuroanatomy and Special Sense Organs. Saunders, Philadelphia 1978

Bostroem, A., H. Spatz: Über die von der Olfactoriusrinne ausgehenden Meningeome und über die Meningeome im allgemeinen. Nervenarzt 2 (1929) 505–521

v. Braitenberg, V.: Gehirngespinste, Neuroanatomie für kybernetisch Interessierte. Springer, Berlin 1973

Braus, H.: Anatomie des Menschen. Springer, Berlin 1960

Brazis, P. W., I. C. Masdeu, I. Biller: Localization in Clinical Neurology. Little Brown & Co., Boston 1985

Broca, P.: Rémarques sur le siège da la faculté du language articulé. Bull. Soc. anat. Paris 36, (1861) 330–357

Broca, P.: Recherches sur la localisation de la faculté du langage articulé. Expose des titres et travaus scintifiques 1868

Broca, P.: Anatomie comparée circonvolutions cérébrales. Le grand lobe limbique et la scissure limbique dans la série des mammifères. Rev. anthropol. Ser. 2, 1 (1878) 384–498

Brock, M., C. Fieschi, D. H. Ingvar, N. A. Lassew, K. Schürmann: Cerebral Blood Flow, Springer, Berlin 1969

Brock, S., H. P. Kriger: The Basis of Clinical Neurology, Williams & Wilkins, Baltimore 1963

Brodal, A.: Neurological Anatomy in Relation to Clinical Medicine, 2nd ed. Oxford University Press, London 1969

Brodmann, K.: Vergleichende Lokalisationslehre der Großhirnrinde in ihren Prinzipien darge-

stellt auf Grund des Zellaufbaus. Barth, Leipzig 1909; Neudruck 1925
Broser, F.: Topische und klinische Diagnostik neurologischer Krankheiten. Urban & Schwarzenberg, München 1975
Brown, B. St. J.: Radiographic studies of the vertebral arteries in cadavers. Effects of position and traction on the head. Radiology 81 (1963) 80–88
Brown, J. G.: Aphasie, Apraxie und Agnosie. Fischer, Stuttgart 1975
Bucy, P. C.: Cortical extirpation in the treatment of involuntary movements, Res. Publ. Ass. nerv. ment. Dis. 21 (1942) 551
Bucy, P. C.: The Precentral Motor Cortex, University of Illinois Press, Urbana/Ill. 1944
Bumke, O., O. Foerster: Handbuch der Neurologie, Springer, Berlin 1935
Buser, P. A., A. Rougal-Buser: Cerebral Correlates of Conscious Experience. Inserm. Symp. 6. North-Holland Publ., Amsterdam 1978
Cajal, S. R.: Histologie du systeme nerveux de l'homme et des vertèbres. Maloine, Paris 1911
Cajal, S. R.: Die Neuronenlehre. Ref. in: Handbuch der Neurologie, Vol. 1, ed. by O. Bumke, O. Foerster. Springer, Berlin 1935
Campbell, A. W.: Histological Studies on the Localisation of Cerebral Function. Cambridge University Press, Cambridge 1905
Cantor, F. K.: Trans. global amnesia and temporal lobe seizures. Neurology (Minneap.) 21 (1971) 857–867
Carpenter, M. B.: Human Neuroanatomy, 7th ed. Williams & Wilkins, Baltimore 1976
Chrast, B., J. Korbicka: Die Beeinflussung der Strömungsverhältnisse in der A. vertebralis durch verschiedene Kopf- und Halshaltungen. Dtsch. Z. Nervenheilk. 183 (1962) 426–448
Christian, W.: Klinische Elektroenzephalographie, 2nd ed. Thieme, Stuttgart 1975; 3rd ed. 1982
Chusid, I. G.: Correlative Neuroanatomy and Functional Neurology, 14th ed. Lange, Los Altos/Calif. 1970
Clara, M.: Das Nervensystem des Menschen. Barth, Leipzig 1942
Creutzfeldt, O. D.: Cortex cerebri, Springer, Berlin 1983
Critchley, M.: The Parietal Lobes (Reprint of 1953), Hafner, New York 1966
Cushing, H.: The field defects produced by temporal lobe lesions. Brain 44 (1922) 341–396
Cushing, H.: Intracranial Tumors: Notes upon a Series of Two Thousand Verified Cases. Thomas, Springfield/Ill, 1932
Darley, F. L.: Aphasia. Saunders, Philadelphia 1982
Dejérine, J., G. Roussy: Le syndrome talamique, Rev. neurol. 14 (1906) 521–532
Denny-Brown, D.: The nature of apraxia. J. nerv. ment. Dis. 126 (1958) 9–32
Denny-Brown, D.: The Basal Ganglia and Their Relation to Disorders of Movement. Oxford University Press, London 1962
Denny-Brown, D.: The Cerebral Control of Movement. Liverpool University Press, Liverpool 1966
Dietz, H.: Die frontal-basale Schädelhirnverletzung. Springer, Berlin 1970
Doane, B. K., K. F. Livingston; The Limbic System. Raven Press, New York 1986
Dusser de Barenne, I. G.: Experimental researches on sensory localisations in the cerebral cortex. Quart. J. exp. Physiol. 9 (1916) 355–390
Dusser des Barenne, I. G.: The mode and site of action of strychnine in the nervous system. Physiol. Rev. 13 (1933) 325–335
Duus, P.: Über psychische Störungen bei Tumoren des Orbitalhirns. Arch. Psychiat. Nervenkr. 109 (1939) 596–648
Duus, P.: Die percutane Arteriographie. Nervenarzt 13 (1940) 350–53
Duus, P.: Über die Arteriographie der Hirngefäße mittels der perkutanen Methode. Techn. Assist. 1 (1943) 10
Duus, P.: Die Einengung der Foramina intervertebralia infolge von degenerativen Prozessen als Ursache von neuralgischen Schmerzzuständen im Bereich des Schulter- und Beckengürtels sowie der Extremitäten. Nervenarzt 19 (1948) 489–503
Duus, P.: Zur neurologischen Differentialdiagnose der Wirbelsäulenerkrankungen. Allg. Z. Psychiat. 124 (1949) 188–217
Duus, P.: Neurologische Syndrome bie Einengung der Foramina intervertebralia. Wien. med. Wschr. 124 (1974) 9–13
Duus, P., K. Speckmann: Über die Grenzen der Encephalographie und Arteriographie in der Diagnostik von Hirntumoren. Zbl. Neurochir. 7 (1943) 122–128
Duus, P., G. Kahlau, W. Krücke: Allgemeinpathologische Betrachtungen über die Einengung der Foramina intervertebralia. Langenbecks Arch. klin. Chir. 268 (1951) 341–62
Duvernoy, H. M.: Human Brainstem Vessels. Springer, Berlin 1978
Eccles, I. C.: Das Gehirn des Menschen. Piper, München 1975
Eccles, J. C., M. Ito, J. Szentàgothai: The Cerebellum as a Neuronal-Machine. Springer, Berlin 1967
v. Economo, C.: Zellaufbau der Großhirnrinde des Menschen, Springer, Berlin 1927
v. Economo, C., G. N. Koskinas: Die Cytoarchitektonik der Hirnrinde des erwachsenen Menschen. Springer, Wien 1925
Edinger, L.: Bau der nervösen Zentralorgane des Menschen und der Tiere, Bd. I und II, 7, Aufl. Vogel, Leipzig 1904
Edwards, C. H.: Neurology of Ear, Nose and Throat Diseases. Butterworths, London 1973

Elliot, F. A.: Clinical Neurology, Saunders, Philadelphia 1964

Elliot, H. C.: Textbook of Neuroanatomie, 2nd ed. Lippincott, Philadelphia 1969

Esslen, E.: The Acute Facial Palsies. Springer, Berlin 1970

Faust, C.: Die zerebralen Herdstörungen bei Hinterhauptsverletzungen und ihre Beurteilung. Thieme, Stuttgart 1955

Feneis, H.: Anatomisches Bildwörterbuch, 5. Aufl. Thieme, Stuttgart 1982

Ferrier, D.: The Function of the Brain. Smith & Elder, London 1876

Feuchtwanger, E.: Die Funktionen des Gehirns. Springer, Berlin 1923

Filimonoff, I. N.: Zur embryonalen und postembryonalen Entwicklung der Großhirnrinde des Menschen. J. Psychol. Neurol. 39 (1929) 323–89

Fisher, C. M., R. D. Adams: Transient global amnesia. Trans. Amer. neurol. Ass. 83 (1958) 143–148

Fitz Gerald, M. T. I.: Neuroanatomy. Basic and Applied. Baillière, Tindall & Cassell, London 1985

Flechsig, F.: Anatomie des menschlichen Gehirns und Rückenmarks auf myelogenetischer Grundlage, Bd. I. Thieme, Leipzig 1920

Flourens, P.: Recherches experimentales sur les propriétés et les fonctions du systéme nerveux dans les animaux vertébrés. Crevot, Paris 1824

Foerster, O.: Motorische Felder und Bahnen. In Bumke, O., O. Foerster: Handbuch der Neurologie, Bd. VI. Springer, Berlin 1936

Foerster, O.: Sensible corticale Felder. In Bumke, O., O. Foerster: Handbuch der Neurologie, Bd. VI. Springer, Berlin 1936

Foerster, O., O. Gagel: Ein Fall von Ependymzyste des 3. Ventrikels. Ein Beitrag zur Frage der Beziehungen psychischer Störungen zum Hirnstamm. Z. Neurol. 149 (1934) 312

Fogelholm, Kivalo, Bergstöem: The transient global amnesia syndrome. An analysis of 35 cases. Brain 13 (1975) 72–84

Foix, C., P. Hillemand: Les artères de l'axe incéphaliques jusqu'au diencéphale inclusivement. Rev. neurol. 2 (1925) 705

Ford, F. R.: Diseases of the Nervous System in Infancy, Childhood and Adolescence, 5th ed. Thomas, Springfield/Ill. 1966

Freeman, W., I. W. Watts: Psychosurgery, Thomas, Springfield/Ill. 1942

Freeman, W., J. W. Watts: Psychosurgery in the Treatment of Mental Disorders and Intractable Pain. Thomas, Springfield/Ill. 1950

Freytag, E.: Fatal rupture of intracranial aneurysms. Arch. Path. 81 (1966) 418–424

Freytag, E.: Fatal hypertensive intracerebral hematomas: a survey of the pathologic anatomy of 393 cases. J. Neuro. Neurosurg. Psychiat. 31 (1968) 616–620

Friede, R. L.: Developmental Neuropathology, Springer, Berlin 1975

Frowein, R. A., M. Brock, M. Klinger (Edit.): Head Injuries. Prognosis, Evoked Potentials, Microsurgery, Brain, Death. Springer Berlin, Heidelberg 1989

Fritsch, G., E. Hitzig: Über die elektrische Erregbarkeit des Großhirns. Arch. Anat. Physiol, (wiss. Med.) 37 (1870) 300–332

Fulton, J.: Physiologie des Nervensystems. Enke, Stuttgart 1952

Gagel, O.: Einführung in die Neurologie. Springer, Berlin 1949

Gänshirt, H.: Der Hirnkreislauf. Thieme, Stuttgart 1972

Gardner, E.: Fundamentals of Neurology. Saunders, Philadelphia 1968

Gastaut, H.: Clinical and electroencephalographical classification of epileptic seizures. Epilepsia 11 (1970) 102

Gazzaniga, M. S., I. E. Bogen, R. W. Sperry: Observations on visual perception after disconnection of the cerebral hemispheres in man. Brain 88 (1965) 221–236

Gazzaniga, M. S., R. W. Sperry: Language after section of the cerebral commissures. Brain 90 1967, 131–148

Gerstenbrand, F.: Das traumatische apallische Syndrom. Springer, Wien 1967

Gerstmann, J.: Fingeragnosie. Wien. klin. Wschr. 37 (1924) 1010–12

Gerstmann, J.: Syndrome of finger agnosia, disorientation for right or left, agraphia and acalculia: local diagnostical value. Arch. Neurol. Psychiat. (Chic.) 44 (1940) 389–408

Geschwind, N.: Disconnection syndrome in animals and man, Part. 1., Part II. Brain 88 (1965) 237–294, 585–644

Geschwind, N., W. Levitsky: Human brain, left-right asymmetries in temporal speech region. Science 16 (1968) 168–187

Geschwind, N.: Language and the brain. Sci. Amer. 226 (1972) 76–83

Gillespie, I. A.: Extracranial Cerebrovascular Disease and its Management, Butterworth, London 1969

Gilman, S., J. R. Bloedel, R. Lechtenberg: Disorders of the Cerebellum. Davis, Philadelphia 1981

Glees, P.: Das menschliche Gehirn., Hippokrates, vensystems. Thieme, Stuttgart 1957

Glees, P.: Das menschliche Gehrin, Hippokrates, Stuttgart 1970

Goldensohn, E. S., St. H. Appel: Scientific Approaches to clinical Neurology, vol. I and II. Lea & Febiger, Philadelphia 1977

Goldstein, K.: Die Lokalisation in der Großhirnrinde. In Bethe-Bergmann, J.: Hand-

buch der normalen und pathologischen Physiologie, Bd. X. Springer, Berlin 1927 (S. 600–842)
Granit, R.: The Basis of Motor Control. Academic Press, London 1970
Green, J. D.: The hippocampus. Physiol. Rev. 44 (1964) 561–608
Grünbaum, A. S. F., C. S. A. Sherrington: Observations on the physiology of the cerebral cortex of some of the higher apes. Proc. roy. Soc. Ser. B. 69 (1901) 206–209
Gudden, B.: Experimentaluntersuchungen über das periphere und centrale Nervensystem. Arch. Psychiat. Nervenkr. 1870, 693–723
Guillain, G., P. Mollaret: Deux cas de myoclonies synchrones et rythmées vélopharyngolaryngo-oculo-diaphragmatiques. Rev. neurol. 2 (1931) 245–566
Guyton, A. C.: Structure and Function of the Nervous System. Saunders, Philadelphia 1972
Hallen, O.: Klinische Neurologie, Springer, Berlin 1973
Hamburger, F. A., F. Hollwich: Augenmuskellähmungen. Enke, Stuttgart 1966; 2, Aufl. 1977
Hansen, K., H. Schliack: Segmentale Innervation. Thieme, Stuttgart 1962
Harmel, M. H.: Neurologic Considerations. Blackwell, Oxford 1967
Hassler, R.: Zur Pathologie der Paralysis agitans und des postencephalitischen Parkinsonismus. J. Psychol. Neurol. 48 (1938) 387–476
Hassler, R.: Anatomie des Thalamus. Arch. Psychiat. Nervenkr. 184 (1950) 249–256
Hassler, R.: Extrapyramidal-motorische Syndrome. Erkrankungen des Kleinhirns. In v. Bergmann, G., W. Frey, H. Schwiejk: Handbuch der Inneren Medizin, Bd. III, 4. Aufl. Springer, Berlin 1953
Hassler, R.: Zum Problem der Alexie (Fall Beringer u. Stein). Nervenarzt 25 (1954) 213
Hassler, R.: Die extrapyramidalen Rindensysteme und die zentrale Regelung der Motorik. Dtsch. Z. Nervenheilk. 175 (1956) 233–258
Hassler, R.: Anatomy of the thalamus. In Schaltenbrand, G., P. Bailey: Introduction to Stereotaxis with an Atlas of the Human Brain. Grune & Stratton, New York 1959
Hassler, R.: Motorische und sensible Effekte umschriebener Reizungen und Ausschaltungen im menschlichen Zwischenhirn. Dtsch. Z. Nervenheilk. 183 (1961) 148–171
Hassler, R.: Spezifische und unspezifische Systeme des menschlichen Zwischenhirns. Progr. Brain Res. 5 (1964) 1–32
Hassler, R.: Zur funktionellen Anatomie des limbischen Systems. Nervenarzt 35, (1964) 386–396
Hassler, R.: Thalamic regulation of muscle tone and the speed of movements. In Purpura, P., M. D. Yahr: Thalamus. Columbia University Press, New York 1966

Hassler, R.: Funktionelle Neuroanatomie und Psychiatrie. In Gruhle, H. W., R. Jung, W. Mayer-Gross, M. Müller: Psychiatrie der Gegenwart, Bd. I. Springer, Berlin 1967
Hassler, R.: Physiopathology of rigidity, In Sigfried, J.: Parkinson Disease, Bd. I. Huber, Bern 1973
Hassler, R.: Fiber connections within the extrapyramidal system. Confin. neurol. 36 (1974) 237–255
Hassler, R., T. Riechert: Klinische und anatomische Befunde bei stereotakischen Schmerzoperationen im Thalamus. Arch. Psychiat. Nervenkr. 200 (1959) 93–122
Hatcher, M. A., G. K. Klintworth: Sylvian aqueduct syndrome. Arch. Neurol. (Chic.) 15 (1966) 215–222
Hausmann, L.: Illustrations of the Nervous System. Atlas III. Thomas, Springfield/III. 1961
Haymaker, W.: Bing's Lokal Diagnosis in Neurological Diseases, 15th ed. Mosby, St. Louis 1969
Head, H.: Studies in Neurology, Oxford University Press, London 1920
Heathfield, K. W., P. B. Croft, M. Swash: The syndrome of transient global amnesia. Brain 96 (1973) 729–736
Hecaen, H.: Right Hemisphere Contribution to Language Function, Cerebral Correlates of Conscious Experience. Inserm Symp. 6 Ed. Buser, P. A., & Rougal-Buser, Elsevier Biomedical Press 1978
Heiss, W. D. et al.: Atlas der Positronen Emissions-Tomographie des Gehirns. Springer, Berlin, Heidelberg 1985
Herrschaft, H.: Die Zirkulationsstörungen der A. vertebralis Arch. Psychiat. Nervenkr. 213 (1970) 22–45
Herrschaft, H.: Die regionale Gehirndurchblutung. Springer, Berlin 1975
Hess, W. R.: Das Zwischenhirn, Schwabe, Basel 1949
Hess, W. R.: The Functional Organization of the Diencephalon. Grune & Stratton, New York 1957
Hess, W. R.: Hypothalamus und Thalamus. Thieme, Stuttgart 1956: 2, Aufl. 1968
Heyck, H., G. Laudahn: Die progressiv-dystrophischen Myopathien. Springer, Berlin 1969
Highstein, M.: Abducens to Medial Pathway in the MLF. Cellular Basis for the Syndrom of Internuclear Ophthalmoplegia, Arvo Symposium 1976. Plenum Press, New York
Holmes, G.: Introduction to Clinical Neurology, 2nd ed. Williams & Wilkins, Baltimore 1952
Horel, J. A.: The Neuroanatomia of Amnesia, Brain 101 (1978) 403–445
House, E. L., B. Pansky: A Functional Approach to Neuroanatomy, 2nd ed. McGraw-Hill, New York 1967

Hubel, D. H., T. N. Wiesel: Ferrier lecture: Functional architecture of macaque monkey visual cortex. Proc. roy. Soc. Serv. B 198 (1977) 1–59

Hubel, D. H., T. N. Wiesel, P. M. Stryker: Anatomical demonstration of orientation columns in macaque monkey. J. comp. Neurol. 177 (1978) 361–397

Huhn, A.: Die Thrombosen der intrakraniellen Venen und Sinus. Fortschr. Neurol. Psychiat. 25 (1957) 440–472

Jackson, J. Hughlings: Loss of speech. Lond. Hosp. Rep. 1864, 388–471

Jacobsen, C. F.: Functions of frontal association areas in primates. Arch. Neurol. Psychiat. (Chic.) 33 (1935) 558–569

Jannetta, P. J.: Arterial compression of the trigeminal nerve at the pons in patients with trigeminal neuralgia. J. Neurosurg. 26 (1967) 150–162

Jannetta, P. J., M. H. Benett: The Pathophysiology of Trigeminal Neuralgia. In "The Cranial Nerves", ed. by M. Samii and P. J. Jannetta, Springer, Berlin 1981, 312–315

Jannetta, P. J.: „Vascular Dekompression in the Trigeminal Neuralgia." The Cranial Nerves, ed. by M. Samii and P. J. Jannetta. Springer 1981, 331–340

Janz, D.: Die Epilepsien, Thieme, Stuttgart 1969

Janzen, R.: Elemente der Neurologie. Springer, Berlin 1969

Janzen, R.: Körper, Hirn und Personalität. Enke, Stuttgart 1973; 2, Aufl 1977

Janzen, R.: Neurologische Diagnostik, Therapie, Prognostik für Arzte und Studierende. Enke, Stuttgart 1975

Jellinger, R.: Zur Orthologie und Pathologie der Rückenmarksdurchblutung. Springer, Wien 1966

Jung, R.: Allgemeine Neurophysiologie. In Bergmann, G. V., W. Frey, H. Schwiegk: Handbuch der Inneren Medizin, Bd. V/1 und III, 4, Aufl. Springer, Berlin 1953

Jung, R.: Einführung in die Bewegungsphysiologie. In Gauer, O. H., K. Kramer, R. Jung: Physiologie des Menschen, Bd. XIV. Urban & Schwarzenberg, München 1976

Kahle, W.: Die Entwicklung der menschlichen Großhirnhemisphaere. In Bauer, H. J., H. Gänshirt, H. Spatz, P. Vogel: Schriftenreihe Neurologie, Bd. I. Springer, Berlin 1969

Kandel, E. R., I. H. Schwarz: Principles of Neural Science, Arnold, London 1981

Kappers, Ariens, C. V.: Die vergleichende Anatomie des Nervensystems der Wirbeltiere und des Menschen, Bohn, Haarlem 1921

Katzmann, R., R. Terry: The Neurology of Aging. Contemporary Neurology Series, vol. XXII, Davis, Philadelphia 1983

Kernohan, I. W., H. Woltmann: Incisura of the crus due to contralateral braintumor. Arch. Neurol. Psychiat. 21 (1929) 274–287

Kessel, F. K., L. Guttmann, G. Maurer: Neuro-Traumatologie mit Einschluß der Grenzgebiete, Bd. II. Urban & Schwarzenberg, München 1969

Klein, R., W. Mayer-Gross: The Clinical Examination of Patients with Organic Cerebral Disease. Cassell, London 1957

Kleist, K.: Gehirnpathologie. In: Handbuch der ärztlichen Erfahrungen im Weltkrieg 1914/18, Bd. IV. Barth, Leipzig 1922–1934

Kleist, K.: Sensorische Aphasien und Amusien auf myeloarchitektonischer Grundlage. Thieme. Stuttgart 1959

Klüver, H.: "The temporal lobe syndrome" produced by bilateral ablations. In: Neurological Basis of Behaviour. Ciba Found. Symp. Churchill, London 1958 (pp. 175–182)

Klüver, H., P. Bucy: Preliminary analysis of functions of the temporal lobes in monkeys. Arch. Neurol. Psychiat. (Chic.) 42, (1939) 979–1000

Kornhuber, H. H.: Motor functions of cerebellum and basal ganglia. Kybernetik 8 (1971) 157–162

Kornhuber, H. H., L. Deecke: Hirnpotentialänderungen bei Willkürbewegungen und passiven Bewegungen des Menschen. Bereitschaftspotential und re-afferente Potentiale. Pflügers Arch. ges. Physiol. 284 (1965) 1–17

Kornhuber, H. H. (Edit.): The Somatosensory System. G. Thieme, Publ. Stuttgart 1975.

Krauland, W.: Verletzungen der intrakraniellen Schlagadern. Springer, Berlin 1982

Krayenbühl, H., M. G. Yarsargil: Die vaskulären Erkrankungen im Gebiet der Arteria vertebralis and Arteria basialis. Thieme, Stuttgart 1957

Krücke, W.: Über das Längsbündel in der Substantia gelatinosa zentralis des Rückenmarkes (Fasciculus parependymalis) und über seine Bedeutung für die Verbindung der vegetativen Zentren des Hirnstammes mit denen des Rückenmarkes. Dtsch. Z. Nervenheilk. 1960 (1948) 196–220

Krücke, W.: Pathologie der cerebralen Venen- und Sinusthrombosen. Radiologe 11 (1971) 370

Kuffler, S. W., J. G. Nicholls: From Neuron to Brain. Sinauer, Sunderland/Mass. 1977

Lance, I. W., I. G. McLeod: A Physiological Approach to Clinical Neurology, 3rd ed. Butterworth, London 1981

Lang, J., H.-P. Jensen, F. Schröder: "Praktische Anatomie", Herausgegeben von J. Lang, W. Wachsmuth. 1. Band, 1. Teil Kopf, Teil A Übergeordnete Systeme. Springer, Berlin 1985

Lang. J.: "Topographical Anatomy of the Cranial Nerves, in "The Cranial Nerves" ed. by M. Samii and P. J. Jannetta, Springer, 1981, 6–15

Lang, J., R. Baldauf: Beitrag zur Gefäßversorgung des Rückenmarks. Gegenbaurs morph. Jb. 129 (1983) 57–95

Lange-Cosack, H.: Anatomie und Klinik der Gefäßmißbildungen des Gehirns und seiner Häute, In Olivecrona, H., W. Tönnis: Handbuch der Neurochirurgie, Bd. IV/2, Springer, Berlin 1966

Larsell, O.: Comparative Anatomy and Histology of the Cerebellum from Myxinoids through Birds. University of Minnesota Press, Minneapolis 1967

Lazorthes, G.: Vascularisation et circulation cerebrales. Masson, Paris 1961

Leiber, B., G. Olbrich: Die klinischen Syndrome, 5. Aufl. Urban & Schwarzenberg, München 1972

Leibowitz, U.: Epidemic incidence of Bell's palsy, Brain 92 (1969) 109–114

Leigh, R. J., D. S. Zee: The Neurology of Eye Movements, vol. XXIII of the Contemporary Neurology Series. Davis, Philadelphia 1983

Lenz, G.: Zwei Sektionsfälle doppelseitiger zentraler Farbenhemianopsie. Z. ges. Neurol. Psychiat. 81 (1921) 135–186

Levy-Agresti, I., R. W. Sperry: Differential perceptual capacities in major and minor hemispheres. Proc. nat. Acad. Sci (Wash.) 61 (1968) 1151

Lewis, A. I.: Mechanisms of Neurological Disease. Little, Brown & Co., Boston 1976

Liepmann, H.: Das Krankheitsbild der Apraxie, Karger, Berlin 1900

Lindenberg, R.: Compression of brain arteries as pathogenetic factor for tissue necroses and their areas of predilection. J. Neuropath. exp. Neurol. 14 (1955) 223–243

Lindenberg, R. Patterns of CNS vulnerability in acute hypoxemia including anestesia accidents. In Schadé, J. P., W. H. McMenemy: Selective Vulnerability of the Brain in Hypoxemia. Blackwell, Oxford 1963 pp. 189–209

Lindenberg, R.: Trauma of meninges and brain. In Minckler, J.: Pathology of the Nervous System, vol. II. McGraw-Hill, New York 1971a

Lindenberg, R.: Systemic oxygen deficiencies. In Minckler, J.: Pathology of the Nervous System, vol. II. McGraw-Hill, New York 1971b

Lindenberg, R.: How they settled for the calcarine cortex. In Glaser, J. S.: Neuro-Ophthalmology, vol. IX. Mosby, St. Louis 1977

Lindenberg, R.: Anoxia does not produce brain damage. Special Communication. Jap. J. Leg. Med. 36 (1982a) 38–57

Lindenberg, R.: Tissue reactions in the gray matter of the central nervous system. In Haymaker, W., R. D. Adams: Histology and Histopathology of the Nervous System, vol. I. Chapter 12. Thomas, Springfield/III. 1982a (pp. 973–1275)

Lindenberg, R.: The Brain in Shock. Chapter 34 (pp. 413–434) in Robert M. Hardaway: Shock: The Reversible Stage of Dying. PSG Publ. Co, Littleton, Mass., 1988.

Lindenberg, R., F. B. Walsh, J. G. Sacks: Neuropathology of Vision: An Atlas, Lea & Febiger. Philadelphia 1973

Lindsay, K. W., J. Bone, R. Callander: Neurology and Neurosurgery Illustrated. Churchill Livingstone, Edinburgh, London 1986

Lockard, J. S., A. A. Ward jr.: Epilepsy – a Window to Brain Mechanisms. Raven Press, New York 1980

Loeb, C., I. S. Meyer: Strokes due to Vertebro-Basilar Disease. Thomas, Springfield/III. 1965

Lorente de No, R.: Cerebral cortex. In Fulton, H. F.: Physiologie des Nervensystems. Enke, Stuttgart 1952

Lou, H. C.: Developmental Neurology Raven Press, New York 1982

Louis, R.: Topographic Relationships of the Vertebral Column, Spinal Cord and Nerve Roots. Anatomia Clinica 1. Springer, Berlin 1978

Luhan, J. A.: Neurology, Williams & Wilkins. Baltimore 1968

Luria, A.: Higher Cortical Function in Man. Basic Books, New York 1966

Luria, A. R.: The Working Brain. Penguin. Harmondsworth/Middlesex 1976

Lyle, D. J.: Neuro-Ophthalmology. Thomas, Springfield/III. 1954

McCormic, D. P.: Herpes simplex as cause of Bell's palsy. Lancet 1972/I, 937–939

McCormick, W. F., S. S. Schochet jr.: Atlas of Cerebrovascular Disease. Saunders, Philadelphia 1976

McDowell, F. H., E. H. Sonnenblick, M. Lesch: Current Concepts of Cerebrovascular Disease. Grune & Stratton, New York 1980

McHenry, L. C.: Cerebral Circulation and Stroke, Green, St. Louis 1978

MacLean, P. D.: Psychosomatic disease and the visceral brain. Psychosom. Med. 11 (1949) 338–353

MacLean, P. D.: The limbic systems with respect to self-preservation and the preservation of the species. J. nerv. ment. Dis. 127 (1958) 1–11

Marie, P., C. Foix, T. Alajonanine: De l'atrophie cérébelleuse tardive à prédominance corticale. Rev. neurol. 38 (1922) 849–885

Magoun, H. W.: The Waking Brain. Thomas, Springfield/III. 1958

Matsui, T., A. Hirano: An Atlas of the Human Brain for Computerized Tomography. Fischer, Stuttgart 1978

Merzbach, A.: Die Sprachiteration und ihre Lokalisation bei Herderkrankungen des Gehirns. J. Psychol. Neurol. (Lpz.) 36 (1928) 211–319

Mifka, P.: Die Augensymptomatik bei der frischen Schädelhirnverletzung. De Gruyter, Berlin 1968

Miller, N., G. Cohen: Clinical Aspect of Alzheimer's Disease and Senile Dementia. Raven Press, New York 1981

Millikan, C. H.: Cerebro-Vascular Disease. Williams & Wilkins, Baltimore 1966

Milner, B.: Intellectual function of temporal lobes. Psychol. Bull. 51 (1954) 42

Milner, B.: Brain mechanisms suggested by studies of temporal lobes. In Millikan, C. H., F. L. Darley: Brain Mechanism Underlying Speech and Language. Grune & Stratton, New York 1967

Milner, B., W. Penfield: The effect of hippocampal lesion on recent memory. Trans. Amer. neurol. Asso. 80 (1955) 42–48

Minkowski, M.: Zur Physiologie der vorderen und hinteren Zentralwindung. Neurol. Zbl. 36 (1917) 572–576

Mishkin, M.: Memory in monkeys severely impaired by combined but not by separate removal of amygdala and hippocampus. Nature 273 (1978) 297–298

v. Monakow, C.: Die Lokalisation im Großhirn. Bergmann, Wiesbaden 1914

Moniz, E.: Tentatives opératoires dans le traitement de certain psychosis. Masson, Paris 1936 (p. 248)

Monnier, M.: Physiologie und Pathophysiologie des vegetativen Nervensystems, vol. I and II. Hippokrates, Stuttgart 1963

Monnier, M.: Functions of the Nervous System, vol. II. Elsevier, Amsterdam 1970

Monrad-Krohn, G. H.: Die klinische Untersuchung des Nervensystems. 2. Aufl. Thieme, Stuttgart 1954

Moruzzi, G., H. W. Magoun: Brainstem reticular formation and activation of the EEG. Electroencephal. clin. Neurophysiol. I (1949) 455–473

Mossy, J., O. Reinmuth: Cerebrovascular Diseases. Raven Press, New York 1981

Mountcastle, V. B.: Modality and topographic properties of single neurons of cats' somatic sensory cortex. J. Neurophysiol. 20 (1957) 408–434

Mumenthaler, M.: Neurologie, 4, Aufl. Thieme, Stuttgart, 1973; 7. Aufl. 1982

Mumenthaler, M., H. Schliack: Läsionen peripherer Nerven, 2 Aufl. Thieme Stuttgart 1973; 4. Aufl. 1982

Munk, H.: Über die Funktionen der Großhirnrinde. Gesammelte Mitteilungen aus den Jahren 1877–1880, vol. X. Hirschwald, Berlin 1881

Murphy, S. M.: Cerebrovascular Disease. Year Book Medical Publishers, Chicago 1955

Myers, R. E.: Function of corpus callosum in interocular transfer. Brain 79 (1956) 353–363

Myers, R. E.: Localization of function in the corpus callosum. Arch. Neurol. (Chic.) 1 (1959) 74–77

Myers, R. E., C. O. Henson: Role of corp. callosum in transfer of tactuokinesthetic learning in chimpanzee. Arch. Neurol. (Chic.) 3 (1960) 404–409

Nadjmi, M. (Editor). Imaging of Brain Metabolisme Spine and Cord. Interventional Neuroradiology. Free Communications. XV. th. Congress of the European Society of Neuroradiology 1988 Springer, 1989

Niedermeyer, E.: Compendium of the Epilepsies. Thomas, Springfield/III. 1974

Nieuwenhuys, R., I. Voogd, C. van Huijzen: The Human Central Nervous System. Springer, Berlin 1978

Nissl, F.: Experimentalergebnisse zur Frage der Hirnrindenschichtung, Mschr. Psychiat. Neurol. 23 (1908) 186–188

Noback, C. R., R. J. Demarest: The Human Nervous System, 2nd ed. McGraw-Hill, New York 1975

Noetzel, H., F. Jerusalem: Die Hirnnerven- und Sinusthrombosen. Springer, Berlin 1965

Ojemann, G. A., P. Fedio, J. M. van Buren: Anomia from pulvinar and subcortical parietal stimulation. Brain 91 (1968) 99–116

Olivecrona, H., H. Urban: Über Meningeome der Siebbeinplatte. Beitr. klin. Chir. 161 (1935) 224

Oppenhelm, H.: Lehrbuch der Nervenkrankheiten, vol. I and II. Karger, Berlin 1927

Papez, J. W.: A proposed mechanism of emotion. Arch. Neurol. Psychiat. (Chic.) 38 (1937) 725–43

Papez, J. W.: Comparative Neurology. Hafner, New York 1961

Patton, J.: Neurological Differential Diagnosis. Springer, Berlin 1977

Patton, H. D., I. W. Sundsten, W. E. Crill, Ph. D. Swanson: Introduction to Basic Neurology. Saunders, Philadelphia 1976

Pavlov, I. P.: Conditioned reflexes. An investigation of the physiological activity of the cerebral cortex. Oxford University Press, London. 1927

Peele, T. L.: The Neuroanatomic Basis for Clinical Neurology, 2nd ed. McGraw-Hill, New York 1961

Penfield, W., H. Jasper: Epilepsie and the Functional Anatomy of the Human Brain. Little, Brown & Co., Boston 1954

Penfield, W., B. Milner: Memory deficit produced by bilateral lesions in the hippocampal zone, Arch. Neurol. Psychiat. (Chic.) 79 (1958) 475–497

Penfield, W., T. Rasmussen: The Cerebral Cortex of Man. Macmillan, New York 1950

Penfield, W., L. Roberts: Speech and Brain Mechanisms. Princeton University Press, Princetown/N. J. 1959

Pernkopf, E.: Atlas der topographischen und angewandten Anatomie des Menschen, vol. I. Urban & Schwarzenberg, München 1963

Peters, G.: Klinische Neuropathologie, 2nd. ed. Thieme, Stuttgart 1970

Pfeiffer, R. A.: Angioarchitektonik der Großhirnrinde, Springer, Berlin 1928

Pfeiffer, R. A.: Die Grundlagen der angioarchitektonischen arealen Hirnkarte. Z. ges. Neuro. Psychiat. 167 (1939) 579–581

Pia, H. W., C. Langmaid, J. Zierski: Cerebral Aneurysms. Advances in Diagnosis and Therapy. Springer, Berlin 1979

Pick, A.: Beiträge zur Pathologie und pathologischen Anatomie des Zentralnervensystems. Karger, Berlin 1898

Piscol, K.: Die Blutversorgung des Rückenmarks und ihre klinische Bedeutung. Springer, Berlin 1972

Plum, F., J. B. Posner: The Diagnosis of Stupor and Coma, 3rd ed. Davis, Philadelphia 1980

Poeck, K.: Einführung in die klinische Neurologie, 2nd ed. Springer, Berlin 1972

Poljakow, G. I.: Entwicklung der Neuronen der menschlichen Großhirnrinde. VEB Thieme, Leipzig 1979

Polyak, S.: The Vertebrate Visual Systems. University of Chicago Press, Chicago 1957

Popper, K. R., J. C. Eccles: The Self and Its Brain. Springer, Berlin 1977

Poser, C. M., D. K. Ziegler: Temporary Amnesia as a manifestation oft cerebrovascular insufficiency. Trans. Am. Neurolog. Ass. 85 (1960) 221–223

Pribram, K. H., D. E. Broadbent: Biology of Memory. Academic Press, New York 1970

Quandt, J.: Die zerebralen Durchblutungsstörungen des Erwachsenenalters. Schattauer, Stuttgart 1969

Rasmussen, A. T.: The Principal Nervous Pathways. Macmillan, New York 1952

Rasmussen, G. L., W. F. Windle: Neurol Mechanisms of the Auditory and Vestibular Systems. Thomas, Springfield/III. 1960

Rauber/Kopsch: Anatomie des Menschen 4 vol., Ed. Leonhardt, H., H. B. Tillmann, G. Töndury, K. Zilles. Thieme, Stuttgart 1988

Rexed, B.: A cytoarchitectonic atlas of the spinal cord in the cat. J. comp. Neurol. 100 (1954) 297–379

Richter, E.: Die Entwicklung des Globus pallidus und des Corpus subthalamicum. Springer, Berlin 1965

Roberts, T. D. M.: Neurophysiology of Postural Mechanisms. Butterworth, London 1967

Rohen, J. W.: Funktionelle Anatomie des Nervensystems. Schattauer, Stuttgart 1971

Rorke, L. B.: Pathology of Perinatal Brain Injury. Raven Press, New York 1982

Rose, F. C., W. F. Bynum Historical Aspects of the Neurosciences. Raven Press, New York 1981

Ross, A. T., W. E. De Myer: Isolated syndrome of the medial longitudinal fasciculus in man. Arch. Neurol. (Chic.) 15, 1966

Rosswell, E., S. Fahn: Advances in Neurology, vol. XIV. Ravens Press, New York 1976

Rowland, L. P.: Merrit's Textbook of Neurology, 7th ed. Lea & Febiger, Philadelphia 1984

Ruch, T. C., H. D. Patton: Physiology and Biophysics, 19th ed. Saunders, Philadelphia 1965

Russell Dejong, N.: The Neurologic Examination, 3rd ed. Harper & Row, New York 1965

Sachsenweger, R.: Augenmuskellähmungen. Edition, Leipzig 1965

Sacks, J. G., R. Lindenberg: Dolicho-ectatic intracranial arteries. Symptomatology and pathogenesis of arterial elongation and distension. Johns Hopk. med. J. 125 (1969) 95–106

Samii, M., P. J. Jannetta, ed.: The Cranial Nerves, Springer, Berlin, Heidelberg, New York 1981

Samii, M.: Pathogenese und operative Therapie des Spasmus facialis. Akt. Neurol. 10, 1983

Sanides, F.: Die Architektur des menschlichen Stirnhirns. Springer, Berlin 1962

Sarkissow, S. A.: Grundriß der Struktur und Funktion des Gehirns. VEB Volk und Gesundheit, Berlin 1967

Schade, J. P.: The Peripheral Nervous Systems. Elsevier, Amsterdam 1966

Schade, J. P., D. H. Ford: Basic Neurology. Elsevier, Amsterdam 1967

Schaltenbrand, G.: Die Nervenkrankheiten. Thieme, Stuttgart 1951

Schaltenbrand, G.: Allgemeine Neurologie, Thieme, Stuttgart 1969

Scheid, W.: Lehrbuch der Neurologie, 1. Aufl. Thieme, Stuttgart 1963; 5. Aufl. 1983

Schiefer, W., H. H. Wiegk: Spinale raumfordernde Prozesse. Straube, Erlangen 1976

Schilder, P.: Das Körperschema. Springer, Berlin 1953

Schmidt, R. M.: Der Liquor cerebrospinalis. VEB Volk und Gesundheit, Berlin 1966

Schürmann, K.: Die Chirurgie der extrapyramidalen Hyperkinesen. In Olivecrona, H., W. Tönnis: Handbuch der Neurochirurgie, vol. I. Springer, Berlin 1957

Schürmann, K., M. Brock, H.-J. Reulen, D. Voth: Cerebello Pontine Angle Tumors. In: Advances in Neurosurgery. Springer, Berlin 1973

Scoville, W. B., B. Milner: Loss of recent memory after bilateral hippocampal lesions. J. Neurol. Neurosurg. Psychiat 20 (1957) 11–21

Sherrington, C. S.: The Integrative Action of the Nervous System. Scribner, New York 1906; Cambridge University Press, London 1947

Smith, A., C. Burklund: Dominant hemisphereectomy. Science 153 (1966) 1280–1282

Smith, E.: A new topographical survey of the cerebral cortex being on the account of the distribution on the anatomical distinct cortical areas and their relationship to the cerebral sulci. J. Anat. Physiol. (Lond.) 41 (1907) 237–254

Spatz, H.: Über Anatomie, Entwicklung und Pathologie des „Basalen Neocortex". Acta med. belg. 1962, 766–779

Spatz, H.: Der basale Neocortex und seine Bedeutung für den Menschen. Ber. phys. med. Ges. Würzburg. 71 (1962–64) 7–17

Speckmann, K.: Über zentrale Schmerzen und Hyperpathie bei Verletzungen des Großhirns, insbesondere der Hirnrinde. Der Nervenarzt, 16, Heft 5, 1943, 208–220

Sperry, R. W.: Cerebral organization and behavior. Science 133 (1961) 1749–1757

Sperry, R. W.: The great cerebral commissure. Sci. Amer. 210 (1964) 42–52

Sperry, R. W., B. Preilowski: Die beiden Gehirne des Menschen. Bild d. Wissenschaft 9 (1972) 920–927

Stöhr, M., J. Dichgans, H. C. Diener, U. W. Buettner: Evozierte Potentiale, Springer, Berlin 1982

Ström-Olsen, R., P. M. Tow: Late social results of prefrontal leucotomy. Lancet 1, 1949, 87

Strub, R. L., F. W. Black: The Mental Status Examination in Neurology, Davis, Philadelphia 1977

Struppler, A.: Elektrophysiologische Diagnostik in der Neurologie. Thieme, Stuttgart 1982

Stumpf, W. E., L. D. Grant: Anatomical Endocrinology. Karger, Basel 1974

Swash, M., C. Kennard: Scientific Basis of Clinical Neurology. Churchill-Livingstone, Edinburgh 1985

Tönnis, W., F. Loew: Raumbeengende Prozesse im Inneren des Schädels. In Bock, H. E., W. Gevoh, F., Hartmann: Klinik der Gegenwart, Bd. IV. Urban & Schwarzenberg, München 1957

Tow, P. M.: Personality Changes Following Frontal Leucotomy. Cumberlege, Oxford 1955

Tower, D. B.: The Nervous System (3 volumes). Raven Press. New York 1975

Travis, A. M.: Neurological defiencies following supplementary motor area lesions in Macaca mulatta. Brain 78 (1955) 174–198

Umbach, W.: Elektrophysiologische und vegetative Phänomene bei stereotaktischen Hirnoperationen. Springer, Berlin 1966

Van der Eecken, H. M., R. D. Adams: The anatomy and functional significance of the meningeal arterial anastomoses of the human brain. J. Neuropath. exp. Neurol. 12 (1953) 132–157

Van Valkenburg, C. T.: Zur fokalen Lokalisation der Sensibilität in der Größhirnrinde des Menschen. Z. ges. Neurol. Psychiat. 24 (1914) 294–312

Victor, M. R. D. Adams, G. H. Collins: The Wernicke-Korsakoff Syndrome. Davis, Philadelphia 1971

Vinken, P. J., G. W. Bruyn: Handbook of Clinical Neurology. North-Holland Publishing Co., Amsterdam 1969

Vogt, O.: Die myeloarchitektonische Felderung des menschlichen Stirnhirns. J. Psychol. Neurol. 15 (1910)

Vogt, O., C. Vogt: Allgemeine Ergebnisse unserer Hirnforschung. J. Psych. 25, Erg. H. 1, 1925

Wada, J. A., J. K. Penry: Advances in Epileptology. The Xth Epilepsy International Symposium. Raven Press. New York 1980

Walker, A. E.: Cerebral Death, 2nd ed. Urban & Schwarzenberg, München 1981

Wall, M., S. H. Wray: The „One and a Half" syndrome. A unilateral disorder of the pontine tegmentum. Neurology (Chic.) 33 (1983) 971–980

Walsh, F. B., W. F. Hoyt: Clinical Neuro-Ophthalmology, vol. I–III, 3rd ed. Williams & Wilkins, Baltimore 1969

Walton I. Introduction to Clinical Neuroscience. Baillière Tindall, London 1987

Warwick, R.: Representation of the extraocular muscles with oculomotorius nuclei of the monkey. J. comp. Neurol. 98 (1953) 449–503

Warwick, R.: Oculomotor organization. In Bender, M. B.: The Oculomotor System. Harper & Row, New York 1964

Wechsler, I. S.: Clinical Neurology, 9th ed. Saunders, Philadelphia 1963

Weisenburg, T., K. McBride: Aphasia. (Reprint of 1935), Hafner, New York 1964

Weitzmann, E. D.: Advances in Sleep Research, vol. 1. Spectrum, Flushing (N.Y.) 1974

Welt, L.: Über Charakterveränderungen des Menschen infolge von Läsionen des Stirnhirns. Dtsch. Arch. klin. Med. 42 (1888) 339–390

Wernicke, C.: Der aphasische Symptomenkomplex, eine psychologische Studie auf anatomischer Basis. Cohn & Weigert. Breslau 1874

Whitehouse, J. M. A., H. E. M. Kay: CNS Complications of Malignant Disease. University Park Press, Baltimore 1980

Whitty, G. W., I. T. Hughes, F. O. MacCallum: Virus Diseases and the Nervous System. Blackwell, Oxford 1968

Wigand, M. E., T. Berg, G. Rettinger: Mikrochirurgische Neurolyse des VIII. Hirnnerven bei cochleo-vestibulären Störungen über einen erweiterten transtemporalen Zugang. HNO 31 (1983) 295–302

Willis, W. D., R. E. Coggeshall: Sensory Mechanisms of the Spinal Cord. Plenum Press. New York 1978

Williams, P. L., P. Warwick: Functional Neuroanatomy of Man. Churchill-Livingstone, Edinburgh 1975

Woolsey, C. N.: Patterns of sensory representation in the cerebral cortex. Fed. Proc. 6 (1947) 437–41

Woolsey, C. V., W. H. Marshall, P. Bard: Representation of cutaneous tactile sensibility in the cerebral cortex of the monkey as indicated by evoked potentials. Bull. Johns Hopk. Hosp. 70 (1942) 339–441

Wüllenweber, R., H. Wenker, M. Brock, M. Klinger (Edit.): Treatment of Hydrocephalus. Computer Tomographie. Springer Berlin, Heidelberg 1978

Zeidel, E.: Lexical Organisation in the right Hemisphere. INSERM Symposium No. 6 ed. Buser, P. A. and Rougal-Buser (1978) 177–197 Elsevier/ North Holland, Biomedical Press

Zülch, K. J., O. Creutzfeld, G. C. Galbraith: Cerebral Localization, on Otfried Foerster Symposium. Springer, Berlin 1975

Index

Note: page numbers in *italics* refer to figures and tables

A
A fibers 17
abasia 170
abducens nerve 71, *78*, 87–90
 paralysis 37, 88, 94
accessory cuneate nucleus 14
accessory nerve 72, *79*, 129, *130*
 causes of damage 132
 impairment 131–2
accessory olives 139
accommodation 97–9
 central pathways *98*
acoustic neurinoma 177–8
acoustic radiation 118, 266
acoustic schwannoma 120
acromegaly 213
action potential 6
activating fibers 35–6
adenohypophysis 194
Adie's syndrome 99
adiposogenital dystrophy 200
adrenal glands 216
adrenocorticotropic hormone 199, *201*
afferent fibers
 autonomic 75
 colaterals 12
 somatic 75
ageusia 112, 126
agnosia
 acoustic 290
 auditory 120
 body-image 286, 288
 dominant hemisphere damage 291–2
 tactile 285
 visual 290
agraphia 288
akinesia 163, 232, 232–3
 paralysis agitans 233
alcoholism 209
alertness, attentive 143
alexia 85, 290, 295
aliquorrhea 249

allocortex 204
alpha 1 fibers 39
alpha motoneurons 39
Alzheimer's disease
 cerebral atrophy 249
 limbic form *206*, 207
 parieto-occipital form 288
amaurosis fugax 312
ambient gyri 77
amimia 110
Ammon's horn 160, 202, *204*, 205, 260, *262*
 arteries 307, *308*
 bilateral loss 205
 cortex 259
 damage 207, 208
 removal 291
 sclerosis 301
amnesia
 global transitory 310, 311
 see also memory
amnestic syndromes 205, 207
amygdaloid nuclear complex 204–5, 225
amyotonia congenita 69
amyotrophic lateral sclerosis 38, 53–4, 134
anarthria 134
angina pectoris 224
angiodysgenic necrotizing myelopathy 66
angiography, digital subtraction/serial 254
angiomatosis, retinal 177
anhidrosis 102
anisocoria 103
anosmia 80, 81, 283, 297
anosognosia 288
ansa hypoglossi 132
ansa lenticularis 231, 233
anterior commissure 80, 268
anterior horn
 alpha cells 32
 neurons *34*, 38–9

and pyramidal tract damage, syndrome of combined 53–4
 syndrome 52–3
anterior nucleus of thalamus 183–4, *186*
anterior and posterior roots and peripheral nerves, syndrome of 54
anterior striate body *228*
antidiuretic hormone *see* vasopressin
Anton's syndrome 288, 315
anulospiral endings 2, 9, 10
anulus fibrosus 59
aortic aneurysm 129
aortic arch receptors 130
apallic syndrome 163
aphasia
 amnestic 295, 296–7
 conduction 295, 296
 cortical motor 279
 dissociative 296
 global 296
 jargon 296
 sensory 119, 290–1, 294–7, 295–6
 subcortical motor 280
 transcortical 297
aphemia 280
apoplectic hematoma *317*, 318–19, 324
apraxia 288, 289
aqueduct of Sylvius 243
aqueductal stenosis 248
arachnoid 240–1
 blood perforation 317
arachnoidal villi 247
archicerebellum 122–3, 164, 170, 171
arcuate fibers 267
area postrema 145
Argyll Robertson pupil 99
Arnold–Chiari syndrome 248

arterial aneurysms 316–18
arterial circle of Willis *see* circle of Willis
arteriovenous angioma, rupture 176
ascending reticular activating system 143, 187
asomatognosia 286
associated movements 228
association fibers 264, 266–8
astasia 170
astereognosis 16, 21
asynergia 170, 171
ataxia 55
   Brown–Séquard syndrome 56
   cerebellar 170
   neocerebellar dysfunction 171
   superior cerebellar artery compression 175
   sylvian aqueduct syndrome 156
   truncal 170, 171
athetosis 234–5
atlanto-occipital fusion 248
auditory association area 290–4
auditory cortex *276*, 277
auditory lateral lemniscus 141
auditory pathway 119, 142
auditory system 114–20
   tonotopic order of fibers 118
Auerbach's myenteric plexus 217
auriculotemporal nerve, neuralgia 108
autonomic accessory nuclei 100
autonomic crisis 163
autonomic nervous system, functions 214–15
autonomic nuclei 85
autotopagnosia 286
axon 3, 6
   wallerian degeneration 48
azygos vein 66

B
Babinski's sign 36
Baillarger's lines 259, 263
ballistic syndrome 236
baroceptors, carotid sinus wall 130
basal cistern 158–9, 160, 242, *242*
basal ganglia 225–6, *227, 228*
   infarct 252
basal vein of Rosenthal 148, 159, 188, 322, *323*

basilar artery 145, 147–8, 172
   embolism 315
   internal carotid artery insufficiency 311
basilar impression 248
basilar membrane 115–16
basket fibers 166
basophilic adenoma 213
Bechterew's nucleus 122, 203
Benedikt syndrome 152
Betz's cells 29, 263
Bing-Horton syndrome 107–8
bipolar cells 81
blepharospasm 110
blindness 315
blink reflex 103, 110
blood pressure control 145
blood–CSF barrier 244
Bochdalek's flower basket 164, 243
boutons terminaux 6
Bowman's glands 77
brachia conjunctiva/pontis 164
brachial plexus 23, *24*, 47
brain
   cisterns 242–3
   displacement of structures 159–60
brainstem 70–4, 80
   arteries 145–8
   blood supply 145–56, *157*, 158–63
   internal steal syndrome 311
   internal structure 134–6
      medulla oblongata 136–40
      mesencephalon 141–3, *144*, 145
      pons 140–1
   lesions causing contralateral hemiplegia 149
   tumors 154–6
   veins 148
   see also reticular formation
Broca's cortex 279–81
Broca's limbic lobe 259
Broca's region, cortex 294
Brodmann's area 20–1, 29, 32
   calcarine fissure 84, 85
   gustatory cortex 277
   visual cortex 276
Brodmann's fields 263, 264
Brodmann's map 260, *261*, 264
Brown–Séquard syndrome 56, 68–9
bulbar paralysis 134
   progressive 54, 114, 134
bulbothalamic tract 15

bundle of Vicq d'Azyr *see* mamillothalamic tract

C
C fibers 17
Cajal's nucleus 96, 123, 143, 156
calcarine artery
   compression 315
   obstruction 308
calcarine cortex 81, 84, 97, 257, 258, 277
   calcarine artery obstruction 308
   damage in spots 315
   ischemia 314
calcarine fissure 84
canalis hypoglossi 132
carbon monoxide poisoning 207
carotid sinus
   baroceptors in wall 130
   branches of glossopharyngeal nerve 125
carotid-cavernous fistula 316
carpal tunnel syndrome 49
cauda equina 21, 62
cauda syndrome 58, 59, 62, *63*
caudal pontine tegmentum syndromes 151, *153*
caudate nucleus 225, 226
causalgia 49
cavernous sinus 88
central nervous system
   CSF changes in disease 245–6
   neurons 6–7
central spastic paralysis, syndrome of 36–8
central sympathetic tract 102, 143
central tegmental tract 137
centromedian nucleus of thalamus 181, *184*, 186
cerebellar angioblastoma 177
cerebellar artery
   inferior
      anterior 148, 174
      posterior 64, 174
   superior 148, 173–4
      compression along tentorial margin 174–5
      obstruction 174
cerebellar astrocytoma 176
cerebellar disease, degenerative 179
cerebellar hematoma 175–6, 318
cerebellar lesions, acute 163
cerebellar peduncle 164

Index

inferior 70, 167
middle 70, 167, 169
superior 70, 169
cerebellar tumors 176–9
cerebellar veins 174
cerebellar vermis 159
cerebellopontine angle 72
cerebellorubral fibers 142
cerebellum 70
  afferent impulses 170
  afferent pathways 167, *168*, 169
  arteries 172–4
  circulatory lesions 174–6
  cortex 165–7
  efferent impulses 170
  efferent pathways 167, *168*, 169
  external architecture 164–5
  function 170–2
  impulse termination 167
  internal architecture 165–7, *168*, 169–70
  metastases 177, *178*
  molecular layer 165–6
  paired nuclei 166–7
  somatotropic order in connections with cerebrum 179
  veins 174
cerebral arteriosclerosis 236–7
cerebral artery 302, 304–8
  anterior 305–6, *309*
    obstruction 314
  compression 160
  middle 306–7, *309*
    obstruction 313, 314
  peripheral anastomoses *306*, *308*, *309*
  posterior 187, 307–8
    obstruction 314–15
    thalamoperforating branches 307
cerebral atrophy 249
cerebral circulatory deficiency 308–20
cerebral cortex
  arterial aneurysms 316–18
  auditory *276*, 277
  basic types *265*
  cell types 263
  central fissures 257
  compression by space-occupying lesion 298
  cortex 259–61, *262*, 263–4
  cryoarchitecture 260, *261*, *262*, 263, 264
  cytoarchitectonic basis of function localization 269, *270*, *271*

deficit localization 269–70
dural sinuses 320, *321*, *323*
electroencephalography 270
external characteristics 256–9
folding pattern 256, *258*
formation 228
frontal lobe 277–84
functional organization 268–71, *272*, 273–301
granule cells 263
gustatory *276*, 277
gyri 256, *258*
hemisphere dominance 291–2, *293*
hemisphere functions 293–4
hypertensive arterial disease 318–20
impulse pathway 187
internal characteristics 259–61, *262*, 263–8
intracerebral bleeding 318–20
Kleist's map 269, *270*, *271*
memory 291
microelectrode recording 271
motor field stimulation *272*
motor speech 279–81
occipital 257, 274–7
  association area 284–94
parietal 274–7
  association area 284–94
prefrontal 281–4
premotor 278–9
pyramidal cells 263
secondary receptive cortical fields 284–94
somatomotor cortex 278
somatosensory *276*
  association area 285
  primary 274–5
stereotactic methods 271
sulci 256, *258*
temporal 257, 274–7, 291
  association area 284–94
tertiary parietal association area 285–9
tumors 298–9
veins
  external 320–2
  internal 322–3
  thrombosis symptomatology 324–7
vestibular 277
visual 273–4, 275–7
white matter 264–8
cerebral ganglia, deep, venous infarction 325
cerebral hematoma 132
cerebral hemisphere, swelling 160–1, 162

cerebral infarct 132
cerebral peduncle 70, 73, 141, 143
  syndrome 152
cerebral veins 321–2, *323*
  acute thrombosis 325–6
  internal 188
  thrombosis 324
cerebromedullary cistern 242
cerebrospinal fluid (CSF) 241, 242, 244, *245–6*, 247–55
  circulation blockage 297–8
  flow blockages 247–55
cerebrum
  arterial supply 301–8
  circulatory system 301–27
  diseases 297–301
cervical ganglia 216
cervical myeloma glioma *252*
cervical nerve roots, syndromes of lesions limited to individual 60–1
cervical plexus *23*, 47
cervical radicular syndrome 59–60
cervical rib syndrome 48–9
cervical vertebra, transverse injuries 58
Charlin's syndrome of neuralgia 107
chemoreceptors 130
chewing 145
chewing muscle, flaccid paralysis 106
chorda tympani 111
chorea 235
choroid plexus
  anterior choroidal artery 305
  cerebrospinal fluid secretion 244, 247
  ventricular 243–4
choroidal artery 187
  anterior 304–5
    obstruction 314
  lateral posterior 307
chromophobe adenoma 213
ciliary ganglion 86, 98, 100
ciliospinal center 101–2
cingulate gyrus 184, 202
  bilateral extirpation 207–8
  compression by space-occupying lesion 298
  displacement 314
cingulum 202, 268
circle of Willis 158, 302–4, *305*
  anomalies in posterior part 311
  arterial aneurysms 209, 316

circle of Willis, internal carotid artery insufficiency 311, 312
circulatory disorders, syndromes 148–54
cistern of the great cerebral vein 158, 242
cisterna ambiens 158, 159, *242*, 243
cisterna magna 242
cisterna vermis 243
Clarke's column 136, 167
claustrum 225, 226
  apoplexy *319*
climbing fibers 166
clonic tic 114
cochlea 114–15
cochlear duct 115, *116*
cochlear nerve 117
  central pathways *118*
  deafness 120
cochlear nucleus 117
cogwheel phenomenon 233
collagen disease 69
coma
  cerebral vein thrombosis 324
  vigil 163
commissural fibers 264, *267*, 268, 292
common pathway, final 39
communicating artery, posterior 187
cones 81
consciousness state 143
constructive apraxia 288
conus
  syndrome of *58*, 59
  terminalis 21, *62*
convergence 97–9
  central pathways *98*
conversation 294, *295*
corneal reflex 106, 110
corona radiata 265–6
corpora restiformia 164
corpus callosum 80, 268
  displacement 314
  rostral 314
  sensory impressions 292
  splenium *229*
  visual information transfer 292
corpus Luysi *see* subthalamic nucleus
corpuscula bulboidea 1
corpuscula lamellosa 1
corpuscula tactus 1
cortex of Heschl's transverse convolutions 257
cortical motor fields 231

corticobulbar tract 32
corticofugal fibers, efferent 264
corticomesencephalic tract 32
corticonuclear bundle 30
corticonuclear tract 32, 106, 139
corticopontine fibers 34
  ipsilateral 140
corticopontocerebellar tracts 32, 171
corticospinal bundle 30
corticospinal fibers 264
corticospinal tract 139
  anterior 32
  lateral 32
  syndrome 54–5
  see also pyramidal tract
Costen's syndrome 108
cranial nerves 74–5, *76*, *77*
  accessory nerve 129, *130*, 131–2
  auditory system 114–20
  components 74, *78–9*
  distribution at base of skull 77
  facial nerve 108–10, 113–14
  fibers 75
  hypoglossal nerve 132–4
  intermediate nerve 108, 110–14
  nuclei *73*
  nucleus ambiguus 129
  oculomotion 85–90, *91–2*, *93*–103
  olfactory system 76–7, *79*, 80–1
  optic system 81–5
  roots *107*
  trigeminal nerve 103–8
  vagal system 125–31
  vagus nerve *127*, 128–9
  vestibular system 120–5
craniopharyngioma 209–12, 254
  third ventricle obliteration 247
crista ampullaris 121, *122*, 124
crura cerebri 70
  see also cerebral peduncle
crus syndrome of Kernohan 130, *161*, 326
crying
  forced 134, 188
  see also tears
cuneate nuclei 136
Curschmann-Steinert syndrome 69
Cushing's syndrome 213

D
Darkschewitsch's nucleus 96, 123, 143
deafness
  acoustic neurinoma 178
  anterior inferior cerebellar artery obstruction 148
  apoplectiform 120
  conduction 119
  nerve 119
decerebrate rigidity 162–3
Deiter's cells 116
Deiter's nucleus 122, 123
Dejerine's syndrome 150, *151*
dendrites 6
  anterior horn neurons 38
dentate nucleus *137*, 142, 166–7, *168*
  feedback circuit 278
dentatothalamocortical pathway 171
dermatome 23, *25*
dermatomyositis 69
diabetes insipidus 161, 198, 209
diencephalon 180–1
diplopia 90
  myasthenia 94
  trochlear nerve paralysis 94
disconnection syndrome 289
dissociated disorder of sensibility 28
dolichoectasia, arterial 318
doll's head maneuver 156
dopaminergic fibers 231
dorsal longitudinal bundle 112–13, 213, 222
dorsolateral medulla syndrome 150
dressing apraxia 288
drop attacks 309
dura 241
  inner meningeal layer 239
  innervation 240
  mater 239–40
dura sinuses 320, *321*, 323
  thrombosis symptomatology 324–7
dural sleeve 239–40, 241
Duret's hemorrhage 160
dysarthria 134
dysdiadochokinesia 171
dysesthesia 26
dysmetria 171
dysphagia 127, 134
dyspraxia 288, 289
dystonia 232
dystrophia myotonica 69

E

Edinger–Westphal nuclei 85, 98, 100, 103, 142, 197
- efferent motor fibers 100
- fiber connections 100

efferent fibers 75
ejaculation 222
electroencephalography 270
emboliform nucleus *137*, 166–7, *168*
emotion, speech 295
emotional exultation 202, 203
emotional liability, thalamic damage 188
emotional outburst, limbic portion of amygdala stimulation 205
empty sella 255
- syndrome 213

endolymph 120
endoneurium 4
enophthalmus 102
enteroceptors 1
entorhinal area 203–4
eosinophilic adenoma 213
ependymitis 248
ependymoma 179
epiconus, syndrome of 58–9
epicritic sensitivity 141
epidural bleeding, spinal 66
epidural hematoma 319–20
epilepsy
- attacks 36
- temporal lobe 120
- resection 205

epileptic seizures 205, 300–1
- cerebral cortex tumors 298–9
- focal motor 301
- generalized 301
- orbital lobe damage 284

epineurium 4
epiphysis 180
epithalamus 181, 192–3
equilibrium system 120–5
Erb-Duchenne paralysis 47
Erb-Goldflam disease 69
erythroprosopalgia 107
esotropia 88
ethmoid bone, osteitis 80
ethmoidal sinus 88
ethmoidal sinusitis 80
evoked potentials 270
external auditory canal 114
exteroceptors 1
extracranial ganglion inferius 125
extrafusal fibers 8, 9
extramedullary tumor 51

extraocular muscle innervation 89
extrapyramidal fibers 34–5
extrapyramidal grisea, lesions 232–6
extrapyramidal motor system 32–8
extrapyramidal pathway
- damage 35–8
- origin 231

extrapyramidal system 226–38
- connection 230
- development 227–8

extrapyramidal tracts 21
eye
- fixation reflex 297
- malignant tumor 241
- pursuit reflex 297
- sympathetic innervation 101–3

eye field
- of Brodmann's area 8 32
- frontal 96

eye movements 94
- conjugate 94, *95*
- basic 89
- rotary 96
- upwards 96
- voluntary 95, 96, 279

eye muscles
- coordination 88–90
- innervation
  - parasympathetic *101*
  - reflex 94–7
  - sympathetic *101*
  - voluntary 94–7
- paralysis 89–90, *91*–*2*, 93–4
  - deviation *91*–*2*
  - diagnosis 90
  - double images *93*
  - peripheral palsy 94

F

facial apraxia 289
facial canal 110
facial colliculus *71*, 73
facial nerve 73, *78*, 108–10, 113–14
- central pathways *109*
- external knee 110
- inner knees 109
- internal knee 87–8
- nuclear paralysis 114
- peripheral paralysis 113–14
- reflex arc 110
- supranuclear paralysis 114

facial pain 106–8
facial palsy, supranuclear 114
facial paralysis 110

facial spasm, tonic 114
fasciculi proprii 21
fasciculus thalamicus 231
fastigial nucleus 122, *137*, 166–7, *168*
fever, central 200
fila olfactoria 77, 80
fixation reflex 95
flexor reflex 13
flight reflex 13
flocculonodular lobe of cerebellum 170
flocculonodular syndrome 170
flower-spray terminals 10–11
Foix-Alajouanine's disease 66
food intake 145, 200
foramen jugulare 125
foramen of Luschka 72, 164, 243, 244
- blockage 247

foramen of Magendie 72, 243, 244
- blockage 247
- obliteration 248

foramen magnum impaction 148, 156, 158–63, 175
foramen of Monro 180, 194, 196, 243
- obstruction 247, *248*

foramen spinosum 239
forehead musculature, supranuclear innervation 110
Forel's axis 180
fornical commissure 196
fornix 195–6
- bilateral interruption 205

Foster Kennedy syndrome 81, 83, 299
free nerve endings 1
Freidreich foot 56
Friedreich's ataxia 51, 55
Froins's CSF loculation syndrome 251
Frölich's syndrome 200
frontal cortical areas 281
frontal eye field 96
frontal lobe, anterior damage syndrome 282
frontopontine fiber bundles 33
frontopontocerebellar tract, feedback circuit 278
funiculus, posterior 15–17
- injury syndromes 16–17

G

GABA-ergic fibers 231
gait, acoustic neurinoma 178
gamma motoneurons 9–10, 39, 41

gamma motor cells 32
gamma neuron-spindle system 10
gamma neurons 10
ganglia of vagus nerve 128
Ganser's ganglion 80
gasserian ganglion 72, 103
gastrointestinal tract, hypothalamic effects 201
gaze, pontine paralysis 96, *97*
geniculate body 85
 lateral/medial 182, 183, *186*
geniculate ganglion 111
genioglossus muscle 132, 134
genital organs, parasympathetic nervous system control 218, 222
Gennari's stripe 84
Gerstmann's syndrome 288
giant pyramidal cells 263
gigantism 213
glaucoma, trigeminal pain 107
glioblastoma *252*
 multiforme *253*
glioma 155
globus pallidus 193
glomus 243
 caroticum 130
 tumor 119
glossopharyngeal nerve 72, 78–9, 125–8, 130–1
 afferent visceral fibers 130–1
 branches 125
 impairment 126–8
  syndrome 126–7
 neuralgia 127–8
 somatic afferent fibers 131
 taste fibers 111
Golgi tendon organs 169
Golgi-Mazzoni's corpuscle *2*, *3*
Gordon's reflex 36
Gradenigo's syndrome 107
grasp reflex 279
gray communicating rami 216
gray matter syndrome 52
great vein of Galen 148, 158, 174, 188, 322, 323
 cistern 243
growth hormone 198, *201*
Gudden's nucleus 203
Guillain-Barré syndrome 48
gustatory cortex *276*, 277
gustolacrimal reflex, paradoxical 114

H
habenular nuclei 192
habenulopeduncular tract 80
Haemophilus influenzae 242

hair cells
 auditory 115
 maculae staticae 120–1
hair cuff 1, *2*
Hallervorden–Spatz disease 235
Hand–Schüller-Christian disease 300
head-dropping test 233
Head's zones 222, *223*, 224
hearing
 impairments 119–20
 temporal lobes 257
 unilateral pathway interruption 120
hearing loss
 acute 120
 sylvian aqueduct syndrome 156
heat metabolism 200
hematoma, intraspinal 66
hematomyelia 51, 52, 53, 66
hemianopsia
 bilateral 315
 binasal 84
 bitemporal 83, 161, 212, 213
 homonymous 84, 85, 276, 277, 324
 upper quadrant 291
hemiataxia 188
hemiballismus 194
hemiconvulsion hemiplegia syndrome 301
hemiparalysis, internal carotid artery insufficiency 312
hemiparesis
 contralateral 188
 flaccid 38
 internal carotid artery insufficiency 312
hemiplegia
 alternate 28
 contralateral 149
  spastic 36–7
 cruciata 28
 supratentorial lesion 160
hemisection of spinal cord, syndrome of 56
hemisphere dominance 291–2, 293
herpes zoster 50
 oticus 112, 113
Heschl's gyrus 142
Heschl's transverse convolutions 118, 257, 259, 277
Hippel's disease 177
hippocampal commissure 268
hippocampal gyrus 202
hippocampus 205, 260, *262*
 function 184

histiocytosis X 300
homeostasis 200, 214
homonymous muscle 9
Horner's syndrome 47, 102, 143
 ipsilateral 217
hourglass tumor 68–9
Huntington's chorea 235
Hunt's neuralgia 113
hydrocephalus
 communicating 247, 318
  internal 248–51
 external ex vacuo 247
 hypersecretion 249
 hypertensive 250
  internal 247
 internal 250–1
  ex vacuo 247
 noncommunicating 178, 190, 247
 normal pressure 248
 occlusive 250
hygroma 320
hyoglossus muscle 132
hypacusis 118, 120
 senile 120
hypalgesia 25
hyperesthesia 224
hyperkinesia 163, 232
 stereotactic treatment 236
hyperkinesia–hypotonia syndrome 234–6
hyperpathia 188
hyperreflexia 36
hypertensive arterial disease 318–20
hypertensive hematoma 318
hypertonia 232
hypesthesia 25
 contralateral 188
hypoglossal nerve 71, *79*, 132–4
hypoglossal nucleus 132–3
hypokinesia 232
hypokinesia–hypertonia syndrome 232
hypoliquorrhea 249
hypomimia 110
hypophysis, anterior lobe *199*
hypothalamus 181, 194–205, *206*, 207–13
 afferent connections 195–6
 blood supply *208*
 caudal 202
 circulatory disorders 208
 damage 208–13
 function 200–2
 homeostatic function 200
 hormones 198–9, *201*
 humoral action 214

inflammatory changes 208–9
limbic system 202–5
nuclei *194*, 195
peripheral autonomic system control 213
rostral 201
structure 194–7
trauma 208
tumors 209–13
visceral afferents 196
visceral efferents 197
hypothalamus–pituitary connection 197–9
hypotonia 172, 232

I
Ia fibers 10, 14
ideational apraxia 289
ideomotor apraxia 289
impotence 222
infantile spastic diplegia 325
inferior anastomotic vein of Labbé *321*, 322
inferior cerebellar peduncle 136
inferior colliculi *71*, 86, 142
inferior oblique muscle 89
inferior plexus paralysis 47
infundibulum 180
inhibiting fibers 35–6
inner ear 114
  deafness 119
innervation apraxia 289
insula 259, 277
intercostal nerves 47
interhemispheric cistern 242–3
intermediate nerve 108, 110–14
  neuralgia 113
internal acoustic canal 109
internal auditory meatus 113
internal carotid artery *88*, 302, 303, 304
  aneurysm 108
  faint pulse 313
  insufficiency 308, 311–13
  thrombosis 312
internal steal syndrome 311
internuncial neurons 12–13
interpeduncular cistern 242
interpeduncular fossa 73
interpeduncular nucleus 80
intervertebral disk
  atrophy 47
  degenerative process 60–1
  osteochondrosis 59
  prolapse 59, 61, *252*
  protrusion 61, *63*
intra-arachnoidal cyst 178, 249–50

intracerebellar hematoma, apoplectic 175
intracerebral bleeding 318–20
intracerebral hematoma 162, 317
intracortical neuronal chains 263, *264*
intracranial carotid, aneurysms 316–18
intracranial ganglion superius 125
intracranial pressure
  acute cerebral vein thrombosis 326
  CSF circulation blockage 250, 298
intrafusal muscle fibers 2, 8, 9
intralaminar nuclei of thalamus 185–6
intramedullary tumor 51, 52
intrasellar cyst 194
  arachnoid 255
intraspinal capillaries 65
intrinsic neuronal system of spinal cord 13
intumescentiae cervicalis/lumbalis 22–3
iritis, trigeminal pain 107
isocortex 204

J
Jacksonian attacks 27, 36, 301
  supranuclear facial palsy 114
Jendrassik's maneuver 233

K
Kernohan's notch 326
Klippel–Feil syndrome 248
Klumpke's paralysis 47
Klüver–Bucy syndrome 202
Korsakoff's syndrome 205, 209
Krause's corpuscles 1, *2*
kyphosis 56

L
labyrinth *116*, 120
  kinetic/static 124
lacrimal nucleus 197
lamina quadrigemina 141
lamina terminalis, rostral 180
Landry's paralysis 48
lateral cistern 242–3
lateral dorsal nucleus of thalamus 184, *186*
lateral femoral cutaneous nerve 26
lateral geniculate body 81, *82*, *83*, 84, 257
lateral lemniscus 117–18
lateral rectus muscle 89

lateral reticular nucleus 136
laughter, forced 134, 188
lens, eye 81
lentiform nucleus 225
leptomeningitis 208, 241–2
licking 145
light reflex 99–101
limb-kinetic apraxia 279, 289
limbic cortex *203*
limbic lobe of Broca 259
limbic system 80, 184, 197, 202–5, *206*
  circuitry mechanisms 205, *206*, 207–8
  emotional behaviour 202
Lindau–von Hippel disease 177
line of Gennari 259
lingual branch of glossopharyngeal nerve 125
liquorrhea 255
Lissauer's zone 104
Little's disease 234–5
lobus pallidus 225
locomotion, sensation loss 16
locus coeruleus 145
logoclonia 236
logorrhea 295
longitudinal fascicle
  inferior 267–8
  superior 267
lumbago, acute 62–3
lumbar plexus 47
lumbar roots, syndromes of lesions limited to individual 61–3
lumbar spinal cord, transverse lesion 58
lumbosacral plexus 23, *24*

M
maculae staticae 120, *122*, 124
  hair cells 120–1
macular fibers 81
  atrophy 82
magnetic resonance imaging (MRI) 251, *252*
mamillary body 160, *161*, 180, 194, 203, *229*
  bilateral damage 205, 207
  destruction in craniopharyngioma 210
mamillotegmental fascicle 197
mamillotegmental tract 213
mamillothalamic fascicle 183
mamillothalamic tract 197, 202
mandibular nerve 103
Marie's hereditary ataxia 56
massa intermedia 180
masseter reflex 106

masticatory muscle innervation 141
mastoiditis, peripheral facial palsy 113
maxillary nerve 103
mechanoreceptors 1
medial forebrain bundle 80, 195, 213
medial geniculate body, impulses to auditory cortex 277
medial lemniscus 16, 18, *19*, 142
medial longitudinal fasciculus 119, 141, 143
medial medulla oblongata syndrome 150, *151*
medial nucleus of thalamus 184, *186*, 196
medulla oblongata 70–2, *134*, *135*, 136–40
  anterior inferior cerebellar artery 148
  arterial supply *147*
medullary striae 72
medulloblastoma 176–7
Meissner's submucosal plexus 217
Meissner's touch corpuscles 1, 2
melanin pigment 143
melanocytoma 241
memory 204, 291
  see also amnesia; amnestic syndromes
Mendel–Bechterew's reflex 36
Ménière's disease 124, 125
meningeal artery 239
meninges 239–43
meningioma 155, 241, 299–300, 327
  epileptiform seizure 299
  multiple 300
  olfactory groove 299, *300*
  parasagittal 299–300
  sphenoid ridge 299, *300*
  tuberculum sellae 299
meningitis 242
  basal 208–9
menisci, tactile 1
meralgia paresthetica 26
Merkel's tactile meniscus 1, 2
mesencephalon *see* midbrain
mesenchephalic tectum, neurons 140
metastases
  cerebellum 177, *178*
  parietal lobe *253*
  temporal lobe *253*
Meyer's loop 85, 258
Meynert's axis 180

microaneurysm 316
midbrain *136*, *137*, *138*, *139*, 141–3, *144*, 145
  arterial supply *147*
  cerebral hemisphere swelling 160–1
  compression 162, 298, 313
  displacement 326
  external structure 73–4
  hemorrhage 160, *161*
  parts 141
  shift 160
  supratentorial space-occupying lesions 160–1
  syndrome of peduncle *157*
  tegmentum 141
  tentorial impaction 163
  tentorial opening *159*
  veins 148
middle ear 114
  deafness 119
midpontine base syndrome 152
Millard-Gubler's syndrome 151, *152*
mimetic facial spasm 110
miosis 102
monoparesis 36
monosynaptic reflex 12
  arc 6, 7, 9
Morvan's disease *252*
mossy fibers 166
motoneurons 7, 29
motor area, feedback mechanism 278
motor cortex, feedback circuit 278
motor end-plates 30, *31*
motor engram 294
motor root, indicator muscles *40*, 42
motor seizure attack 27
motor speech cortex 279–81
motor system 29–30
motor unit 39
  disorder 43, 46–63
multiple sclerosis 38, 179, 209
  mono-ocular nystagmus 99
muscle
  agonist 12
  antagonist 12
  contraction 279
  disorders 69
  feedback systems 9, *10*, 11
  length feedback circuit 9, 11, 35
  resting tone 12
  spindle 10
  tension 10, 11
  tone 11–12

  see also neuromuscular junction; neuromuscular spindle
muscular dystrophy, progressive 69
myasthenia
  diplopia 94
  gravis pseudoparalytica 69
  ptosis 94
mydriasis 101, 103
myelin sheath 3, 4, 6
  wallerian degeneration 48
myelitis 53
myelography 251
myoclonias 138
myoclonic movements 236
myopathy 69
myorhythmias 138
myotactic reflex 2
myotonia congenita 69

N

Naffziger's syndrome 48–9
neocerebellar dysfunction 171–2
neocerebellum 164–5, 171
neopallium isocortex 261, *262*
  layers 263
neostriatum 225, 227
nerve fiber, myelinated 4
nerve plexus 23
  damage 23, 47–8
nerve roots *25*
neural muscular atrophy 54
neurinoma, pontocerebellar angle 300
neurofibromatosis 300
neurohypophysis 194, 195, 197
neuromuscular junction disorders 69
neuromuscular spindles 2, 7–8, 9, *10*
  nerve fibers 5–6
neuronal hamartoma 212
neurons
  anterior horn 34, 38–9
  first 33
  interconnection in medulla oblongata 140
  second 14, 17, 21, 34
  spinal nucleus 104
  third 15, 16, 17, 18, 20
  trigeminal pathway 105
nigrostriatal fibers 231
nociceptors 1, 13
nodes of Ranvier 4
nuclear bags 8
nuclear paralysis 94
nuclear-bag fibers 2–3, 10

nuclear-chain fibers 3
  secondary endings 10
nucleus ambiguus 125, 129
nucleus cuneatus 15
nucleus gracilis 15, 136
nucleus pulposus 59
nystagmus 124, 125
  cerebellar tumors 176
  mono-ocular 99
  optokinetic 97
  peripheral 125

O

obesity, craniopharyngioma 210, 211
occipital association area 284–94
occipital fascicle, vertical 268
occipital fields 96
occipital lobe 257
  alexia 290
occipito-frontal fascicles 268
oculomotion 85–90, *91–2*, *93*–103
  posterior fossa space-occupying lesions 163
oculomotor nerve 71, 73, *78*, 85–6, *87*, *88*, *89*
  brain structure displacement 159–60
  interruption 86
  nuclei 142
  paralysis 93–4
oculomotor nucleus complex 85, *86*
oculomotor palsy 93–4
odors 80
olfaction disorders 80–1
olfactory area, glioma *253*
olfactory aura 81
olfactory bulb 77
  destruction 80
olfactory groove meningioma 80, 299, *300*
olfactory hallucinations 81
olfactory mucosa 76–7
  diseases 80
olfactory nerve *78*, *79*
olfactory stimuli, emotions 80
olfactory system 76–7, *79*, 80–1
olfactory tracts 77
  agenesis 80
olfactory trigones 77
oligodendrocytes 6
olivary complex 136–8
olivary nuclei 136, 138
  inferior 70–1
olives, accessory 139

olivocerebellar tract 136–8, 167, 171
ophthalmic arteries 302
ophthalmic nerve 103
ophthalmoplegia
  interna/externa 94
  internuclear 99
  totalis 94
opisthotonus 162
Oppenheim's disease 69
Oppenheim's reflex 36
optic agnosia 85, 269
optic atrophy
  primary 82
  secondary 83
optic axis 89
optic chiasm 81, *83*
  damage 83
optic nerve *78*, 81, *82*, *83*
  glioma 255
optic radiation 81, 84, 95, 265–6
  interruption of fibers 85
optic system 81–5
optic tract 81
optical aura 85
optical memory fields 85
optokinetic process 97
oral ventral nucleus 183
orbital axis 89
orbital lobe 259
  damage 282–4
organ of Corti 114, 115, *116*, 119
  deafness 120
  pathological rearrangement 119
osteochondrosis 59, 60
otitis media
  conduction deafness 119
  peripheral facial palsy 113
otoliths 121
otosclerosis, conduction deafness 119
oxycephaly 300
oxytocin 195, 197, 198

P

pacchionian granulations 241
pain, referred 222, *223*, 224
pain sensation 17, 18–20
  loss 27
palatal reflex absence 126
paleocerebellum 14, 164
paleocerebrum 170–1
paleostriatum 225
palikinesia 236
palinphrasia 236
pallidum 181, 225, 227, *228*

bilateral destruction 234
  infarct 314
  tumor *237*
palpebral fissure, narrowing 102
Pancoast's tumor 47
Papez circuit 202, *206*
papilledema 250
  acute cerebral vein thrombosis 326
para-aortic bodies 130
paragrammatism 295
parahippocampal cortex 203, *204*
parahippocampal gyrus 77, 260, *262*
  displacement 160
  herniation 160, *161*
parallel fibers 166
paralysis
  flaccid 35, 42
    meningioma 155
    syndrome 46–7
  inferior plexus 47
  ipsilateral spastic 56
  peroneal nerve 48
  progressive bulbar 54
  radicular pattern 42
  somatomotor cortex destruction 278
  spastic 35, 36–8
  superior plexus 47
  tibial nerve 48
  ulnar with claw hand 49
paralysis agitans 232, 232–4
  akinesia 232–3
  antagonist tremor 234
  rigor 233
  sine agitatione 233
  tremor 233
paraphasia 291, 295
paraplegia 38
parasagittal meningioma *253*
parasympathetic motor nuclei 129–30
parasympathetic nerves 215
parasympathetic nervous system 217–19, *220–1*, 222, *223*, 224
  referred pain 222, *223*, 224
  sacral component 217–19, 222
parependymal fascicle 222
paresthesia 26–7
parietal abscess *252*
parietal association area 284–94
parietal lobe, metastases *253*
parieto-occipital region, malacic demarcation 287

Parinaud's syndrome 96, 156, *158*, 193
Parkinson's disease 232–4
paroxysmal paralysis 69
peduncular arteries 307
periaqueductal astrocytoma 156
perikaryon 6
perilymph 120
perineurium 4
peripheral autonomic nervous system
  function 213–15
  homeostasis 214
  hypothalamic control 213
  parasympathetic nerves 215
  sympathetic nerves 215
peripheral innervation 21–3, *24, 25*–8
  conus terminalis 21, *62*
peripheral motor nerves, course *41*
peripheral muscle innervation 43, *44*–*5*, *46*–63
  damage syndrome 48–9
  flaccid paralysis 46–7
  function *43*–6
  plexus damage 47–8
  spinal cord and peripheral nerve damage syndrome 49–59
  spinal radicular systems 59–63
peripheral nerve 3–6
  branches 47
peripheral nerve damage 25
  syndromes 48–9
peripheral nerve fiber
  classification 4, *5*
  impulse transmission 5
peripheral neurons 38–9, *40*, *41*–3
peripheral servo mechanism 7, 9
Perlia's nuclei 98, 142
  parasympathetic 85–6
peroneal nerve 47–8
  paralysis 48
personality disorder, orbital lobe type 81
petrous bone fracture, peripheral facial palsy 113
pharyngeal branches of glossopharyngeal nerve 125
pia mater 241
Pick's disease 249, 281, 282, 297
pilocytic astrocytoma 209
pineal germinoma 154, 193
pineal gland 180
pinealocytes 192

pinealoma 156, *158*, 193
  ectopic 209
pineocytoma 193
pituitary 181
  adenoma 81
  apoplexy 213
  releasing hormones 198
  tumors 212–13
plexus
  brachialis *43*–*5*
  cervicalis *43*
  lumbalis *45*, 47
  sacralis *45*–*6*
pneumocele 255
pneumoencephalography 252–3
pneumotactic nuclei 145
poikilothermy 200
polioencephalitis 114
poliomyelitis 134
polydipsia 198
polymyositis 69
polyneuropathy 48
polyneuroradiculitis 48
polysynaptic circuits 7
polyuria 198
pons 72–3, *136, 137, 138, 139*, 140–1
  arterial supply *147*
  base 140
  basilar artery 147–8
  feedback circuit 141
  focal cystic softenings *157*
  hematoma *157*
  syndrome of miniature infarcts of base 153
  tegmentum 141
  tumors 155
  veins 148
pontine apoplexy syndrome 153–4
pontine nuclei 140, 141
pontocerebellar angle, neurinoma 300
pontocerebellar fissure, rostral 86
pontocerebellum 165
pontomedullary cisterns 242
pontomedullary junction 72, 145
postcentral gyrus 18, *19*, 20
postcommissural fornix 196
posterior central cortex 257
posterior communicating arteries 302
  branches 304
posterior fossa, space-occupying lesions 163
posterior funiculi
  and corticospinal tracts, syndrome of combined degeneration 52, *53*

spinocerebellar pathways and possibly pyramidal tracts, syndrome of combined disease 55–6
posterior horn syndrome 51–2
posterior nucleus 184–5, *186*
posterior root fibers 4, *5*
  entrance zone 6
posterior roots syndrome 50–1
posterior tracts syndrome 51
postganglionic fibers
  parasympathetic 217
  sympathetic 216
posture, loss 16
precentral gyrus 20, 278
precommissural fornix 196
prefrontal cortex 281–4
  orbital lobe damage 282–4
  syndrome of anterior frontal lobe damage 282
preganglionic fibers
  parasympathetic 217
  sympathetic 216, 217
premotor cortex 278–9
  muscle contraction 279
pressure sella 251
prestitial nucleus 96
pretectal nuclei 100, 142
progressive muscular dystrophy 69
progressive spastic spinal paralysis 54–5
progressive spinal muscular atrophy 53
projection fibers 264–6
prolactin 198, *201*
proprioception 6, 7, 7–17
proprioceptive reflex, monosynaptic 7–10
proprioceptors 1
pseudobulbar paralysis 134
pseudotumor cerebri 326
pseudounipolar spinal ganglion neurons 3, 4
psychosurgery 281–2
pterygopalatine ganglion 112
ptosis 93
  myasthenia 94
pubertas praecox 193, 200
puberty, precocious 212
pudendal nerves 222
pulvinar 181, 184–5, *186*
pupil
  constriction 97–9
  dilator muscle 101, *102*
  contraction 101
  sphincter muscle paralysis 100
  width 101, 102

pupillary light reflex 99–100
pupillary reflex, accommodation 98
pupillary sphincter, paralysis 103
pupillosensory bundle, medial 84
Purkinje cell layer 166
Purkinje cells 166, 167
pursuit reflex 96
putamen 225, 227
pyocephalus 248
pyramidal pathway, damage 35–8
pyramidal tract 29, 30–2, 70

Q
quadrigeminal plate 73, 141
quadrigeminal root of aqueduct *158*
Queckenstedt's test 251

R
rabies 108
radicular nerve damage syndrome 42–3
radicularis magna artery 65
ramus externus 131
Rathke's pouch 194
Raynaud's disease 217
rebound phenomenon 171–2
receptors 1–3
　aortic arch 130
　kinetic of crista ampullaris 121
　muscle 2–3
　pain 13
　semicircular canal 123
　skin 1
　spindle 10
　see also stretch receptors
rectum
　incontinence 222
　parasympathetic nervous system control 219, 222
recurrent laryngeal nerve damage 129
red nucleus 193, 227
　cortex connections 230
　fibers from dentate nucleus 169
　mesencephalon 142
　syndrome 152, *156*
Redlich–Obersteiner area 6
reflex arc
　acoustic impulses 110
　afferent fibers 100
Reissner's membrane 115
releasing hormones 198–9, *201*

Renshaw cells 41
　paralysis agitans 233
respiration, paralysis 163
retching
　center 145
　reflex absence 126
reticular formation 80, 140, 143, *144*
　autonomic function of neurons 145
　cortex connections 230
　fibers 167
　mamillary body connection 203
　nuclei 136, 143
　　controlling blood pressure 145
reticular pathway, descending 143, 145
reticular thalamic nucleus *181*, 182
reticulospinal tracts 143, 145
retina *82*, *83*
　angiomatosis 177
　light effect 99
retinoblastoma 241
retinotopic order of cells 85
rhombencephalon 72
rigidity 232
　activated 233
rigor 233
Rinne test 119
rods 81
Roller's nucleus 122
Romberg's sign 16
　posterior tracts syndrome 51
Romberg's test, cerebellar tumors 176
root damage syndromes *40*
rostral foramen cecum 147
rostral pontine tegmentum syndrome 151, *154*
rubrospinal tract 139–40
Ruffini's corpuscles 1, *2*

S
saccades 94
sacculus 120
sacral plexus 47
St Vitus's dance 235
salivation
　control 145
　reflex 80, 113
salivatory nucleus 112, 197
　superior 129
scalenus syndrome *47*, 48–9
Scarpa's ganglion *see* vestibular ganglion
Schütz's bundle 213, 222

Schwabach test 119
Schwalbe's nucleus 122, 123
Schwann cell, nucleus 4
scleroderma 69
scoliosis 56
scotoma 315
segmental muscle innervation 43, *44–5*, 46–63
　damage syndrome 48–9
　flaccid paralysis 46–7
　function *43–6*
　plexus damage 47–8
　spinal cord and peripheral nerve damage syndrome 49–59
　spinal radicular systems 59–63
seizure state 205
sella turcica 251
semicircular canals 120, 121
　receptors 123
semilunar gyri 77
sensory apraxia 289
sensory disorder, dissociated 51
sensory impressions, corpus callosum 292
sensory pathway interruption syndromes 26–8
septum pellucidum 250
　glioma 247
servo mechanism 11–12
sexual development
　early 193
　precocious 200, 212
shaking palsy 232
singultus 138
skin reflex, spastic palsy 36
skull fracture 319
sleep
　reticular formation 143
　salivation cessation 145
　see also somnolence
Sluder's neuralgia 113
smooth pursuit movement 96
sneezing reflex 106
solitary tract nucleus 111, 125, 140
somatic motor neurons 216
somatomotor cortex 278
somatosensory association area 285
somatosensory cortex 274–5, *276*
somatostatin 201
somatotropic hormone 213
somesthesia, cortical areas *272*
somnolence
　bilateral ventromedial thalamic syndrome 189–90

somnolence, craniopharyngioma 210, 211
thalamoperforating artery obstruction 315
see also sleep
sound wave conductance 114
spastic paraparesis of legs 55
spastic paraplegia 234
spastic spinal paralysis, progressive 54–5
spasticity 232
speech 292–3
    development 294–5
    disorder in progressive bulbar paralysis 134
    scanning 172
    temporoparietal area 296
sphenoid ridge, meningioma 299, *300*
sphenoid sinus 88
spinal arteries 63, 64
    anterior
        occlusion *65*, 66
        syndrome of thrombosis *65*
    circumferential branch 65
    posterior 66
    sulcocommissural branch 65
spinal automatisms 57
spinal canal, venous plexus 321
spinal cord 21–3, *24*, 25–8
    arterial supply 63–5
    circulation disorders 53
    diameter 22–3
    lateral pyramidal tracts 136
    segments 21, *22*
    subacute combined degeneration 51, 52, *53*
    syndrome of complete transection 56–8
    syndrome of hemisection 56
    transverse lesions 58
    venous drainage 65–6
spinal ganglion 46
    syndrome 49–50
spinal motor neurons, hypothalamic impulses 197
spinal muscular atrophy, progressive 53
spinal nerves 47
spinal nucleus 103, 104
spinal peripheral nerve 39
spinal radicular syndromes 59–60
spinal reticular formation 136
spinal root damage 25
spinal shock 56–7
spinal trigeminal nucleus 141
spinal trigeminal tract 103
spinal tumors 66–9

extramedullary 66–8
intramedullary 66, 68
spinal vascular lesions, syndromes caused by 66
spinal veins 65
spindle receptor 10
spino-olivary tract 21
spinocerebellar tract 14, 136, 167
spinocerebellum 165
spinoreticular tract 21
spinotectal tract 21
spinothalamic tract 136, 142
    anterior *16*, 17
    lateral 17–21, 141
spinovestibular tract 21
spiral ganglion 117
spondylosis deformans 61
status epilepticus 301
status lacunaris 236
status marmoratus 234
stellate ganglion 216
stereocilia 115, 116
sternocleidomastoid muscle 132
strabismus, convergent 88
stretch receptors 8, 9
    hypersensitivity 35
stretch reflex 2
stria terminalis 195, *196*, 204, 205
striate body 225, *228*
striatum 229–30
    artery obstruction 313
strionigral tract 231
Strümpell–Lorrain syndrome 56
styloglossus muscle 132
stylopharyngeal branches of glossopharyngeal nerve 125
subarachnoid angioma 67, 68
subarachnoid hemorrhage 316, *317*
subarachnoid space 241–3
    cerebrospinal fluid 244
    hydrocephalus 248
    leaking aneurysm blood collection 317
subclavian artery, stenosis 309–10
subclavian steal 309
subdural hematoma 159, *161*, 298, 320
substantia gelatinosa 13, 17
substantia nigra 141, 143, 193, 227
    cortex connections 230
    neuron loss 233
    tumor *237*
subthalamic nucleus 181, 193–4, 227, 236

cortex connections 230
subthalamus 181, 193–4
sucking 145
Sudeck–Lariche syndrome 49
sulcomarginal fasciculus 123
    superior cerebellar artery, trigeminal neuralgia 107
superior colliculi 140, 142
superior oblique muscle 87
superior petrosal sinus 148
superior plexus paralysis 47
superior rectus muscle 89
supraopticohypophyseal tract 195, 197
supratentorial hematoma 318
supratentorial lesion 160, *161*
    impaction 159, 160
    space-occupying 160–1
swallowing 145
Sydenham's chorea 235
sylvian aqueduct syndrome 156, *158*
sympathetic apraxia 289
sympathetic nerves 215, 217
synapses 6
    impulse 7
syperior anastomotic veins of Trolard *321*, 322
syphilis 209
    thalamic inflammatory disease 191
syringobulbia 114, 134
syringomyelia 51, 52, 53, *252*

T
tabes dorsalis 6, 50, 51
tactile engram 294
tangential fibers 166
taste
    buds 111
    fibers 111
    impulse 140
    sensation pathways *111*, 112
tears 113
    crocodile 114
    see also crying
tectonuclear tract 142
tectospinal tract 142
tectum 73
tela choroidea 180
teleceptors 1
telencephalon *see* cerebral cortex
temperature regulation 200
    hypothalamic impulses 197
temperature sensation 17, 18–20
    loss 27
temporal arteritis, rheumatic 108
temporal association area 284–94

temporal lobe 257
    association areas 291
    isthmus 84
    metastases *253*
    resection in epilepsy 205
temporomandibular joint, pain 108
temporoparietal speech area 296
tendon organ of Golgi 2, 3, *10*, 11
Tensilon test 69
tentorium
    cerebelli 158
    impaction 148
    syndrome 156, 158–63
terminal nerve endings 3
tetanus 108
tetraplegia 36
thalamic astrocytoma *190*, 192
thalamic medullary striae 80
thalamic oligodendroglioma 190
thalamic posterolateral ventral nucleus 15
thalamic syndrome 189–90
thalamo-cingulate radiation 202
thalamocortical connections, reciprocal 231
thalamocortical tract *15*, 16
thalamoperforating artery obstruction 315
thalamostriate vein 322–3
    thrombosis 324
thalamus 181–8, *229*
    afferent impulse coordination 187
    blood supply 187–8
    circulatory disorders 189–90
    disorders 188–92
    extrapyramidal system connections 187
    feedback circuit 278
    function 187
    hand 188
    impulses to facial nuclei 110
    inflammatory disease 191–2
    necrotic foci *189*
    neurons 183
    nuclei 181, 183–6
    somatosensory neuron arrangement *182*
    somatosensory pathways 183, *185*
    syndrome 187, 188, 192
    tumors 190–1
    ventral posteromedial nucleus 104
thermoceptors 1
Thomsen's disease 69
thoracic spinal cord 58

Thorkildsen drainage 250
thyreocostocervical trunk 64
thyroid-stimulating hormone 199, *201*
tibial nerve 47–8
tinnitus 120
Todd's paralysis 301
Tomberg's sign 55
tongue
    muscles 132
    supranuclear paralysis 134
    unilateral spastic paresis 133–4
tonotopic order of auditory fibers 118
torcular Herophili 158
torsion dystonia 235–6
torticollis, spasmodic 235
touch sensation 21
    dermatomic area 25
    transmission 131
toxoplasmosis 191–2
transection of spinal cord, complete 56–8
transient ischemic attack 312
transverse cistern 158, 159, *242*, *243*
transverse myelitis 56
transverse myelopathy 66
transverse sinus 148
trapezius muscle 132
trapezoid fibers 117
trauma 51
tremor 233
    antagonist 234
    intention 171, 179, 188
triangle of Guillain–Mollaret 169, 236
trigeminal ganglion 88, 103
trigeminal lemnisci 142
trigeminal mesencephalic tract nucleus 103
trigeminal nerve 72, *78*, 88, *89*, 103–8
    central connections of nuclei *105*
    ipsilateral paralysis 37
    motor portion 106
    principal sensory nucleus 104–5
    skin areas supplied by 103
    spinal division 141
    spinal nucleus 107
trigeminal neuralgia 106–7
trigeminal pain, symptomatic 107
trigeminal pathway, third neurons 105

trigeminal tract, mesencephalic 142
trismus 108
trochlear nerve 71, 73, *78*, 86–7
    nuclei 142
    paralysis 94
tuber cinereum 180
    damage 200
tuberculosis 209
    thalamic inflammatory disease 191
tuberculum cinereum 72
tuberculum sellae, meningioma 299
tuberoinfundibular tract 198
two-point discrimination loss 16
tympanic canal 115
tympanic cavity 114
tympanic nerve 125

U

U-fibers *see* arcuate fibers
ulnar nerve damage syndrome 49
ulnar paralysis with claw hand 49
uncinate fasciculus of Russell 122, 167, 268
uncinate fits 291, 299
uncinate process 59–60
urinary bladder
    automatic 219
    control disorder 324
    filling perception 219
    parasympathetic nervous system control 217, 218–19
    reflex emptying 219
utriculus 120, 121

V

vagal system 125–31
vagus nerve 72, *79*, *127*, 128–9
    bilateral complete paralysis 129
    branches *126*, 128–9
    dorsal nucleus 129, 130, 140
    ganglia 128
    impairment syndrome 129
    parasympathetic portion 217
    somatic afferent fibers 131
    taste fibers 111
    unilateral complete interruption 129
vagus trigone 140
vasocorona 65
vasopressin 195, 197–8
Vater-Pacini lamellar corpuscles 1, 2, 3

velum medullare superius 73, 86
venae flocculares 148
ventral tegmental decussation 142
ventricle 243–4
　distension with CSF flow blockage 247
　ependymoma 247, *248*
　fourth 243
　　obstruction 248
　lateral 243
　　metastases *253*
　third 243
　　tumor 247
ventriculography 253–4
ventrocaudal pons syndrome 151, *152*
vermis 164, 166
　rostral 174
vertebral artery 145, 146–7, 172, 302
　hypoplasia 310
　stenosis 310
vertebral bodies *22*
vertebral venous plexus
　external 66
　internal 65, 239
vertebrobasilar insufficiency 148, 308, 309–11
vertigo 124, 125
vestibular canal 115
vestibular cortex 277
vestibular ganglion *121*, 122, *123*

vestibular nerve, central pathways *121*
vestibular nuclear complex 122, 123, 141
　central connections *123*
vestibular system 120–5
　cerebral cortex connections 124
　impairment 124–5
　receptor organs 120–1
vestibulocerebellum 165
vestibulocochlear nerve *78*, 113
vestibulocochlear organ 114
vestibulospinal tract 145
　lateral 123
vestibulum 114
vibratory sense loss 16
Virchow–Robin perivascular spaces 241
visceroceptors 1
vision, occipital lobes 257
visual association area 290
visual cortex 81, *83*, 273–4
　bilateral infarction 277
　orientation slab 274
　primary 275–7
visual imprint, association areas 85
visual information transfer 292
visual pathway 81–5
visual stimulus, reflex arc 142
vocal cord paralysis 129
Vogt's syndrome 235
voluntary fixation 98

voluntary motor actions 34
voluntary movement loss 36
vomiting center 145
von Recklinghausen's disease 300

W
wakefulness 143
Wallenberg's syndrome 150, 174, 217, 288
water metabolism regulation 200
　see also vasopressin
Weber's syndrome 37, 152, *157*
Weber's test 119
weight, inability to discriminate 172
Wernicke's aphasia 294–7
Wernicke's encephalopathy 209
Wernicke's sensory aphasia 290–1
Westphal–Strümpell disease 235
white communicating branches, somatic motor neurons 216
white matter 264–8
　association fibers 264, 266–8
　commissural fibers 264, *267*, 268
　projection fibers 264–6
　venous infarction of deep cerebral ganglia 325
Wilson's disease 235